Dual Diagnosis Nursing

**Dedicated to Safian, Hassim, Yasmin Soraya,
Adam Ali Hussein & Reshad Hassan.**

Dual Diagnosis Nursing

Edited by

Professor G. Hussein Rassool
MSc, BA, RN, FETC, RCNT, RNT MILT, FRSH
Cert. Ed., Cert. Couns., Cert in Supervision & Consultation

Professor of Addiction & Mental Health, Departamento de Psiquiatria e Ciências Humanas da Escola de Enfermagem de Ribeirão Preto da Universidade de São Paulo, São Paulo, Brazil. Visiting Professor Federal University of Minas Gerais, Brazil. Formerly Senior Lecturer in Addictive Behaviour, Department of Addictive Behaviour & Psychological Medicine, Centre for Addiction Studies, St George's Hospital, University of London, UK.

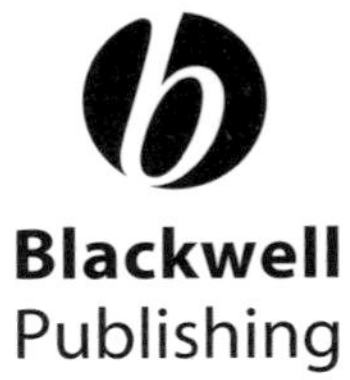

Blackwell
Publishing

Addiction
Press

Editorial offices:
Blackwell Publishing Ltd, 9600 Garsington Road, Oxford OX4 2DQ, UK
Tel: +44 (0)1865 776868
Blackwell Publishing Inc., 350 Main Street, Malden, MA 02148-5020, USA
Tel: +1 781 388 8250
Blackwell Publishing Asia Pty Ltd, 550 Swanston Street, Carlton, Victoria 3053, Australia
Tel: +61 (0)3 8359 1011

First published 2006 by Blackwell Publishing Ltd

ISBN-13: 978-14051-1902-3
ISBN-10: 1-4051-1902-0

Library of Congress Cataloging-in-Publication Data
Dual diagnosis nursing / edited by G. Hussein Rassool.
p. ; cm.
Includes bibliographical references and index.
ISBN-13: 978-1-4051-1902-3 (pbk.: alk. paper)
ISBN-10: 1-4051-1902-0 (pbk.: alk. paper)
1. Dual diagnosis. 2. Psychiatric nursing. 3. Substance abuse – Nursing.
I. Rassool, G. Hussein.
[DNLM: 1. Diagnosis, Dual (Psychiatry) 2. Mental Disorders – therapy.
3. Substance-Related Disorders – therapy. WM 270 D8126 2006]
RC564.68.D793 2006
616.89′0231—dc22

2006007828

A catalogue record for this title is available from the British Library

Set in 9.5/11.5pt Palatino
by Graphicraft Limited, Hong Kong
Printed and bound in Singapore
by COS Printers Pte Ltd

The publisher's policy is to use permanent paper from mills that operate a sustainable forestry policy, and which has been manufactured from pulp processed using acid-free and elementary chlorine-free practices. Furthermore, the publisher ensures that the text paper and cover board used have met acceptable environmental accreditation standards.

For further information on Blackwell Publishing, visit our website:
www.blackwellpublishing.com

Contents

Contributors vii
Foreword ix
Preface xi
Acknowledgements xiii

Part 1 Background **1**

1 Understanding Dual Diagnosis: an Overview 3
G.H. Rassool

2 Policy Initiatives in Substance Misuse and Mental Health: Implications for Practice 16
A. Hammond

3 Understanding Drug Use and Misuse 25
G.H. Rassool & J. Winnington

4 Psychoactive Substances and their Effects 34
G.H. Rassool & J. Winnington

5 Mental Health: an Introduction 45
G.H. Rassool & J. Winnington

6 Alcohol and Dual Diagnosis 54
K. Moore

7 Eating Disorders and Dual Diagnosis 62
M. Abuel-Ealeh & R. Barrett

8 Problem Drug Use and Personality Disorders 73
P. Phillips

Part 2 Special Populations **79**

9 Black and Ethnic Minority Communities: Substance Misuse and Mental Health: Whose Problems Anyway? 81
G.H. Rassool

10 Vulnerable Young People and Substance Misuse 97
M. Epling & J. McGregor

11 Meeting Multiple Needs: Pregnancy, Parenting and Dual Diagnosis 107
F. Macrory

Part 3 Context and Approaches **117**

12 Addiction and Mental Health Nursing: a Synthesis of Role and Care in the Community 119
K. Moore & G.H. Rassool

13 Shared Care and Inter-professional Practice 130
A. Simpson

14 Primary Care and Dual Diagnosis 140
R. Lawrence

15 Dual Diagnosis in Acute In-patient Settings 150
J. Gallagher & S.J. Scott

16 Dual Diagnosis in a Forensic Setting 161
P. Ford & P. Woods

17 Models of Care and Dual Diagnosis 169
D. Gallivan

Part 4 Intervention and Treatment Strategies 175

18 Framework for Multidimensional Assessment 177
G.H. Rassool & J. Winnington

19 Dealing with Intoxication, Overdose, Withdrawal and Detoxification: Nursing Assessment and Interventions 186
G.H. Rassool & J. Winnington

20 Prescribing Authority and Medication Management in Mental Health and Addiction Nursing 196
G.H. Rassool & J. Winnington

21 Spiritual and Cultural Needs: Integration in Dual Diagnosis Care 209
A. Hammond & G.H. Rassool

22 Dual Diagnosis: Interventions with Carers 222
D. Manley & L.M. Rayner

23 Psychological Approaches in the Treatment of Dual Diagnosis 232
K. Barry

24 A Person Centred Approach to Understanding and Helping People with a Dual Diagnosis 240
R. Bryant-Jefferies

25 Motivational Interviewing 253
P.G. Mason

26 Relapse Prevention in Dual Diagnosis 261
D. Manley & J. McGregor

Part 5 Professional Development 271

27 Educational Development and Clinical Supervision 273
G.H. Rassool

28 The Role and Competencies of Staff in the Treatment of Coexisting Problems of Mental Health and Substance Misuse 285
R. Edwards

Index 297

Contributors

M. Abuel-Ealeh. Previously Associate Dean, School of Community Health Studies, Head of Mental and Learning Disability Studies, Anglia Ruskin University, Essex.

R. Barrett. Senior Lecturer in Mental Health, School of Community Health Studies, Mental and Learning Disability Division, Anglia Ruskin University, Essex.

K. Barry. Nurse Consultant, Partnerships in Care Ltd, Llanarth, Wales.

R. Bryant-Jefferies. Sector Manager (Kensington and Chelsea sector), Substance Misuse Service, Central and North West London Mental Health NHS Trust, London.

R. Edwards. Consultant Nurse and Senior Lecturer for Coexisting Mental Health and Substance Misuse Problems (Dual Diagnosis), Joint post between Avon and Wiltshire Mental Health Partnership NHS Trust and the University of the West of England.

M. Epling. Lecturer in Mental Health, Faculty of Medicine and Health Sciences, School of Nursing, the University of Nottingham.

P. Ford. Consultant Psychologist (Substance Misuse), Psychology Department, Kneesworth House Hospital, Bassingbourne, Royston.

J. Gallagher. Senior Lecturer in Mental Health, School of Community Health Studies, Mental and Learning Disability Division, Anglia Ruskin University, Essex.

D. Gallivan. Substance Misuse Worker, Kent and Medway NHS and Social Care Partnership Trust, Dartford, Kent.

A. Hammond. Locality Manager, Kent and Medway NHS and Social Care Partnership Trust, Dartford, Kent.

R. Lawrence. Senior Substance Misuse Worker, Kent and Medway NHS and Social Care Trust, Substance Misuse Service, Medway Towns, Kent.

F. Macrory. MBE. Zion Community Resource Centre, Hulme, Manchester.

D. Manley. Lead Clinician/Team Leader, Nottingham Dual Diagnosis Team (part of NADT), Nottingham.

P.G. Mason. Director Pip Mason Consultancy, Kings Norton, Birmingham.

J. McGregor. Lecturer in Substance Misuse, Nottingham Education Centre, Mapperley, Nottingham.

K. Moore. Manager Dual Diagnosis Service, the Maple Unit, Q1 Block, St Ann's Hospital, Tottenham, London.

P. Phillips. Lecturer in Mental Health & Social Care (Learning Disability), City University, Department of Mental Health & Learning Disability, St Bartholomew's School of Nursing & Midwifery, London.

G.H. Rassool. Professor of Addiction & Mental Health, Departamento de Psiquiatria e Ciências Humanas da Escola de Enfermagem de Ribeirão

Preto da Universidade de São Paulo, São Paulo, Brazil. Visiting Professor Federal University of Minas Gerais, Brazil. Formerly Senior Lecturer in Addictive Behaviour, Department of Addictive Behaviour & Psychological Medicine, Centre for Addiction Studies, St George's Hospital, University of London.

L.M. Rayner. Lecturer in Health, University of Nottingham School of Nursing, Nottingham.

S.J. Scott. Senior Lecturer in Mental Health, School of Community Health Studies, Mental and Learning Disability Division, Anglia Ruskin University, Essex.

A. Simpson. Research Fellow, City University, Department of Mental Health & Learning Disability, St Bartholomew's School of Nursing & Midwifery, London.

J. Winnington. Team Leader, Alex House, Bethlem Royal Hospital, Beckenham, Kent.

P. Woods. Associate Professor, College of Nursing, University of Saskatchewan, Saskatchewan, Canada.

Foreword

It is a pleasure and privilege to be invited to write the Foreword for Hussein Rassool's book on Dual Diagnosis Nursing. I got to know Professor Rassool when we both worked at St George's Hospital Medical School – he ran the postgraduate programme in addiction studies and occasionally I would help by supervising student projects or sitting on the board of examiners.

I always admired the way in which he managed the programme – coordinating the activities of a diverse group of contributors to produce something coherent that is of real practical value. I was not surprised, therefore, to see those same skills applied to this volume. Professor Rassool and the other contributors show a very clear understanding of the needs of their target readership and they present the material without unnecessary embellishment. This volume quite simply contains information that nurses must know if they are to help patients with substance use and psychological problems. The field of addiction, in my opinion, suffers from too many 'manuals' that present waffle and speculation dressed up as fact. This book provides information in the most straightforward terms that will be of practical value to the reader.

The chapters on management of patients with dual diagnosis no doubt presented the greatest challenge because the scientific basis for particular treatment approaches is lacking. We don't know whether approaches such as motivational interviewing give better results than cognitive behavioural approaches or pragmatic, commonsense based approaches – and we may never know because these kinds of issue are extremely difficult to study scientifically. As long as we recognise that the ideas we put forward for managing patients are pragmatic solutions to difficult problems, and do not turn them into articles of faith, no one can ask more of us. Professor Rassool's writing seems to me to fit this ethos very nicely.

Robert West
University College London

Preface

Dual diagnosis, that is the coexistence of substance misuse and mental health problems, is the premise of the book, which is interwoven in all the chapters. The increase in the number of individuals with substance misuse and mental health problems has attracted considerable interest in recent years and will be one of the most important challenges facing both mental health and addiction nurses. It is estimated that 30% of people with mental health problems also have drug and/or alcohol problems, which are highly prevalent across a range of service and treatment settings. Common examples of dual diagnosis include the combination of psychosis with amphetamine use, depression with alcohol dependence, anxiety and alcohol dependence, alcohol and polydrug use with schizophrenia, and borderline personality disorder with episodic polydrug use. Research shows that individuals with a dual diagnosis are at an increased risk of suicide, violent behaviour and non-compliance with treatment. Given the prevalence, and the limited resources available to support individuals with dual diagnosis and their carers, a wide range of professionals from health and social care, including employment, housing and the criminal justice system may be involved in dealing with the complex needs associated with this condition. The prevalence, clinical implications, service provision and the effectiveness of intervention strategies are now becoming more apparent.

This book draws together and synthesises the body of knowledge and clinical nursing practice within the UK framework of working with individuals with dual diagnosis. It focuses on the approaches and intervention strategies that nurses and other health and social care professionals have used to respond to this new challenge in specialist and non-specialist settings. The book does not profess to be a complete dual diagnosis compendium, rather it aims to introduce the reader to the key issues and concerns that surround the coexistence of substance misuse and mental health problems. The book underpins a number of current policy initiatives, as applied to current practice, and covers, practically, most aspects relating to dual diagnosis including an overview of dual diagnosis, the conceptual examination of dual diagnosis and substance misuse and its psychopathology. An added dimension is the coverage of needs of special populations, dual diagnosis in different care and treatment settings, multidimensional assessment, dealing with emergencies, spiritual needs, prescribing and medication management, nursing and psychological interventions, carers' interventions and professional development.

The book is practice oriented and written by

experienced, mostly nursing, academics and clinicians from the field of addiction and mental health nursing. It provides practitioners with awareness, knowledge of addiction and mental health, and skills required to respond effectively to those individuals they encounter in their practice. Whilst the book will address issues related to practitioners in dealing with the coexistence of substance misuse and mental health problems, it will be of interest and act as an excellent resource for other health and social care professionals who are unfamiliar with the 'dual diagnosis' phenomenon. It will be of relevance to students in medicine, nursing, psychology, social work and the criminal justice system, and those attending undergraduate and postgraduate courses in addiction and mental health studies. It will also be beneficial to anyone who has little or no experience in mental health, substance misuse or dual diagnosis.

Dual diagnosis, like substance misuse, is not the sole property of one particular discipline. It is everybody's business (Rassool, 2002)[1].

Structure of the book

This book is presented in five sections. Part 1 introduces the background in providing current literature on dual diagnosis, drug use and misuse, mental health, alcohol and mental health, personality disorders and eating disorders. Part 2 deals with special populations: black and ethnic minority groups, young people and women (parenting and pregnancy). Part 3 covers aspects of a synthesis of role, shared care, dual diagnosis in acute in-patient and forensic settings and models of care. Part 4 focuses on a framework for multidimensional assessment, dealing with overdose, intoxication and withdrawals, prescribing authority and medication management, integrating spiritual needs in holistic care, psychological interventions: cognitive behaviour therapy, motivational interviewing and person centred counselling, and relapse prevention. Part 5 concludes with the role and competencies of staff, educational development and clinical supervision.

---

[1] Rassool G. Hussein (2002) *Dual Diagnosis: Substance Misuse and Psychiatric Disorders*. Blackwell Publishing, Oxford.

Acknowledgements

I would like to thank all the contributors, and the staff at Blackwell Publishing, Oxford, for their support in the preparation of this book. I also would like to thank Beth Knight at Blackwell Publishing for her support and patience throughout the process of writing and the publication of this book.

I am also particularly grateful to Professor James P. Smith, Professor John Strang, Professor A. Hamid Ghodse and the Florence Nightingale Research Foundation for their guidance in my professional development. Special thanks also goes to Professor Margarita Villar-Luis, Deputy Dean, Escola De Enfermagem de Ribeirão Preto, Universidade de São Paulo, Brazil for our collaboration and development in teaching and research activities in addiction and mental health. Thanks also to colleagues and friends at USP and in Ribeirao Preto, especially to Carlos and Roselyne.

My thanks go to Mariam and Muhsinah for smoothing the path and providing me with the necessary support and help during my sabbatical and subsequent stay in Mauritius. Thanks also goes to all those at Al-Furqan, Les Guibies, for their friendship and support. I would like to acknowledge the contribution of my teachers who enabled me, through my own reflective practices, to follow the path.

My special thanks also to Julie for all the help and support over the years. Finally, I owe my gratitude to my children, Yasmin, Adam and Reshad, who keep me going and active in various endeavours.

Part 1

Background

Chapter 1 Understanding Dual Diagnosis: an Overview
Chapter 2 Policy Initiatives in Substance Misuse and Mental Health: Implications for Practice
Chapter 3 Understanding Drug Use and Misuse
Chapter 4 Psychoactive Substances and their Effects
Chapter 5 Mental Health: an Introduction
Chapter 6 Alcohol and Dual Diagnosis
Chapter 7 Eating Disorders and Dual Diagnosis
Chapter 8 Problem Drug Use and Personality Disorders

1 Understanding Dual Diagnosis: an Overview

G.H. Rassool

Introduction

In the past decade, there has been a growing interest in the concept of dual diagnosis or coexisting problems of substance misuse and mental health problems. Dual diagnosis has gained prominence partly due to the closure of long-stay psychiatric institutions, increasing emphasis on care and treatment in the community and the increasing prevalence of substance misuse amongst the general population. Individuals with mental health problems are perhaps becoming more exposed to a wider range of illicit drugs than previously. Furthermore, some individuals with mental health problems who are socially isolated may be drawn into a drug-using culture that appears more attractive and less stigmatised for social interactions.

However, there is still no consensus or common understanding of what is meant by 'dual diagnosis'. The concept 'dual diagnosis' has been applied to a number of individuals with two coexisting disorders or conditions, such as a physical illness and mental health problems, schizophrenia and substance misuse, or learning disability and mental health problems. The concepts of 'dual diagnosis', and 'co-morbidity' are now used commonly and interchangeably. The concept of complex or multiple needs is also associated with those with two existing conditions, which include medical, psychological, social or legal needs or problems. This chapter aims to examine the concept of dual diagnosis and describe its prevalence, treatment models, principles of treatment and issues for service delivery.

Concepts and classifications

There is no operational definition of dual diagnosis. However, dual diagnosis per se does not formally exist as a definitive diagnosis and the concept itself could be interpreted as being misleading and cumbersome (Rostad & Checinski, 1996). Nevertheless the same authors do concede that the 'label' is useful in so far as it draws attention to 'a real problem which is not being addressed'. The diagnostic labels have value in defining a client group and enabling the commissioning and delivery of care but the labels of 'dual diagnosis' should not be perceived as problematic (Rethink & Turning Point, 2004). Health care professionals have used the term dual diagnosis to refer to individuals who were mentally retarded or had a learning disability and who also had a coexisting psychiatric disorder (Evans & Sullivan, 2001). More recently, clinicians have begun to use the term to refer to an individual with a substance use problem and a coexisting psychiatric disorder. The term covers a broad spectrum of mental health and substance misuse problems that an individual might experience concurrently

Table 1.1 Substance use and psychiatric syndromes.

- Substance use (even single dose) may lead to psychiatric syndromes/symptoms.
- Harmful use may produce psychiatric syndromes.
- Dependence may produce psychological symptoms.
- Intoxication from substances may produce psychological symptoms.
- Withdrawal from substances may produce psychological symptoms.
- Withdrawal from substances may lead to psychiatric syndromes.
- Substance use may exacerbate pre-existing psychiatric disorder.
- Psychological morbidity not amounting to a disorder may precipitate substance use.
- Primary psychiatric disorder may lead to substance use disorder.
- Primary psychiatric disorder may precipitate substance disorder, which may, in turn, lead to psychiatric syndromes.

Source: based on Crome (1999).

(Department of Health, 2002). In the context of this book, the concept of dual diagnosis is defined as the coexistence of substance misuse and mental health problems.

The misuse of psychoactive substances, including alcohol, may result in the individual developing a wide range of mental health problems depending on the drug being used. For example, a cocaine user may experience depressive symptoms and paranoid delusions. It is stated that with dual diagnosis patients, the psychiatric disorders and the substance misuse are separate, chronic disorders, each with an independent course, yet each able to influence the properties of the other (Carey, 1989).

The dual diagnosis individual meets the Diagnostic and Statistical Manual of Mental Disorders (DSM-IV) criteria for both substance abuse or dependency and a coexisting psychiatric disorder. The DSM-IV (American Psychiatric Association, 1994), defines a mental disorder as 'a clinically significant behavioural or psychological syndrome or pattern that occurs in an individual and that is typically associated with present distress (a painful symptom) or disability (impairment in one or more areas of functioning)'. Substance misuse, according to DSM-IV (APA, 1994), is the maladaptive pattern of use not meeting the criteria for dependence that has persisted for at least one month or has occurred repeatedly over a long period of time. The dual diagnosis patient meets the DSM-IV criteria for both substance abuse or dependency and a coexisting psychiatric disorder.

The nature of the relationship between these two conditions is complex. Dual diagnosis can be categorised into several subgroups and relationships defined by presumed aetiological mechanisms. The relationship between substance misuse and mental health problems can manifest itself in the following ways as shown in Table 1.1 (Crome, 1999).

Individuals with dual diagnosis, like most substance misusers, are a heterogeneous group and any defining features or diagnostic profiles evident may change over time. A more manageable and clinically relevant interrelationship between psychiatric disorder and substance misuse has been described in the *Dual Diagnosis Good Practice Guide* (Department of Health, 2002). The four possible relationships are:

- A primary psychiatric illness precipitating or leading to substance misuse
- Substance misuse worsening or altering the course of a psychiatric illness
- Intoxication and/or substance dependence leading to psychological symptoms
- Substance misuse and/or withdrawal leading to psychiatric symptoms or illnesses

Figure 1.1 presents the scope of coexistent psychiatric and substance misuse disorders (Department of Health, 2002). The horizontal axis represents severity of mental illness and the vertical axis the severity of substance misuse. Intervention strategies would need to focus on those whose severity falls within the top right hand and bottom right hand quadrants.

Prevalence

Despite certain methodological difficulties, especially with earlier studies, there is now strong research evidence that the rate of substance misuse

Severity of problematic substance misuse

For example, a dependent drinker who experiences increasing anxiety	For example, an individual with schizophrenia who misuses cannabis on a daily basis to compensate for social isolation
Low **Severity of mental illness**	High
For example, recreational misuser of 'dance drugs' who has begun to struggle with low mood after weekend use	For example, an individual with bipolar disorder whose occasional binge drinking and experimental misuse of other substances destabilises their mental health

Figure 1.1 The scope of coexistent psychiatric and substance misuse disorders.
Source: Department of Health (2002).

is substantially higher among the mentally ill compared with the general population. The prevalence rate of substance use disorder among individuals with mental health problems ranges from 35% to 60% (Mueser *et al.*, 1995; Menezes *et al.*, 1996). The Epidemiological Catchment Area (ECA) study (Anthony & Helzer, 1991), a large American population survey, found a lifetime prevalence rate for substance misuse disorder of 16.7% (13.5% alcohol, 6.1% drug) for the general population. Rates for patients with schizophrenia, affective disorders and anxiety disorders were 47%, 32% and 23.7% respectively. For persons with any drug (excluding alcohol) disorder, more than half (53%) had one other mental disorder, most commonly anxiety and affective disorders.

The UK study (Menezes *et al.*, 1996) of 171 inner city London patients in contact with psychiatric services found that the one-year prevalence rate amongst subjects with psychotic illness for any substance misuse problem was 36.3% (31.6% alcohol, 15.8% drug). The National Treatment Outcome Research Study (NTORS) (Gossop *et al.*, 1998) found evidence of psychiatric disorders amongst individuals with primary substance use disorders. The NTORS found that 10% of substance misuse patients entering treatment had a psychiatric admission (not related to substance dependence) in the previous two years. Suicidal thoughts are commonly reported by drug dependent patients (29%) in treatment, and substance misuse is known to increase by 8–15-fold the risk of suicide (Shaffer *et al.*, 1996; Gossop *et al.*, 1998; Oyefeso *et al.*, 1999). Some of this increased risk may be explained by the presence of co-morbid psychiatric conditions such as depression or personality disorder in substance misusers (Neeleman & Farrell, 1997). The Office of Population Censuses and Surveys household survey estimated the prevalence of alcohol and drug dependence amongst the general population to be 5% and 2% respectively (Farrell *et al.*, 1998). Consumption of drugs was particularly high amongst adults with a phobic disorder, panic disorder and depression. Mental health problems are highly prevalent amongst the homeless population, making the chances of dual diagnosis in this population very high. A study of a sample of 124 individuals aged 18–65, who had remained in contact with the mental health team (Wright *et al.*, 2000), showed that 33% of patients fulfilled the study criteria for substance misuse. Those individuals (23%) with psychosis had 19 admissions in the two years prior to interview, while 18% of individuals with dual diagnosis had 11 admissions. In a study of 1075 adults, of whom 90% were opiate dependent (Marsden *et al.*, 2000), anxiety, depression, paranoia and psychoticism were found, with polydrug use closely linked to psychiatric symptoms. The use of illicit psychoactive substances, including alcohol, by individuals with psychiatric disorders increases the risk for those individuals to have an alcohol or drug-related problem or dependence. Individuals with schizophrenia for instance, have a three-fold risk of developing alcohol dependence compared with individuals without a mental illness (Crawford, 1996).

A study of the prevalence and management of co-morbidity amongst adult substance misuse and mental health treatment populations (Weaver *et al.*, 2002) showed that some 74.5% of users of drug services and 85.5% of users of alcohol services experienced mental health problems. Most had affective disorders (depression) and anxiety disorders and psychosis. Almost 30% of the drug treatment population and over 50% of those in treatment for alcohol problems experienced 'multiple' morbidity (co-occurrence of a number of psychiatric disorders or substance misuse problems). Some 38.5% of drug users with a psychiatric disorder were receiving no treatment for their mental health problem. Some 44% of mental health service users reported drug use and/or were assessed to have used alcohol at hazardous or harmful levels in the past year.

In summary, UK data from one national survey and from local studies (Department of Health, 2002) generally show that:

- Increased rates of substance misuse are found in individuals with mental health problems
- Alcohol misuse is the most common form of substance misuse
- Where drug misuse occurs it often coexists with alcohol misuse
- Homelessness is frequently associated with substance misuse problems
- Community mental health teams typically report that 8–15% of their clients have dual diagnosis problems, although higher rates may be found in inner cities
- Prisons have a high prevalence of substance misuse and dual diagnosis

Complex problems, complex needs

Individuals with substance misuse and mental health problems are a vulnerable group of people with complex needs. While it is true that each disorder alone may have major implications for how an individual functions, the disorders together may have interactive and overwhelming effects when they coexist. Individuals with this combination of problems often have a lot of additional difficulties that are not purely medical, psychological or psychiatric. They are more likely to have a worse prognosis with high levels of service use, including emergency clinic and in-patient admissions (McCrone *et al.*, 2000). In addition, they have problems relating to social, legal, housing, welfare and 'lifestyle' matters. In summary, the major problems associated with individuals with dual diagnosis are:

- Increase likelihood of self-harm
- Increased risk of HIV infection
- Increased use of institutional services
- Poor compliance with medication/treatment
- Homelessness
- Increased risk of violence
- Increased risk of victimisation/exploitation
- Higher recidivism
- Contact with the criminal justice system
- Family problems
- Poor social outcomes, including impact on carers and family
- Denial of substance misuse
- Negative attitudes of health care professionals
- Social exclusion

In addition, those individuals from black and ethnic minority groups with dual diagnosis face the compounded pressure of stigma, prejudice, institutional racism and ethnocentric intervention strategies. These complex needs cannot be dealt with by a single approach and require a more holistic approach from several different agencies or services in order to meet the medical, psychological, social, spiritual and/or legal needs of the individual.

Aetiological theories: reasons why individuals with mental health problems use psychoactive substances

There are a variety of models and theories that hypothesise why individuals with mental health problems are vulnerable to the misuse of psychoactive substances. These are the self-medication hypothesis, the alleviation of dysphoria model, the multiple risk factor model and the supersensitivity model.

Self-medication hypothesis

Self-medication refers to the motivation of patients to seek a specific drug for relief of a particular set of symptoms. Khantzian (1985; 1997) proposed a model of self-medication and suggested that individuals misuse psychoactive substances adaptively to cope with painful affective states and related psychiatric disorders that may predispose them to addictive behaviours. He stated that potential addicts do not select specific psychoactive substances at random but for their unique effects. Khantzian argues that an opiate user may self-medicate with, or have a preference for, opiates because of their powerful action in dealing with rage, aggression and/or depression. Cocaine has its appeal because of its ability to relieve distress associated with depression, hypomania and hyperactivity.

However, there is available evidence that does not support this hypothesis: no specific substances were found to alleviate specific symptoms of a particular psychiatric disorder (Dixon *et al.*, 1990; Noordsy *et al.*, 1991). The most common substances used by individuals with mental health problems are alcohol, nicotine, amphetamines, cannabis, and hallucinogens (Schneider & Siris, 1987). These have been shown to increase severity of positive symptoms of psychosis (auditory and visual hallucinations, delusional beliefs and other thought disorders) so would not be used to decrease distress or to alleviate such symptoms. However, the self-medication theory may still retain some credence. For example, opiates, cannabis or alcohol may reduce the agitation and anxiety associated with mental illness, whilst stimulants may be used as self-medication for negative symptoms or depression. Psycho-stimulants may help counteract extrapyramidal side effects of antipsychotic medication (Smith & Hucker, 1994) especially akathisia. There is no evidence in support of the self-medication hypothesis as a necessary reinforcer of continued drug use (Castaneda *et al.*, 1994).

Alleviation of dsyphoria

This model put forward that severely mentally ill patients are prone to dysphoric experiences (feeling bad) that make them susceptible to use psychoactive substances (Birchwood *et al.*, 1993). The rationale for using psychoactive substances initially is for the relief of bad feeling and to feel good (Leshner, 1998) and the literature supports this notion that dysphoria motivates initial alcohol and drug use (Carey & Carey, 1995; Pristach & Smith, 1996; Addington & Duchak, 1997). Most of the studies generally support the alleviation of dysphoria model.

Multiple risk factor model

According to Mueser *et al.* (1995), in addition to the dysphoric experiences, there are other underlying risk factors that may motivate the severely mentally ill patient to use psychoactive substances. The risk factors include social isolation, deficit in interpersonal skills, poor cognitive skills, educational failure, poverty, lack of adult role responsibility, association with drug subcultures and availability of illicit psychoactive substances (Anthony & Helzer, 1991; Berman & Noble, 1993; Jones *et al.*, 1994). However, there is no direct evidence for this model, but the rationale for using psychoactive substances is related to the identified factors (Dixon *et al.*, 1990; Noordsy *et al.*, 1991).

The supersensitivity model

According to this model, 'psychobiological vulnerability, determined by a combination of genetic and environmental events, interacts with environmental stress to either precipitate the onset of a psychiatric disorder or to trigger relapse' (Mueser *et al.*, 1995). Mueser *et al.* (1995) argue that the sensitivity to psychoactive substances (increased vulnerability) may cause patients with severe mental illness to be more likely to experience negative consequences from using relatively small amounts of psychoactive substances. There are several studies that provide evidence for this model: lower levels of physical dependence (Drake *et al.*, 1990; Corse *et al.*, 1995); trigger of clinical symptoms by low dose of amphetamine (Lieberman *et al.*, 1987); and negative clinical effects, such as relapse, with small quantities of alcohol or drugs (Drake *et al.*, 1989). The supersensitivity model, according to Mueser *et al.* (1995), provides a useful theoretical framework in the understanding of how low level use of psychoactive substances often results in negative consequences in severely mentally ill patients and also the increased prevalence of drug dependence in this population.

There may be other explanations as to why individuals with mental health problems may use certain psychoactive substances. They may be doing it for the same reasons as the rest of the population. For example, to relax, to relieve boredom, to get high, or because of increased availability or acceptability. Whilst this contention may be true, it fails, however, to explain the observed increased prevalence of substance use compared with the general population. A number of possible explanations can therefore be advanced. The individual with mental health problems may experience downward drift to poor inner city areas (social drift hypothesis) where drug availability is increased. With the advent of deinstitutionalisation, more of the individuals with mental health problems may be finding themselves exposed to an increased availability of drugs in the community (Williams, 2002). Equally, an increased availability of illicit drugs in psychiatric institutions may be a contributory factor (Laurence, 1995; Williams & Cohen, 2000).

Principles of treatment

The accurate assessment and treatment of individuals with dual diagnosis requires time, adequate resources and relevant experience. Drake *et al.* (1993) described nine principles in the treatment of drug misuse in individuals with dual diagnosis. These principles are applicable in most settings and within a shared care framework. A summary of the principles of treatment of substance misuse in individuals with mental health problems is presented in Table 1.2.

Assertive outreach

This group of individuals have a tendency not to engage with treatment agencies or disengage from treatment and they are poor at attending appointments. A more assertive approach will enable supervision and work towards the reinstatement of engagement with the appropriate services. The individuals may require practical assistance with basic needs, such as housing, state benefits or welfare, in which there is some tangible gain for the individual. Contact with the individuals may be

Table 1.2 Principles of treatment of substance misuse in individuals with mental health problems.

Assertiveness	Outreach in the community Practical assistance with basic needs Working with family members
Close monitoring	Intensive supervision Voluntary and at times involuntary
Integration	Integrated treatment programmes in which the same clinician provides mental health and substance misuse treatment in same setting
Comprehensiveness	Addresses living skills, relationships, vocational and interpersonal skills in addition to clinical treatments
Stable living conditions	Access to housing, support and companionship in the community
Flexibility and specialisation	Successful clinicians modify previous beliefs, learn new skills and try new approaches empirically
Stages of treatment	Treatment proceeds in stages: engagement, persuasion, active treatment and relapse prevention
Longitudinal perspective	Recognises that substance misuse and mental illness are chronic relapsing conditions and treatment occurs over years rather than episodically or during crisis
Optimism	Encourages hope and counters demoralisation amongst patients, family and clinicians

Source: based on Drake *et al.* (1993).

made at various locations, for example at the social security department, chemist, family home or probation service. Working with family members is an important aspect for assessment and support of carers.

Close monitoring

There should be intensive supervision at least three times a week, initially, to establish a therapeutic relationship and engage the client for other intervention strategies. Close monitoring, voluntary and at times involuntary, must be made on the mental/psychological state of the individual and on compliance with prescribed medications (methadone, antipsychotics, antidepressants, disulfiram, etc.).

Integration

The treatment programme is based on integrated care pathways in which there is concurrent and coordinated treatment. The use of the care programme approach (CPA) would enhance and facilitate better liaison between mental health and substance misuse services and other appropriate agencies. Virtual teams can be formed across teams and organisations and this has the advantage of flexibility but lacks the cohesion of a single 'physical team' (Checinski, 2002). A strong key worker system would enable the coordination of the network of care and treatment required.

Comprehensiveness

Individuals with dual diagnosis often have complex needs in other areas of their lives. This means addressing living skills, relationships, vocational and interpersonal skills, in addition to routine screening (dental, ophthalmology, cervical smears) and clinical treatments.

Stable living situation

Links with housing services and associations is essential in the provision of accommodation for the individual. Access to appropriate supportive housing may be necessary in the overall support system, as attending hostels or night shelters may expose the individual to alcohol and/or drug environments.

Flexibility with specialisation

Successful practitioners will need to modify previous beliefs, learn new skills and try new approaches. Practitioners need to re-evaluate and modify traditional therapeutic approaches to be effective in engaging individuals with dual diagnosis. Directive 'counselling' and confrontational challenges may be counterproductive and may heighten the risk of disengagement with the treatment services. Overtly self-abusive behaviour, particularly when it involves illicit psychoactive substances, is dealt with in a suppressive and moralistic way by many health care workers, not least of all nurses, probably out of a sense of frustration or inadequacy about their ability to effect any change (Gafoor, 1985). This needs to change.

Stages of treatment

The treatment of individuals with dual diagnosis proceeds in stages: engagement, persuasion, active treatment and relapse prevention. However, in clinical practice treatment rarely proceeds in a linear pathway. Each individual will be different and will typically enter the cycle of change and move through the stages intermittently. Individuals will move back and forward between the stages and specific interventions will be required for particular stages.

Longitudinal perspective

It is important to recognise that substance misuse and mental disorder are chronic relapsing conditions and treatment occurs over years rather than episodically or during crisis.

Optimism

Individuals with dual diagnosis are likely to feel hopeless about the future due to the combined effects and consequences of both conditions. This may be perceived as having poor or a lack of motivation to engage in treatment. However, practitioners need to view motivation as a dynamic process that can be undermined or enhanced by different therapeutic techniques and approaches. The best treatment outcome may depend upon staff who have therapeutic optimism towards the individual, treatment and recovery.

Models of treatment: whose patient anyway?

Dual diagnosis patients are a heterogeneous population and the demands they make on services pose huge challenges to the models of intervention and the health care delivery system. Models of intervention are based on whether the services are identified as serial, parallel, integrated or shared care. The serial or sequential model is where one treatment follows the other, but they are not offered simultaneously. The parallel model is based on treatment being delivered by both substance misuse teams and the mental health teams concurrently. In both models, expertise is not shared across teams and they have difficulties engaging patients in treatment and reducing non-compliance, which in turn is associated with poor service coordination, and fragmentation of the care delivery process (Edeh, 2002). However, dual diagnosis services with this liaison role have begun to emerge in the UK (Department of Health, 2002).

The integrated treatment model is based on a single treatment system (or dual team) whereby an individual's substance misuse and mental health problems are treated simultaneously by the same practitioner. This model is designed to offer a comprehensive range of interventions, which include pharmacological, psycho-educational, behavioural, case management and self-help approaches. However, this model views dual diagnosis as a static condition where the needs and problems of the individual remain the same constantly. It is regarded as an expensive service provision and isolated from mainstream services. The components of an integrated model are presented in Table 1.3.

The shared care model (joint liaison/collaborative approach) involves the delivery of parallel treatment with close collaboration and communication between teams and the careful timing of interventions. This model is expected to reduce non-compliance, poor service coordination, the fragmentation of the care delivery process and enhance the engagement of dual diagnosis individuals with treatment services. However, the skills and expertise of those in substance misuse and mental health services need to be utilised effectively to provide effective treatment. There is no clear evidence supporting the advantage of any model as a preference over others (Health Advisory Service, 2001; Ley *et al.*, 2001). Each local area needs to identify the appropriate model and approach based on health care needs and service configurations. For a comprehensive review of dual or separate services see Edeh (2002).

The National Treatment Agency (2002) guidance on models of care provides a treatment framework for the commissioning of an integrated drug treatment system for adult drug misusers in

Table 1.3 Common components of integrated treatment.

Case management	Multidisciplinary case management with assertive outreach
Close monitoring	Medication supervision (including urine drug screening)
Substance misuse treatment	Motivational interviewing; harm reduction and cognitive behavioural; self-help group (twelve-step programmes) and social skills training
Rehabilitation	Provision of long-term support: day care or residential care, to enable restoration of social and occupational function (supported education and employment)
Housing	Supported and independent
Pharmacotherapy	Provision of antipsychotic medication (particularly clozapine) in those with schizophrenia, and improvement of compliance by providing education and medication supervision

Source: adapted from Drake & Mueser (2000).

England. The models of care framework is intended to support the move towards an integrated care pathway in the development of the essential components of specialist substance misuse services and the importance of links with other health, social care and criminal justice agencies. The integrated care pathways provide a means of agreeing local referral and treatment protocols to define where and when a particular service user needs to be referred.

An optimal model of care for patients with dual diagnosis could be developed in the context of current service models and structures, provided minimum standards for quality are established. This has been suggested by Abou Saleh (2000; 2004). The quality standards for service planning should include:

- Access to relevant services (crisis, support, housing, aftercare, therapeutic and legal services)
- Responsive and flexible approaches (assessment, engagement, retention, managing chaos and crisis, individual responses)
- Continuous care and management (monitoring, liaison, involvement of carers, risk assessment and management)
- Adequately trained staff (access to mental health trained staff)

Intervention strategies

An assessment of substance misuse should form an integral part of standard assessment procedures for mental health problems. For further information on screening and assessment see Chapter 18 on a Framework for Multidimensional Assessment. Osher & Kofoed (1989) provide a useful framework for utilising therapeutic interventions with individuals who have coexisting substance misuse and mental health problems. They identified four stages of intervention:

- Engagement
- Motivation for change (persuasion)
- Active treatment
- Relapse prevention

Within these stages exist various cognitive approaches to the care and treatment of individuals with dual diagnosis, such as harm reduction, motivational interviewing, individual cognitive behavioural counselling, lifestyle change, relapse planning and prevention, and family education.

Engagement

Engagement is concerned with the development and maintenance of a therapeutic alliance between staff and client. Attempts to establish a therapeutic relationship prematurely may exacerbate the potential for clients to disengage from treatment services. The aim at this stage is to understand the client and their view, to respond to their behaviour and language, to recognise their often unspoken needs, and thereby to develop some trust and genuineness (Price, 2002). This can be enhanced by the style of interaction, which should be non-confrontational, empathic and respectful of the client's subjective experiences of substance misuse. The strength of this alliance will depend upon the value a client attributes to the service, the social marketing of the services by the staff and meeting the client's immediate needs. Substance misuse is not addressed directly until the end of the engagement process when a working alliance has developed.

The following guidelines (Rethink & Turning Point, 2004) will help to promote engagement:

- Motivate clients to see the benefits of the treatment process: this requires a clear idea of what they need and value
- Have a non-confrontational, empathic and committed approach
- Offer help with meeting initial needs such as food, shelter, housing, clothing
- Provide assistance with benefit entitlements
- Provide assistance with legal matters
- Involve family or carers wherever possible
- Meet clients in settings where they feel safe: this may be more constructive than expecting them to come to services

Motivation

This stage draws upon the principles of motivational interviewing (see Chapter 25 on Motivational Interviewing) to effect change and is contingent upon regular contact and a working alliance between staff and client. In this context, its purpose is to empower the client to gain insight into their problems and to strengthen a client's motivation and commitment to change whilst avoiding confrontation and resistance. A variety of simple techniques (Department of Health, 2002) can be used for this purpose including:

- Education about substances and the problems that may be associated with misuse, including the effects on mental health
- Presentation of objective assessment data (for example liver function tests, urinalysis)
- Balance sheets on which the client lists the pros and cons of continued use/abstinence
- Exploration of barriers to the attainment of future goals
- Reframing problems or past events, emphasising the influence of substance misuse
- Reviewing medication and the use of an optimal medication regime

Active treatment

This stage involves the persuasion of the client of the value and benefits of treatment, although it may take a few months before a client is ready to receive active treatment interventions for their substance misuse. It is important at the outset to agree the anticipated goal of treatment and to integrate treatment of mental health problems and substance misuse. This should entail the active involvement of the client in formulating goals and a care plan. If it is unrealistic to aim for abstinence it may be more appropriate to consider intermediate goals that represent reductions in the harm incurred from drug and alcohol misuse, whilst not focusing prematurely on complete cessation (Department of Health, 2002). A number of interventions have been identified for the effective treatment of dual diagnosis, but these lack specificity (Department of Health, 2002). The interventions are:

- Integrated treatment
- Staged interventions
- Assertive outreach
- Motivational interventions
- Individual counselling
- Social support interventions
- Long-term perspective

Cognitive behavioural therapy has been shown to be a potent therapeutic tool for a range of mental health problems (Dattilio & Freeman, 1992). This is no less true in dually diagnosed clients, where the skilful use of analysis, disputing cognitions, combined with realistic homework tasks can enhance the skills that promote abstinence, including increasing self-efficacy in finding, establishing and maintaining appropriate support networks (Price, 2002). Other interventions as part of the holistic approach should be provided in relation to pharmacological management, social support and building self-esteem, social skills, occupational therapy, welfare advice and employment services.

Relapse prevention

Substance misuse and mental health problems are chronic relapsing conditions. Given the relapsing nature of substance misuse it is important, once a client has reduced their misuse, or become abstinent, to offer interventions aimed at the prevention and management of future relapses. It is also crucial that both clients and staff accept relapse and do not perceive it as a weakness or failure. If the substance use is sustained, a return to the motivation for change stage is necessary and attention should be given to the development of new action plans. The principles and strategies of 'relapse prevention' for substance misuse (see Chapter 26) and the management of relapses to psychosis are recommended for this purpose. This approach aims to identify high-risk situations for substance misuse and rehearse coping strategies proactively.

Conclusion

The term dual diagnosis is often used to describe this coexistence and these patients tend to be more problematic to treat and manage in view of higher rates of non-compliance, violence, homelessness and suicide. The relationship between substance misuse and mental health problems is complex. Intoxication and withdrawal from drugs and alcohol can produce psychiatric symptoms, while on the other hand some individuals with psychiatric disorders, such as antisocial personality disorders and schizophrenia are more susceptible to substance misuse. The mental state of the patient may act as a barrier to recognition as some patients may not be able to understand the nature of the symptoms they experience or adequately describe them in a way that enables clinical staff to make an accurate assessment. This task of diagnosis is further compounded if the patient is a polydrug user and is taking a combination of psychoactive substances at the same time. Even when substance misuse is identified it is often difficult to distinguish between symptoms that are related to substance misuse or a psychiatric disorder. Failure to recognise and treat substance misuse at an early stage will not only lead to ineffective management and treatment outcomes, but may also result in a deterioration of the patient's symptomatology.

The national guidance on good practice in dual diagnosis (Department of Health, 2002) is a step in the right direction. It focuses on the complex needs of patients with coexistence of substance misuse and mental health problems. However, the document fails to address important issues relating to social care, the resource implications of this major service development, and the interface between mainstream mental health services and addiction services, as well as implications for the future and the scope of addiction services (Abou Saleh, 2004). The involvement of service users, families and carers is central in the care planning and treatment process, and must not be tokenistic or superficial. The involvement should take place at all stages: in treatment, in the planning, delivery and development of existing services, and in the planning and commissioning of future services (Rethink & Turning Point, 2004). Attention also needs to be focused on special populations (see Part 2) in relation to dual diagnosis, such as black and ethnic minority groups, homelessness, older people (alcohol and tranquillisers), young people and women (Health Advisory Service, 2001).

There is also the need to address the training and continuing professional development (Chapter 27) of staff to working with coexistence of substance misuse and psychiatric disorders. There is evidence to suggest that mental health service workers lacked the knowledge and skills for assessment and treatment of substance misuse and were insufficiently aware of the available resources and how to access substance misuse services (Maslin *et al.*, 2001). Dual diagnosis is often not picked up by substance misuse or mental health services, indicating a need for improvement in staff training and routine assessment and recording (Weaver *et al.*, 2002).

The changing patterns and prevalence of the coexistence of substance misuse and psychiatric disorders in the UK necessitate new and innovative responses from health and social care workers and service providers. Dual diagnosis, like substance misuse, is not the sole responsibility of one discipline or specialist. It requires a multidimensional approach and involves inter-agency collaboration in the ownership of common goals in meeting the complex physical/medical, social, psychological and spiritual needs of the individual. There is cause for optimism.

References

Abou Saleh, M.T. (2000) Substance misuse and co-morbid psychiatric disorders. *CPD Bulletin in Psychiatry*, 2, 61–7.

Abou Saleh, M.T. (2004) Dual diagnosis: management within a psychosocial context. *Advances in Psychiatric Treatment*, 10, 352–60.

Addington, J. & Duchak, V. (1997) Reasons for substance use in schizophrenia. *Acta Psychiatrica Scandinavica*, 96, 329–33.

American Psychiatric Association (1994) *DSM-IV: Diagnostic and Statistical Manual of Mental Disorders*, 4th edn, pp. 75–90. American Psychiatric Association, Washington, DC.

Anthony, J.C. & Helzer, J.E. (1991) Syndromes of drug abuse and dependence. In: *Psychiatric Disorders in America: the Epidemiologic Catchment Area Study* (Robins, L.N. & Regier, D.A., eds), pp. 116–54. Free Press, New York.

Berman, S. & Noble, E.P. (1993) Childhood antecedents of substance misuse. *Current Opinion in Psychiatry*, 6, 382–7.

Birchwood, M., Mason, R., MacMillan, F. & Healy, J. (1993) Depression, demoralisation and control over psychotic illness: a comparison of depressed and non-depressed patients with chronic psychosis. *Psychological Medicine*, 23, 387–91.

Carey, K.B. (1989) Emerging treatment guidelines for mentally ill chemical abusers. *Hospital Community Psychiatry*, 40, 341–2.

Carey, K.B. & Carey, M.P. (1995) Reasons for drinking among psychiatric outpatients: relationship to drinking patterns. *Psychology of Addictive Behaviours*, 9, 251–7.

Castaneda, R., Lifshutz, H., Galanter, M. & Franco, H. (1994) Empirical assessment of the self-medication hypothesis among dually diagnosed in-patients. *Comprehensive Psychiatry*, 35 (3), 180–4.

Checinski, K. (2002) Treatment strategies and interventions. In: *Dual Diagnosis: Substance Misuse and Psychiatric Disorders* (Rassool G.H., ed.). Blackwell Publishing, Oxford.

Corse, S.J., Hirschinger, N.B. & Zanis, D. (1995) The use of the Addiction Severity Index with people with severe mental illness. *Psychiatric Rehabilitation Journal*, 19, 9–18.

Crawford, V. (1996) Co-morbidity of substance misuse and psychiatric disorders. *Current Opinion in Psychiatry*, 9, 231–4.

Crome, I.B. (1999) Substance misuse and psychiatric co-morbidity: towards improved service provision. *Drugs: education, prevention and policy*, 6, 151–74.

Dattilio, F.M. & Freeman, A. (1992) Introduction to cognitive therapy. In: *Comprehensive Casebook of Cognitive Therapy* (Freeman, A. & Dattilio, F.M., eds), pp. 3–11. Plenum, New York.

Department of Health (2002) *Mental Health Policy Implementation Guide. Dual Diagnosis Good Practice Guide.* Department of Health, London.

Dixon, L., Haas, G., Weiden, P., Sweeney, J. & Frances, A. (1990) Acute effects of drug abuse in schizophrenic patients: clinical observations and patients' self reports. *Schizophrenia Bulletin*, 16, 69–79.

Drake, R.E. & Mueser, K.T. (2000) Psychosocial approaches to dual diagnosis. *Schizophrenia Bulletin*, 26, 105–117.

Drake, R.E., Banels, S.J., Teague, G.B., Noordsy, D.L. & Clarke, R.E. (1993) Treatment for substance misuse in severely mentally ill patients. *Journal of Nervous and Mental Diseases*, 181, 606–11.

Drake, R.E., Osher, F.C., Noordsy, D.L., Hurlbut, S.C., Teague, G.B. & Beaudett, M.S. (1990) Diagnosis of alcohol use disorders in schizophrenia. *Schizophrenia Bulletin*, 16, 57–67.

Drake, R.E., Osher, F.C. & Wallach, M.A. (1989) Alcohol use and abuse in schizophrenia: a prospective community study. *Journal of Nervous and Mental Disease*, 177, 408–14.

Edeh, J. (2002) Dual or separate services? In: *Dual Diagnosis: Substance Misuse and Psychiatric Disorders* (Rassool G.H., ed.). Blackwell Publishing, Oxford.

Evans, K. & Sullivan, J.M. (2001) *Dual Diagnosis: Counselling the Mentally Ill Substance Abuser*, 2nd edn. Guilford Press, New York.

Farrell, M., Howes, S., Taylor, C. *et al.* (1998) Substance misuse and psychiatric co-morbidity: an overview of the OPCS National Psychiatric Morbidity Study. *Addictive Behaviours*, 23 (6), 909–18.

Gafoor, M. (1985) Nurses' attitudes to the drug abuser. Letter to *Nursing Times*, 30 Oct.

Gossop, M., Mardsen, J. & Steward, D. (1998) *NTORS at One Year: The National Treatment Outcome and Research Study.* Department of Health, London.

Health Advisory Service (2001) Substance misuse and mental health co-morbidity (dual diagnosis). *Standards for Mental Health Services.* Health Advisory Service, London.

Jones, P., Guth, C., Lewis, S. & Murray, R. (1994) Low intelligence and poor education achievement precede early onset of schizophrenic psychosis. In: *Neuropsychology of Schizophrenia* (David, A.S. & Cutting, J.C., eds), pp. 131–44. Erlbaum, East Essex.

Khantzian, E.J. (1985) The self-medication hypothesis of addictive disorders: focus on heroin and cocaine dependence. *American Journal of Psychiatry*, 142 (11), 1259–64.

Khantzian, E.J. (1997) The self-medication hypothesis of addictive disorders: a reconsideration and recent applications. *Harvard Review of Psychiatry*, 4, 231–44.

Laurence, J. (1995) Mental hospitals are 'paradise for drug-pushers.' *The Times*, 14 June, p. 6.

Leshner, A.I. (1998) *Bridging the Disconnect Between Research and Practice.* The National Conference on Drug and Drug Addiction Treatment: From Research to Practice. National Institute on Drug Abuse, Washington, DC.

Ley, A., Jeffery, D., Aclaren, S. & Siegfried, N. (2001) Treatment programmes for people with both severe mental illness and substance misuse. *Cochrane Review, Issue 3.* The Cochrane Library.

Lieberman, J.A., Kane, J.M. & Alvir, J. (1987) Provocative tests with psychostimulant drugs in schizophrenia. *Psychopharmacology*, 91, 415–33.

McCrone, P., Menezes, P.R., Johnson, S. *et al.* (2000) Service use and costs of people with dual diagnosis in South London. *Acta Psychiatrica Scandinavica*, 101, 464–72.

Marsden, J., Gossop, M., Stewart, D. *et al.* (2000) Psychiatric symptoms among clients seeking treatment for drug dependence. Intake data from the National Treatment Outcome Research Study. *British Journal of Psychiatry*, 176, 285–9.

Maslin, J., Graham, H.L., Cawley, M.A.C. *et al.* (2001) Combined severe mental health and substance use problems: what are the training and support needs of staff working with this client group? *Journal of Mental Health*, 10 (2), 131–40.

Menezes, P., Johnson, S., Thornicroft, G. *et al.* (1996) Drug and alcohol problems among individuals with severe mental illnesses in South London. *British Journal of Psychiatry*, 168, 612–19.

Mueser, K., Bennett, M. & Kushner, M. (1995) Epidemiology of substance use disorders among persons with chronic mental illness. In: *Double Jeopardy: Chronic Mental Illness and Substance Use Disorders* (Lehman, A. & Dixon, L., eds). Harwood Academic, Chur, Switzerland.

National Treatment Agency (2002) *Models of Care.* Parts 1 and 2. National Treatment Agency, London.

Neeleman, J. & Farrell, M. (1997) Suicide and substance misuse. *British Journal of Psychiatry*, 175, 303–4.

Noordsy, D.L., Drake, R.E., Teague, G.B. *et al.* (1991) Subjective experiences related to alcohol use among schizophrenics. *The Journal of Nervous and Mental Disease*, 1179, 410–14.

Osher, F.C. & Kofoed, L.L. (1989) Treatment of patients with psychiatric and psychoactive substance abuse disorders. *Hospital Community Psychiatry*, 40, 1025–30.

Oyefeso, A., Ghodse, H., Clancy, C. & Corkey, J. (1999) Suicide among drug addicts in the UK. *British Journal of Psychiatry*, 175, 277–82.

Price, P. (2002) Nursing Interventions in the Care of Dually Diagnosed Clients. In: *Dual Diagnosis: Substance Misuse and Psychiatric Disorders* (Rassool G.H., ed.), Blackwell Publishing, Oxford.

Pristach, C.A. & Smith, C.M. (1996) Self-reported effects of alcohol use on symptoms of schizophrenia. *Psychiatric Services*, 47, 421–3.

Rethink & Turning Point (2004) *Dual Diagnosis Toolkit Mental Health and Substance Misuse. A Practical Guide for Professionals and Practitionery.* Rethink & Turning Point, London.

Rostad, P. & Checinski, K. (1996) *Dual Diagnosis: Facing the Challenge*. Wynne Howard Books, Surrey.

Schneider, F.R. & Siris, S.D. (1987) A review of psychoactive substance use and abuse in schizophrenia: patterns of drug choice. *Journal of Psychiatry*, 165, 13–21.

Shaffer, D., Gould, M.S., Fisher, P. *et al.* (1996) Psychiatric diagnosis in child and adolescent suicide. *Archives of General Psychiatry*, 53, 339–48.

Smith, J. & Hucker, S. (1994) Schizophrenia and substance abuse. *British Journal of Psychiatry*, 165, 13–21.

Weaver, T., Charles, V., Madden, P. & Renton, A. (2002) Co-morbidity of substance misuse and mental illness collaborative study (COSMIC). National Treatment Agency, London.

Williams, H. (2002) Dual diagnosis – an overview: fact or fiction? In: *Dual Diagnosis: Substance Misuse and Psychiatric Disorders* (Rassool G.H., ed.). Blackwell Publishing, Oxford.

Williams, R. & Cohen, J. (2000) Substance use and misuse in psychiatric wards: a model task for clinical governance? *Psychiatric Bulletin*, 24, 43–6.

Wright, S., Gournay, K., Glorney, E. & Thornicroft, G. (2000) Dual diagnosis in the suburbs: prevalence, need, and in-patient service use. *Social Psychiatry Psychiatric Epidemiology*, 35, 297–304.

2 Policy Initiatives in Substance Misuse and Mental Health: Implications for Practice

A. Hammond

Introduction

Mental health and substance misuse policy has evolved gradually and separately over time. To understand the action plans set down in policy documents we need to explore the various influences that have impacted on the decision makers who develop these policies. According to Palmer & Short (1989) economic, political, sociological, epidemiological and public health issues of the day are important predictors of policy formation. Also, scientific and medical discoveries, psychological understanding, and philosophical and religious beliefs all underpin policy frameworks. This chapter will explore some of these influences in the context of history, before looking at some of the most recent documents and concerns that have led to the present interest in policy development for those with a dual diagnosis.

Historical context

Before the eighteenth century, policy, if there was such a thing, was underpinned by a belief that God or the gods were responsible for all illness, mental and physical (Escohotado, 1999; Porter, 2002). The ancients knew the link between mental health and drug use; they knew that some drugs used in excess could cause hallucinations and delirium, including alcohol (Escohotado, 1999). During the Dark Ages religion dictated policy. The belief in the supernatural culminated in the witch hunts. This had enormous implications for those with a mental illness and for those who made, took, sold or dispensed drugs that were thought of as diabolic; they were at risk of being drowned or burned at the stake. In his book, *De Praestigiis Daemonum* (1563) (On the Conjuring Tricks of Demons) Johannes Weyer suggested that hallucinations were caused by either dreams or drugs and not witchcraft. He was also branded a sorcerer for his words. With the renaissance the tide turned, and the ideas first put forward by Hippocrates, that mental illness is organic in origin and pharmacology was not inspired by the devil, grew (Porter, 2002), putting the supernatural into the background.

Years of asylum

By the eighteenth century, those whose behaviour was not considered normal were increasingly being cared for in madhouses; these became known as asylums, later mental hospitals and then psychiatric hospitals. Some were concerned about the quality, treatment and civil liberties of those in the institutions as well as the safety of the general public. As a result, several acts of Parliament were passed addressing some of these issues (Rogers &

Pilgrim, 2001; Porter, 2002). Institutions continued to be thought to be the best place to treat patients, and it is only now in the twenty-first century that we are seeing the last of the great asylums being demolished.

Shift in ideology

The twentieth century brought a shift in the understanding of mental illness. The degeneration theory proposed that people had a genetic vulnerability to mental illness, evidenced by a family history of neurasthenia, nervous hysteria, alcohol and opiate addiction, prostitution, insanity proper and idiocy (Porter, 2002). This model was discredited following the First World War when it was found that the officer soldier was experiencing mental health problems, as this ran counter to the theory. Also, women who were working prolonged hours in the ammunitions factory were presenting with anxiety, miscarriages and exhaustion; this led to a renewed interest in the environmental theory first put forward by the pioneers in moral therapy, such as Philippe Pinel and William Tuke of the late eighteenth and early nineteenth century, who believed that the traditional approach was inhuman. The difference being that rather than the institution being thought of as the best place to give refuge and therapy the best place and choice of treatment was outpatient psychotherapy (Rogers & Pilgrim, 2001; Porter, 2002).

Concern about drugs

Prior to the First World War, North American prohibitionists were warning of the physical and moral dangers of opium use to the individual and society. This is not surprising considering the degeneration theory described above. Concern led to the 1909 Shanghai International Opiate Commission and the 1911 and 1913 Hague Conferences. The Americans won over other world leaders and the signatories agreed to curb production, distribution and consumption of opiates, morphine, heroin and cocaine, and to restrict their use for medical purposes only. The regulations would be bound by international law. Ratification of the agreement was postponed until after the First World War, though those countries that had already signed could begin making them law in their own countries. In 1919, it was ratified in the Treaty of Versailles. These regulations underpin modern British legislation (Release, 2005). The Misuse of Drugs Act 1971 classifies drugs into three classes, A, B and C. The class of drug determines the sentence the offender is given. The legislation also laid down the prescribing responsibilities of the doctor. The Misuse of Drugs Regulations 1973 and 2001 place classes of drug under five schedules. The schedule determines who can produce, supply and prescribe; drugs found under schedule 1 require a Home Office licence, whereas those under schedule 5 include those that can be sold over the counter (Home Office, 2005).

The first indications of prohibition in Britain arrived with the 1916 Defence of the Realm regulations that made it an offence to give or sell cocaine to soldiers, though this was modified allowing members of the medical profession and those on a prescription to be in possession. In 1920 and then in 1923 the Dangerous Drugs Acts were passed, which meant a prescription would be needed to obtain opium, its derivatives and cocaine. In 1926 the Rolleston Committee decided that drug addiction was not a deviant activity to be dealt with by the criminal justice system as in the USA, but was a disease and should be treated accordingly with opiates. Unlike the Harrison Act in the USA, the British system allowed the prescribing of maintenance doses of opiates to those who could lead a normal life on such a dose and had previously tried but failed detoxification (Release, 2005).

Buds of community care

After the First World War the medical profession turned their attention to psychotherapy to treat what was now termed the more neurotic conditions caused by environmental issues rather than psychosis. The 1930 Mental Treatment Act opened the asylum door to voluntary admissions. Rather than being placed in the asylum, outpatient treatment was becoming established for those with a mental illness as well as drug addicts. Mental health came under the umbrella of the National Health Service (NHS) when it was established in 1948 and the move toward outpatient treatment continued (Rogers & Pilgrim, 2001).

The 1960s brought Enoch Powell's famous water tower speech, where he presented the ideas laid down in his hospital plan, which was published in 1962. The plan promoted community care, recommending that asylums be run down, community service be developed and psychiatric wards be attached to general hospitals. By the 1970s community care was becoming a reality despite the oil crisis of 1973 that reduced the spending on health by successive governments. Community mental health teams were on the increase between 1977 and 1987, growing from one to fifty four (Rogers & Pilgrim, 2001).

This period also saw an increase in trends of drug misuse. The Brain Committee had been established between 1958 and 1959 to look into this apparent increase. They did not support the claim, but by 1964 a sudden rise in the number of addicts known to the Home Office prompted the second Brain Committee to reform and their findings formed the basis of the Dangerous Drugs Act of 1967 (Release, 2005). With more clients being treated in the community there was also increased drug availability, indicated by numbers of convictions. By 1982 between 17 000 and 20 000 people were convicted of possession of all types of drug, and by 1992 between 40 000 and 45 000 people were convicted (Ghodse, 1995). It is therefore not surprising that dual diagnosis and co-morbidity were being recognised and reported in the literature.

Foundations of modern policy

Internal market

The 1980s and 1990s saw the introduction of the internal market into the NHS. Commissioners or GP fundholders were given the responsibility of purchasing services from providers on behalf of their patients. These principles rely on availability of choice and the freedom to choose (Rogers & Pilgrim, 2001). It may be said that there is very little choice in mental health or drug services because these are determined by postcode system and GP. Mental health services usually have the monopoly because of their authority under the Mental Health Act to detain and treat clients. It is slightly different with drug and alcohol services where there is sometimes more than one provider in a location, giving clients and commissioners more choice. The freedom to choose is sometimes more complex; it is limited to the client being included or excluded in the decision making process. Clients with dual diagnosis have no choice, are at greater risk of relapse, have increased number of hospital admissions, are more likely to be involved in criminal justice issues, including violence, homelessness and infections such as HIV and hepatitis, and often fall through the net between services (Drake *et al.*, 2001).

Drake *et al.* (2001) outlined the possible reasons for this: fragmented services, funding barriers, administrative barriers, no outcome measures or quality assurance, judgemental attitude and poor training by those making the diagnosis; they may not make a diagnosis if they think it will pull on their budget, or they may not have the training to recognise a dual diagnosis and may make a wrong diagnosis. Other reasons for lack of opportunities for choice are that staff in mental health services may lack understanding of the effect of drugs on mental health and appropriate physical and psychological treatments, and those in drug services may not recognise someone with a serious mental illness. Different philosophies mean that mental health services offer outreach but that substance misuse services do not.

1997 and beyond

When the Labour Government came to power in 1997 they set out to modernise the NHS, keep what was good about previous policy and address its limitations. They set out their agenda in the following White Papers: *The New NHS: Modern and Dependable* (Department of Health, 1997) and *The NHS Plan* (Department of Health, 2000). The ideas from the former paper were developed in the paper *A First Class Service: Quality in the New NHS* (Department of Health, 1999a). Out of this came the *National Service Framework for Mental Health* (NSF) (Department of Health, 1999b). The NHS plan has built on these former policies and is currently used in the delivery of mental health services and further supported by the NSF for mental health. The delivery of the NHS Plan and NSF is found in the *Mental Health Implementation Guide* (Department of Health, 2001). The relevant aspects of the strategy are embedded in the *Models of Care* (Department of Health, 2002a, 2005), which specifies how services for drug users should be planned, delivered and monitored.

The main theme of the Government's policy was to remove the internal market by abolishing GP fundholding and replace it with primary care groups and then trusts. To mend the fragmentation and minimise the risk of people falling through the net of services they expect the NHS and Social Services to pool their budgets by merging and becoming NHS and Social Care trusts.

Both mental health and substance misuse services have a responsibility to ensure that the Government's strategy is put in place to improve services and stop the postcode lottery. The Government's policy is founded in social inclusion not exclusion. The following is a summary of the Government's strategy for improving the quality of the health service. We then focus on those policies specific to mental health and substance misuse, including published guidelines that give the framework for how mental health, substance misuse and dual diagnosis services can be delivered according to local need.

A First Class Service: Quality in the New NHS (1999a) is a tripartite framework encompassing:

(1) Standard setting
  (a) The National Institute of Clinical Excellence
  (b) The National Service Framework
(2) Delivering system
  (a) Clinical governance
  (b) Quality improvement by ensuring service is cost effective and accessible
  (c) Raising performance by clinical audit
  (d) Evidence based practice
  (e) Risk assessment and management risk of client to self and others, plus iatrogenic risk
  (f) Continuous professional development
(3) Monitoring systems
  (a) Commission for Health Improvement
  (b) The National Performance Assessment Framework
  (c) The national survey of patients

This framework underpins the following strategies and service guidelines.

Strategy for mental health and substance misuse

National service framework for mental health

In 1999, the Government published a ten-year mental health strategy in the *National Service Framework* (Department of Health, 1999b), relevant to all statutory and non-statutory services. The framework sets out how services should be planned, delivered and monitored; it also sets out seven standards in five areas:

1	Mental health promotion
2 and 3	Primary care and access to services
4 and 5	Effective services for people with severe mental illness
6	Caring about carers
7	Preventing suicide

Reference to dual diagnosis is implicit in the following NSF standards.

Standard one
Mental health promotion

- Development of programmes to combat discrimination and social exclusion in vulnerable groups such as those with mental health and drug and alcohol problems
- Brief interventions offered to alcohol users that could dramatically decrease intake in those drinking over the recommended limits
- Strengthen links between drug, alcohol and mental health services that could reduce suicides

Standards two and three
Primary care and access to services

Staff should:

- Consider the role of drugs and/or alcohol in those presenting with mental health problems, and mental health problems in those presenting with drug and alcohol problems
- Recognise that substance misuse increases risk of suicide in those with mental health problems
- Have a clear understanding of how to access drug, alcohol and mental health services

Standards four and five
Effective services for those with severe mental illness

- Mainstreaming of those with a dual diagnosis into existing mental health and drug and alcohol services
- Clients to have a care plan under the care programme approach (CPA). (This is a framework that supports inter-agency working, including the service user and carers. It consists of assessment, making a care plan, identifying a care coordinator and at least six-monthly reviews. A client with a severe mental illness would be placed on enhanced CPA and those with less severe problems under standard CPA)
- Assertive outreach and crisis resolution teams; recognition that working with this client group is long-term work; staff from these teams should be trained to work with this client group

Standard six Caring for the carers
Standard seven Reducing suicide

Tackling drugs to build a better Britain

In 1995, *Tackling Drugs Together* (Home Office, 1995) was published to address drug issues. By focusing on crime, young people and public health the need was recognised for services to work together and it brought together the Department of Health, Home Office and Department of Education. It introduced drug action teams to implement the strategy, depending on local need. They set up local multi-agency reference groups. The Government has built on this policy with the publication of *Tackling Drugs to Build a Better Britain* in 1998; they updated this in 2002 and again in 2004 with the publication of *Tackling Drugs: Changing Lives* (Home Office, 2004). This aimed:

- To help young people resist drugs misuse to achieve their full potential
- To protect communities from antisocial and criminal behaviour
- To enable people with drug problems to overcome them and live healthy and crime free lives
- To stifle availability of illegal drugs on our streets

Harm reduction/minimisation

Safety of the public has also been the theme in drug services, whether by the prevention of crime or the spread of blood-borne viruses into the general population. The Government's policy on drugs in the 1980s and 1990s was more about public health than that of individual drug users. The fear of the spread of HIV into the non-drug using population prompted the Advisory Council on Drug Misuse to advise services that the threat of HIV is greater than drug misuse itself. The goal of services was to aim towards stopping clients acquiring or transmitting HIV through harm reduction, and maintenance if abstinence is not possible. Community needle exchanges were introduced with the aim of stopping injections with unsterile equipment (Laffan & Gerada, 2005). This policy continues to be successful and underpins today's treatment strategy.

Guidelines

Mental Health Policy Implementation Guide

The *Mental Health Implementation Guide* (Department of Health, 2001) is a framework for delivering mental health services via crisis resolution teams, assertive outreach, early intervention in psychosis, primary care and gateway workers, women only services, break for carers services, strengthening carers support networks, secure accommodation, personality disorder and prison inreach. Clients with a drug or alcohol problem may present at any of these services.

Models of care plus drug misuse and dependency guidelines on clinical management

To enable services to deliver the National Service Framework (NSF) and *Tackling Drugs to Build a Better Britain* (Home Office, 1998) the National Treatment Agency was set up in 2001 as a new health authority to oversee the Government's strategy to double the numbers in treatment by 2008. They published the *Models of Care* (Department of Health, 2002a) that defines how services across the country should be planned, delivered and monitored (see Chapter 17).

Once clients are in the system, the *Drug Misuse and Dependency – Guidelines on Clinical Management* (Department of Health, 1999c) recommends a range of treatment options that have been found to be cost effective. The National Treatment Outcome Research Study (Gossop *et al.*, 2001) found that treatment works. It was a prospective, longitudinal, cohort study and monitored the progress of individuals recruited into one of four treatment settings. At the five-year follow-up they reported that drug treatment reduced drug use by 40–60% and reduced arrest for violent and non-violent criminal behaviour by as much as 50%. Following this, the researchers published the following hierarchy of treatment goals:

- Reduction of psychological, social and other problems related to drugs
- Reduction of psychological, social or other problems not related to drug use
- Reduction of harmful or risky behaviour related to drugs, including the sharing of equipment
- Attainment of controlled, non-dependent or non-problematic drug use
- Abstinence from main problem drug
- Abstinence from all drugs

This recognises that treatment works and saves the country £9.50 to £18 in the cost of crime for every £1 spent on treatment (Godfrey *et al.*, 2004). Treatment and criminal justice therefore come together in the drug requirement and rehabilitation (DRR) programmes and the criminal justice intervention programmes (Home Office, 2005). Clients presenting with a first episode of mental illness, drug induced or otherwise, or established mental illness, may come through any of these services.

QuADS

The Government is keen to improve standards and monitor that services are delivering what is expected of them. Drug and alcohol services have a measuring tool called QuADS (quality in alcohol and drug services) (Alcohol Concern, SCODA, 1999) to enable them to do this. It helps services to monitor themselves but it is also a useful tool to be used by the drug and alcohol action team during the inspections. It outlines a range of standards that each service should be delivering and can be measured against.

Social control

Safety of the general public, civil liberties and quality of care has always proved to be challenging for politicians. In the past, asylums acted as places of social control for all those thought to be deviant or who had mental health problems. Today, the challenge is how these can be balanced and clients managed in the community. For those with a mental health problem, section 117 of the 1983 Mental Health Act, and the care programme approach (CPA), established in 1991 as a framework for planning, reviewing and monitoring care, were designed to address these problems. But a number of care in the community enquiries found that these were poorly implemented and the enquiry also found failures around poor communication between services. This resulted in the *Building Bridges* (Department of Health, 1995) strategy which gave guidance on coordination and communication between services and in 1998 the CPA was reviewed. The 1983 Mental Health Act has been found to be unsatisfactory to address the needs of clients in the community and is currently being revised to give more powers to treat such clients. The proposed new Mental Health Bill has prompted a lot of concern from statutory and non-statutory organisations. Two of the contested issues are, first, the plans propose dropping exclusion clauses with the risk of a greater number of service users becoming eligible for enforced treatment; the fear is that this will alienate service users who may avoid asking for help for fear of being placed on an order, so, as in the past, clients who are most vulnerable may fall through the net. The second concern around the community treatment orders (CTO) is who is going to enforce removing a person to a clinical setting when this does not comply with treatment health and safety issues as well as the law on human rights (Rogers & Pilgrim, 2001)?

All of the above agendas and policies came together in the *Dual Diagnosis Good Practice Guide* (Department of Health, 2002b). Although choice and the freedom to choose may continue to be limited for those with a dual diagnosis, the Government has published a good practice framework that is underpinned by the policies from mental health and substance misuse services that have already been discussed. In these the Government has attempted to address issues of civil liberties, quality of care and social inclusion, services for diverse groups such as black and minority ethnic (BME), women, gay, lesbian and transgender groups. When money was divided between health and social care many clients were at risk of falling through the net and not having their needs met. The *Dual Diagnosis Good Practice Guide* (Department of Health, 2002b) has recommended joined-up thinking if the policies from mental health and substance misuse services are to inform the development of an integrated dual diagnosis service.

The main points of the delivery of this service are:

- There should be mainstreaming of clients, meaning that the responsibility for delivering this service lies with mental health services so as to reduce the risk of clients falling between services.
- The client group will have severe mental health problems with combined substance misuse problems.
- Assertive outreach teams are the likely service to manage this client group.
- Substance misuse services should offer specialist support to the mental health services.
- Mental health services should offer specialist support to substance misuse services to enable them to support those with less severe mental health problems.
- There should be clear care pathways between services.
- There should be inter-agency collaboration and training between all agencies involved.
- The service should be underpinned by clinical governance.
- All clients should be under the care programme approach and have a risk assessment.

The document addresses issues of assessment and treatment and presents a number of established models.

Training needs

The Government hopes to drive up standards by having a highly trained and skilled workforce. To aid this and to support the training needs of staff, occupational standards have been developed in the substance misuse field as well as for the NHS. Drug and alcohol national occupational standards, known as DANOS (Skills for Health, 2005), have been published that outline the skills substance misuse workers need to inform their practice. Staff in the NHS will also be expected to be trained to the occupational standard set down in the KSF (*Knowledge and Skills Framework*, Department of Health, 2004). Specific training will be necessary for services to work with this client group. The dual diagnosis guidelines recommend inter-agency training where good practice can be shared.

Conclusion

History has shown that mental health has always been at the mercy of politics and economics. People with drug and/or alcohol and combined mental health problems have always been around, yet it is only recently with the publication of the *Dual Diagnosis Good Practice Guide* (Department of Health, 2002b) that services are able to respond to those clients with complex needs in a more unified way. This is in keeping with the Government's ambition to make sure that the most vulnerable people are not excluded from services.

The central theme running through the ages has been quality and the civil liberties of those being treated, versus the safety of the general public. This has specific implications for those presenting with a dual diagnosis who for too long have been marginalised from services. Focusing on the needs of this client group means that clients are more likely to be socially included and have all their psychological, social and physical, medical and spiritual needs met. What we must guard against, though, is social control at the expense of social inclusion, and it is this that is causing concern with the review of the Mental Health Act. MIND (2005) has suggested that if more money is put into community support, housing and education, there may be less reliance on medication and less need for the new proposed community treatment orders.

Community care is now being realised, albeit with limited resources. Mental health and substance misuse is about the interrelationship between the individual and their internal as well as their external environment. It is therefore foolhardy to rely only on the Western reductionist scientific tradition to inform practice. Research into a range of treatments from medicinal, to psychological, sociological and complementary approaches would lead the way to more holistic forms of treatment. We are beginning to listen to service users; this is a move in the right direction.

Quality for service users has always been of concern to some. Clinical governance, monitoring of services and the standardisation of services according to local need is to be welcomed, but the Government must realise that services have moved beyond the mechanistic view of the seventeenth century; there is now a move amongst clinicians towards a more holistic bio-psychosocial and spiritual approach in the understanding and care of those with mental health and substance misuse problems; this runs contrary to a target setting, form filling approach. The challenge is how to measure quality, standards and effectiveness without being reductionist, but by being person centred.

References

Alcohol Concern, SCODA (1999) *Quality in Alcohol and Drug Services (QuADS). Organisational Standards for Alcohol and Drug Services.* Alcohol Concern. SCODA, London.

Department of Health (1995) *Building Bridges.* HMSO, London.

Department of Health (1997) *The New NHS: Modern and Dependable.* HMSO, London.

Department of Health (1999a) *A First Class Service: Quality in the New NHS.* HMSO, London.

Department of Health (1999b) *National Service Framework for Mental Health.* HMSO, London.

Department of Health (1999c) *Drug Misuse and Dependency – Guidelines on Clinical Management.* HMSO, London.

Department of Health (2000) *The NHS Plan. A Plan for Investment a Plan for Reform.* HMSO, London.

Department of Health (2001) *Mental Health Implementation Guide.* HMSO, London.

Department of Health (2002a) *Models of Care for Substance Misuse Treatment.* HMSO, London.

Department of Health (2002b) *Dual Diagnosis Good Practice Guide.* HMSO, London.

Department of Health (2004) *The NHS Knowledge and Skills Framework and the Development Review Process.* HMSO, London.

Department of Health (2005) *Models of Care for the Treatment of Adult Drug Misusers. Update.* Department of Health, London.

Drake, R.E., Essock, S.M., Shaner, A. *et al.* (2001) Implementing dual diagnosis services for clients with severe mental illness. *Psychiatric Services*, 52 (4), 469–76.

Escohotado, A. (1999) *A Brief History of Drugs: From the Stone Age to the Stoned Age.* Park Street Press, Rochester, Vt.

Gerada, C. (2005) *RCGP Guide to The Management of Substance Misuse in Primary Care.* Royal college of General Practitioners, London.

Ghodse, H. (1995) *Drugs and Addictive Behaviour. A Guide To Treatment*, 2nd edn. Blackwell Science, Oxford.

Godfrey, C., Stewart, D. & Gossop, M. (2004) Economic analysis of costs and consequences of the treatment of drug misuse: two-year outcome data from the National Treatment Outcome Research Study (Norse) *Addiction*, 99 (6), 697.

Gossop, M., Marsden, J., Stewart, D. & Treacy, S. (2001) Outcomes after methadone maintenance and methadone reduction treatments: two-year follow-up results from the NTORS. *Drug and Alcohol Dependence*, 62, 255–64.

Home Office (1995) *Tackling Drugs Together.* HMSO, London. www.homeoffice.gov.uk

Home Office (1998) *Tackling Drugs to Build a Better Britain.* HMSO, London. www.homeoffice.gov.uk

Home Office (2002) *Tackling Drugs to Build a Better Britain Updated Strategy.* HMSO, London. www.homeoffice.gov.uk

Home Office (2004) *Tackling Drugs: Changing Lives.* HMSO, London. www.homeoffice.gov.uk

Home Office (2005) *Tackling Drugs. Changing Lives.* www.homeoffice.gov.uk

Laffan, A. & Gerada, C. (2005) Drug Policy in the United Kingdom. In: *RCGP Guide to The Management of Substance Misuse in Primary Care* (Gerada, C., ed.). Royal College of General Practitioners, London.

MIND (2005) *History of Mental Health.* www.mind.org.uk

Palmer, G. & Short, S. (1989) Health care and public policy: an Australian analysis. In: *Mental Health Policy in Britain* (Rogers, R. & Pilgrim, D., eds), 2nd edn. Palgrave Macmillan, Basingstoke.

Porter, R. (2002) *Madness: a Brief History*. Oxford University Press, Oxford.

Release (2005) *Drug Law History*. www.release.org.uk

Rogers, R. & Pilgrim, D. (2001) *Mental Health Policy in Britain*, 2nd edn. Palgrave Macmillan, Basingstoke.

Skills for Health (2005) *Drug and Alcohol National Occupational Standards* (DANOS). www.skillsforhealth.org.uk

Weyer, J. (1563) *De Praestigiis Daemonum* (On the Conjuring Tricks of Demons) In: *Madness: A Brief History* (Porter, R., ed.). Oxford University Press, Oxford.

3 Understanding Drug Use and Misuse

G.H. Rassool & J. Winnington

Introduction

Psychoactive drugs are substances that have an effect on the central nervous system in altering mood, cognitive process and behaviour. Psychoactive drugs are considered to be illicit as a result of social custom and law, both of which change depending on worldview, culture and societies. In most societies there is no dovetailing of interest in the use and misuse of tranquillisers, barbiturates, heroin, volatile substances, stimulants such as amphetamines and cocaine and its derivatives, cannabis and hallucinogens. Legal drugs such as alcohol, caffeine and nicotine are used as a social lubricant and as a self-medication, to relieve tension and anxiety or to facilitate social intercourse. Despite the increasing risk of morbidity and mortality, alcohol is actively encouraged and socially reinforced in some societies, especially in the Northern hemisphere. Some individuals with dual diagnosis who have become acquainted with psychoactive substances through legitimate medical use are engaging in self-medication for the relief of a particular set of symptoms or to counterbalance the effects of other psychoactive substances.

According to the *UK Drug Report on Trends in 2001* (Jeffery *et al.*, 2002), cannabis was by far the most widely consumed drug, but usage has more or less stabilised in all age groups. Heroin use remained low in 2001 for all ages, with no clear trends. The most marked development was a decline in the availability of amphetamine, but the increase in cocaine and ecstasy use has continued. HIV prevalence among injecting drug users in London has remained at, or near, 4%, and prevalence among injectors in the rest of England and Wales was extremely low, at less than 1%. In 2001, hepatitis C prevalence among injectors was just under 50% in London, compared with about 30% for the rest of England and Wales, but the rate increases with the number of injecting years. Hepatitis B was also higher in London compared with elsewhere in England and Wales.

It is estimated that over 3 million people in the UK use illegal drugs every year, with more than half a million using the most serious drugs such as heroin and crack. There are 280 000 heroin and/or crack users: at any one time, only 20% of high harm causing users are receiving treatment (80% are not) (Cabinet Office, 2003). Drugs such as heroin and crack are by far the most addictive and result in social harm to users and society as a whole. Alcohol misuse is linked to over 30 000 hospital admissions annually for alcohol dependence syndrome and causes up to 22 000 premature deaths per annum. It is reported that at peak times, up to 70% of all admissions to accident and emergency (Cabinet Office, 2004) are related to alcohol. In Great Britain, there were 16 800 casualties in traffic accidents involving illegal alcohol levels, 5% of all traffic accident casualties (Statistical Bulletin, 1999). Currently, more than 120 000 people die each year in the UK from tobacco smoking (Department of Health, 1998a).

The aim of this chapter is to examine the key concepts related to drug use and dependence. The drug experience, patterns of substance use and misuse, how people take drugs and the effects of psychoactive drugs are also presented.

The policy and service framework for drugs

The policy initiatives in substance misuse and mental health have been addressed in the previous chapter. This section seeks briefly to summarise the policy and service framework for drugs. The document *Tackling Drugs to Build a Better Britain* (Department of Health, 1998b) represents current UK drug policy. Efficient delivery mechanisms all need to be in place, including effective UK and regional coordination, partnerships across agencies and rigorous audit and evaluation. Drug action teams (DATs), consisting of senior representatives of health, social services, criminal justice, education and housing agencies, have been established to ensure the strategy is translated into practice. The *Guidelines on Clinical Management* (Department of Health, 1999) for drug misuse and dependence, which underpin the UK drug strategy, placed its emphasis on the rights of individual drug users to receive appropriate treatment and on the responsibility of all doctors to address drug-related problems. This should include the provision of 'shared-care' arrangements, evidence based interventions, such as hepatitis B vaccinations, and providing harm reduction advice. The UK drug strategy is also supported by legislative developments such as The Criminal Justice and Court Services Act (2001) and requires all offenders, including suspects, to be liable for drug testing at each stage of the criminal process. The Act requires the court to take positive drug test results into account when determining whether or not to grant bail. Drug treatment and testing orders (DTTOs) have been introduced to those offenders, or suspects, who are identified as having a drug problem. This legislation also provides a potential mechanism for individuals with a dual diagnosis to enter mental health and/or substance misuse services. The National Treatment Agency, a new special health authority, was created with the aim of increasing the number of drug misuse clients treated and raising the effectiveness of their treatment. The Agency aims to:

- Develop and promulgate evidence based standards for treatment provision and commissioning
- Take action to reduce variations in the availability and standards of treatment
- Ensure the treatment field is able to deliver these improvements
- Develop providers and commissioners
- Promote policy management and development

An *Updated Drug Strategy* (Home Office, 2002) builds on the foundations laid and lessons learned from previous drug strategies. This updated strategy sets out a range of policies and interventions, which concentrate on the most dangerous drugs, the most damaged communities and the individuals whose addiction and chaotic lifestyles are most harmful, both to themselves and others. Implicit in the strategy is the fact that the Government has no intention of legalising any illicit drug.

A recent publication from the National Treatment Agency is the *Models of Care for Substance Misuse Services* (NTA, 2002), a national service framework for substance misuse. The guidance on models of care provides a treatment framework and process intended to support the move towards consensus about the essential components of specialist substance misuse services and the importance of links with other health, social care and criminal justice agencies. The *Alcohol Harm Reduction Strategy for England* (Cabinet Office, 2004) sets out the Government's strategy for tackling the harm and cost of alcohol misuse. The strategy recognises the need for coordination of services and commits to working within the models of care framework on integrated care pathways. It also has a series of measures that aim to tackle alcohol-related disorder in town and city centres, improve treatment and support for people with alcohol problems, clamp down on irresponsible promotions by the industry and provide better information to consumers about the dangers of alcohol misuse.

Under the Road Traffic Act 1988 it is an offence to drive or be in charge of a motor vehicle when unfit through drugs, and disqualifications, stiffer fines and imprisonment can apply. It is also an offence to be drunk whilst in charge of a vehicle. The Misuse of Drugs Act 1971 outlined the degree of severity of penalties for possession, dealing and trafficking of drugs in the UK. It divides drugs into three classes, A–C. Class A drugs are regarded as the most dangerous and so carry the heaviest penalties. Some drugs, for example ketamine, are not yet classified and are regulated through the Medicines Act.

The classes of drug are outlined below:

(1) Class A drugs
Include: ecstasy, LSD, heroin, cocaine, crack, magic mushrooms (if prepared for use), amphetamines (if prepared for injection).
Penalties for possession: up to seven years in prison or an unlimited fine, or both.
Penalties for dealing: up to life in prison or an unlimited fine, or both.

(2) Class B drugs
Include: amphetamines, methylphenidate (Ritalin), pholcodine.
Penalties for possession: up to five years in prison or an unlimited fine, or both.
Penalties for dealing: up to 14 years in prison or an unlimited fine, or both

(3) Class C drugs
Include: cannabis, tranquillisers, some painkillers, GHB (gammahydroxybutyrate).
Penalties for possession: up to two years in prison or an unlimited fine, or both.
Penalties for dealing: up to 14 years in prison or an unlimited fine, or both.

Drugs, drug misuse and dependence

There are various elements of what constitute a drug (food is considered a drug), as the concept is heavily influenced by the socio-cultural context and purpose of its use. The therapeutic use of drugs means a pharmacological preparation used in the prevention, diagnosis and treatment of an abnormal or pathological condition, whereas the non-therapeutic use of drugs is commonly referred to as the use of illegal or socially disapproved substances (Rassool, 1998). However, drugs can be either therapeutic or non-therapeutic, or both. According to the World Health Organization (1981), a drug is 'any substance or chemical that alters the structure or functioning of a living being'. Despite the broadness of the concept, which limits its use for clinical and for certain practical purposes, it provides some perspective to its pervasive nature. A drug, in the broadest sense, is a chemical substance that has an effect on bodily systems and behaviour. This includes a wide range of prescribed drugs, illegal and socially accepted substances.

The term 'drug misuse' may be seen as the use of drugs in a socially unacceptable way that is harmful or hazardous to the individual or others (Royal College of Psychiatrists & Royal College of Physicians, 2000). Drug misuse also implies use outside the therapeutic use that harms health or functioning. It may take the form of physical or psychological dependence or be part of a wider spectrum of problematic or harmful behaviour. The World Health Organization recommends the use of the following terms:

- Unsanctioned use: a drug that is not approved by society
- Hazardous use: a drug leading to harm or dysfunction
- Dysfunctional use: a drug leading to impaired psychological or social functioning
- Harmful use: a drug that is known to cause tissue damage or psychiatric disorders

The term 'drug dependence' refers to behavioural responses that always include a compulsion to take the drug in order to experience its physical or psychological effects, and sometimes to avoid the discomfort of its absence. Dependence is often described as either physical or psychological. Physical dependence is a common and often important, but not a necessary, element of drug dependence. This highlights the core features of dependence, such as tolerance, psychological and physical dependence. These concepts need further explanation and are examined in the next section. Dependence, according to Diagnostic and Statistical Manual of Mental Disorders (DSM-IV) (APA, 1994), requires that three out of seven criteria occur at any time in the same 12-month period. The DSM-IV criteria for dependence are briefly presented in Table 3.1.

The terms 'problem drug user' and 'problem drinker' have been used to refer to those who are dependent on psychoactive substances. A problem drug user has been described as 'any person who experiences social, psychological, physical or legal

Table 3.1 DSM-IV diagnostic criteria for substance dependence.

A maladaptive pattern of substance use leading to clinically significant impairment or distress, as manifested by three or more of the following occurring during the same twelve-month period:

(1) Tolerance, as defined by either of the following:
   (a) Need for markedly increased amounts of the substance to achieve intoxication or desired effect.
   (b) Markedly diminished effect of continued use of the same amount of the substance.

(2) Withdrawal, as manifested by either of the following:
   (a) The characteristic withdrawal syndrome for the substance.
   (b) The same (or a closely related) substance is taken to relieve or avoid withdrawal symptoms.

(3) The substance is often taken in larger amounts or over a longer period than was intended.

(4) A persistent desire or unsuccessful efforts to cut down or control substance use.

(5) A great deal of time is spent in activities necessary to obtain the substance (for example visiting multiple doctors or driving long distances), using the substance (for example chain-smoking) or recovering from its effects.

(6) Important social, occupational or recreational activities are given up or reduced because of substance use.

(7) The substance use is continued despite knowledge of having a persistent or recurrent physical or psychological problem that is likely to have been caused or exacerbated by the substance (for example current cocaine induced depression or continued drinking despite recognition that an ulcer was made worse by alcohol consumption).

problems related to intoxication and/or regular excessive consumption and/or dependence as a consequence of his own use of drugs or other chemical substances' (ACMD, 1982). This definition was widened to include any form of drug misuse that involves, or may lead to, sharing of injecting equipment (ACMD, 1988). The above definition focuses on the needs and problems of the individual and places less emphasis on the substance oriented approach. It is a holistic definition in acknowledging that the problem drug user has social, psychological, physical and legal needs, and the definition could be expanded to incorporate the spiritual needs of the individual problem drug user or problem drinker (Rassool, 2002).

Psychological and physical dependence

Tolerance

Tolerance is a behavioural state and refers to the way the body usually adapts to the repeated presence of a drug. Higher quantities or doses of the psychoactive substance are required to reproduce the desired or similar cognitive, affective or behavioural effects. Tolerance may develop rapidly in the case of LSD, or slowly in the case of alcohol or opiate. The drug must be taken on a regular basis and in adequate quantities for tolerance to occur. For example, amphetamines can produce considerable tolerance and strong psychological dependence with little or no physical dependence, and cocaine can produce psychological dependence without tolerance or physical dependence. Furthermore, in certain medical applications, morphine has been reported to produce tolerance and physical dependence without a significant psychological component.

Psychological dependence

Psychological dependence can be described as a compulsion or a craving to continue to take the drug because of the need for stimulation, or because it relieves anxiety or depression. Psychological dependence is recognised as the most widespread and the most important. This kind of dependence is not only attributed to the use of psychoactive drugs but also to food, sex, gambling, relationships or physical activities.

Physical dependence

Physical dependence is characterised by the need to take a psychoactive substance to avoid physical disturbances or withdrawal symptoms following cessation of use. The withdrawal symptoms depend on the type or category of drugs. For example, for nicotine, the physiological withdrawal symptoms may be relatively slight. With other dependence inducing psychoactive substances, such as opiates and depressants, the withdrawal experience can range from mild to severe. The withdrawal from alcohol for instance can cause hallucinations or epileptic fits and may be life threatening. Physical withdrawal syndromes are not, however, the essence of dependence. It is possible to have dependence without withdrawal and withdrawal without dependence (Royal College of Psychiatrists, 1987). However, it is argued that many of the supposed signs of physical dependence are sometimes psychosomatic reactions triggered off not by the chemical properties of psychoactive drugs but by the user's fears, beliefs and fantasies about what withdrawal entails (Plant, 1987).

The dependence syndrome

The original framework of the dependence syndrome related specifically to alcohol dependence, but this has been expanded to include other psychoactive substances. According to Edwards & Gross (1976), there are seven components of the syndrome:

- Increased tolerance to the drug
- Repeated withdrawal symptoms
- Compulsion to use the drug (psychological state known as craving)
- Salience of drug-seeking behaviour (obtaining and using the drug becomes more important in the person's life)
- Relief or avoidance of withdrawal symptoms (the regular use of the drug to relieve withdrawal symptoms)
- Narrowing of the repertoire of drug taking (pattern of drinking may become an everyday activity)
- Rapid reinstatement after abstinence

The dependence syndrome, derived from the disease, biological and behavioural models, has provided a common language for academics and clinicians to talk about the same phenomena.

Why do people use drugs?

Many models and theories have been put forward to explain why people use or misuse psychoactive substances and about the causes of substance misuse. The theories provide explanations for the initiation into substance misuse or why individuals begin to use drugs, and the process of addiction. It will become apparent that no single theory is sufficient to explain substance use and misuse per se, and that a range of 'risk factors' have to be considered. Most of the studies are retrospective in design and more research has been conducted in relation to alcohol than any other substances. For a more comprehensive review of the theories and models of substance misuse see Rassool, 2001.

There is a myth that individuals use illicit psychoactive substances because they are having problems. This is usually not true. They may be attracted to illicit drugs for similar reasons as they are to alcohol:

- To enjoy the experience
- To get the same experience as alcohol
- To enjoy the short-term effects
- To feel confident
- To 'break the rules'
- To be part of the subculture
- To be curious about the effects
- Because the drugs are easily accessible and available
- Because their friends use them
- To lose weight
- To escape from stress
- To avoid unpleasant feelings
- To enhance work performance
- To continue the habit
- Because it is part of their home/social life
- To relieve boredom
- To allieviate pain
- To satisfy cravings
- To avoid withdrawal symptoms
- To counter the withdrawal effects of other drugs (use of benzodiazepines after stimulants)
- To counter the unpleasant effects of prescribed medications

However, the reason why people start using drugs may not be the same reason why they continue to use drugs. The reasons why people continue to use drugs may be related to a combination of factors, such as dependence, chaotic use, fear of withdrawal symptoms, social exclusion, mental health problems and other psychosocial and environmental conditions.

Patterns of substance use and misuse

The patterns of drug or alcohol use and misuse for some individuals sometimes vary over a period of time. The patterns of substance misuse are often described as experimental, recreational and problematic. Other patterns of substance misuse include binge drinking or drug taking and chaotic use.

Experimental users

Experimental users can be described as those who have used drugs, legal or illicit, on a few occasions. By definition, anyone's initial use of a drug, alcohol or tobacco is experimental (Rassool, 1998). The motivating factors include curiosity, anticipation of effects and availability. This usually forms part of the desire among adolescents to experiment and try new risky experiences and can be seen as a normal developmental pattern. There is no 'pattern' in the use of psychoactive substances, but the choice of the drug misused is indiscriminate. The choice of drug depends on factors such as availability, social marketing and reputation of the drug, subculture, fashion and peer-group influence. Experimental use of illicit psychoactive substances is usually a short-lived experience and the majority of people may confine the consumption to drugs that are socially acceptable. Experimental users, however, are in the highest category of risk for infections (if injecting), medical complications or overdose, due to the indiscriminate use of adulterated psychoactive substances. It has been suggested that the likelihood of 'their future significant engagement with, or disengagement from, further drug use has not yet been firmly determined' (RCP & RCP, 2000).

Recreational users

Experimental users may or may not become recreational users of illicit psychoactive substances. The term 'recreational' refers to a form of substance use in which pleasure and relaxation are the prime motivations. There is a strict adherence to the pattern of use so that the drug is only used on certain occasions such as weekends, and is less likely to be used on consecutive days. There is usually a preference for a particular drug (drug of choice), because the user has learnt how to use it and appreciate its effects. Drug or alcohol use is one aspect of the user's life and tends to complement social and recreational activities. There are usually no adverse medical or social consequences as a result of the recreational use as in the case of controlled drinking.

Dependent users

By definition and its very nature, a dependent user has progressed to regular and problematic use of a psychoactive drug or become a polydrug user (multiple drug use). There is the presence of psychological and/or physical dependence and it is distinguished from experimental and recreational use. The pattern of use is more frequent and regular, but less controlled. The process of obtaining the drug is more important to the user than the quality of experience. This tends to displace rather than complement social activities. Injecting drugs is common, and the frequent use creates problems of intoxication, infections, if sharing needles and syringes, and other medical complications. Personal, social, psychological and legal problems may be present in this group.

Binge

In recent years the term 'binge drinking' has gained currency as referring to a high intake of alcohol in a single drinking session. Binge drinking is often defined as the consumption of more than a certain number of drinks over a short period of time, a single drinking session or at least during a single day (men consuming at least eight, and women at least six standard units of alcohol) (Institute of Alcohol Studies, 2004). The features of binge drinking (MCM Research Limited, 2004) are:

- Drinking with the intention of getting drunk, often mixing drinks
- Drinking to the point at which the individual loses control

- Drinking as much as possible in a short space of time
- Occasional, heavy drinking

Binge drinking and severe intoxication can cause muscular incoordination, blurred vision, stupor, hypothermia, convulsions, depressed reflexes, respiratory depression, hypotension and coma. Death can occur from respiratory or circulatory failure or if binge drinkers inhale their own vomit (Institute of Alcohol Studies, 2003). It is well known that binge drinkers are at increased risk of accidents and alcohol poisoning. These patterns of behaviour are also relevant to the episodic use of a psychoactive drug, other than alcohol, in large quantities over a period of time, followed by limited use or abstinence.

Chaotic use

Chaotic use is referred to when an individual is regarded as taking a drug or drugs in a spontaneous way that tends not to follow any typical drug-using pattern. It is generally associated with problematic bouts of heavy use that may cause the user harm (Drugscope, 2002). This is often the excessive use of multiple drugs or polydrug use over a prolonged period of time. The individual's life is circumscribed by their drug use in completely unordered and unpredictable ways, and is combined with other significant health issues such as HIV, liver damage and mental health problems.

Routes of drug administration (how people take drugs)

The absorption of a drug is in part dependent upon its route of administration. Since psychoactive drugs must enter the bloodstream to reach their site of action, the route of administration is very important in the speed of influencing the physical and psychological effects of the drug. The routes of taking drugs are orally, smoking, inhalation and by injection. The most common route of administration is orally, in either liquid or tablet form. When a drug is required to act more rapidly the preferred route of administration is by injection. Drugs of misuse, such as heroin, are often administered intravenously, for example directly into a vein. Certain drugs are smoked, for example cannabis, crack cocaine, heroin. Some psychoactive drugs, for example cocaine and amphetamines, are also taken by the intranasal route.

Oral

The oral route (swallowing) is the most popular method of drug administration although effectively the slowest route because of the slow absorption of the drug into the bloodstream. There is no stigma attached, compared with smoking and injecting, to taking a psychoactive substance orally either in tablet form or in the form of beverages containing alcohol or caffeine.

Smoking

Smoking is also a very effective route as the drug is inhaled, as in the case of tobacco or heroin smoking (chasing the dragon). Cannabis or marijuana is also smoked in the form of a 'joint', which is usually mixed with tobacco.

Inhalation

The inhalation route (sniff) is also used to self-administer drugs. Absorption of the drug is through the mucous membrane of the nose and mouth. The types of drug that are inhaled include cocaine, tobacco snuff and volatile substances and solvents. Inhalation may also produce rapid absorption and response as in the case of crack cocaine.

Injecting

The methods of drug injecting include intramuscularly or subcutaneously/intravenously. Injection of drugs is less widespread than other routes of drug administration but also the most hazardous. The major danger of injecting is the risk of overdose because of the concentrated effect of this method. There is also the risk of infection from non-sterile injection methods, including hepatitis B and HIV infections, abscesses, gangrene and thromboses.

Table 3.2 Complications of injecting.

Equipment	The drug	Site of injection	Effects
Environment	Drug	Trauma and infection	Overdose
Cooker	Drug Interactions	Skin abscess	Poisoning
Water	Allergy	Fat necrosis	Infection
Filter	Contaminants	'Simple' miss	Thrombosis
Syringe	Infectious agents	Connective tissue	Embolism
Needle		Arterial injection	
		Nerves	
		Lung, breast, penis, neck	

Source: adapted from Pates *et al.* (2005).

The onset of the effect of the drug is rapid when it is administered intravenously and is a major reason why drugs are often self-administered by injecting. Drugs that are mainly injected include heroin, cocaine, amphetamines and some hypno-sedatives. Table 3.2 summarises the complications of injecting.

Intervention strategies: harm reduction to abstinence

The most important factors in intervention approaches are to ensure that management and treatment of substance misusers or individuals with dual diagnosis address a broad range of complex needs. These include physical or health needs, social, psychological, spiritual or legal needs or problems of the individual. Intervention strategies range from total abstinence to harm reduction.

Whilst abstinence as a goal of treatment may be an appropriate target for some individuals with dual diagnosis or those who are not dependent upon the drugs, for others, who are dependent or are chaotic users, it may be unrealistic for abstinence to be their immediate short-term goal. A harm reduction approach may be more appropriate for this group of individuals. Proponents of harm reduction recognise that there will always be illicit psychoactive drug use and that many individuals are unable or lack the readiness to change to be drug free, but nonetheless could benefit from intervention.

Harm reduction means trying to reduce the harm that people do to themselves, or other people, from their drug use. It can be contrasted with primary prevention, which tries to stop people using drugs in the first place or to stop using them if they have already started. Harm reduction focuses on 'safer' drug use and has also been developed as a way of educating young people about drug use (Drugscope, 2002). Harm reduction has also been described as a set of practical strategies that reduce negative consequences of drug use, incorporating a spectrum of strategies from safer use, to managed use to abstinence. Harm reduction strategies meet drug users 'where they're at', addressing conditions of use along with the use itself (Harm Reduction co.uk, 2003). The principles of Harm Reduction (Harm Reduction co.uk, 2003) are outlined below:

- Accepts psychoactive substances are a part of our society, and chooses to minimise its harmful effects rather than to ignore or condemn them.
- Understands that substance use is a complex and multifaceted phenomenon that encompasses a continuum of behaviours, ranging from dependence to total abstinence, and acknowledges that some ways of using drugs or alcohol are clearly safer than others.
- Calls for the non-judgemental, non-coercive provision of services and resources to individuals who use drugs and to the communities in which they live, in order to assist them in reducing attendant harm.
- Ensures that substance misusers and those with a history of substance misuse routinely have a real voice in the creation of programmes and policies designed to serve them.
- Affirms substance misusers themselves as the primary agents of reducing the harm of their substance use, and seeks to empower users to share

information and to support each other in strategies that meet their actual conditions of use.

- Recognises that the realities of poverty, class, racism, social isolation, past trauma, sex-based discrimination and other social inequalities affect people's vulnerability to and capacity for effectively dealing with substance related harm.
- Does not attempt to minimise or ignore the real and tragic harm and danger associated with licit and illicit drug use.

Working with substance misusers from a harm reduction perspective opens the door to helping these individuals to reduce harm in some way that wouldn't otherwise occur. Small reductions of harm are better than no reduction. An open door policy can result in a harm reduction snowball effect: small improvement can pave the way for further reduction of drug use and an improved lifestyle in other ways. This snowball effect can continue, eventually to the point of abstinence (Westermeyer, 2002). Harm reduction programmes include supervised consumption of medication, needle exchange programmes, programmes to reduce the risk associated with HIV and hepatitis, and health information about safer drug use and safer sex.

References

Addiction Foundation Research (1986) *Essential Concepts and Strategies*. Canadian Government Publishing Centre, Supply and Services, Toronto, Canada.

Advisory Council on the Misuse of Drugs (1982) *Treatment and Rehabilitation*. HMSO, London.

Advisory Council on the Misuse of Drugs (1988) *Aids and Drug Misuse: Part 1*. HMSO, London.

American Psychiatric Association (1994) *DSM-IV: Diagnostic and Statistical Manual of Mental Disorders*, 4th edn, pp. 75–90. American Psychiatric Association, Washington, DC.

Cabinet Office (2003) *Drug Report Phase One*. Strategy Unit, London. www.strategy.gov.uk

Cabinet Office (2004) *Alcohol Harm Reduction Strategy for England*. Strategy Unit, London. www.strategy.gov.uk

Department of Health (1998a) *Smoking Kills*. Department of Health, London. www.doh.gov.uk

Department of Health (1998b) *Tackling Drugs to Build a Better Britain. The Government's Ten-year Strategy for Tackling Drugs Misuse*. Stationery Office Publication, London.

Department of Health (1999) *Drug Misuse and Dependence – Guidelines on Clinical Management*. Department of Health, London.

Drugscope (2002) *Drug Terms*. Drugscope, London. www.drugscope.org.uk

Edwards, G. & Gross, M. (1976) Alcohol dependence: provisional description of a clinical syndrome. *British Journal of Addiction*, 81, 171–3.

Harm Reduction co.uk (2003) *Harm Reduction*. http://www.harmreduction.co.uk/index3.html

Home Office (2002) *Updated Drug Strategy*. http://drugs.homeoffice.gov.uk/drug-strategy/drug-strategy-publications

Institute of Alcohol Studies (2003) *Binge Drinking: Medical and Social Consequences*. Institute of Alcohol Studies, St Ives.

Institute of Alcohol Studies (2004) *Binge Drinking: Nature, Prevalence and Causes*. Institute of Alcohol Studies, St Ives.

Jeffery, D., Klein, A. & King, L. (2002) *UK Drug Report on Trends in 2001. Report from the UK Focal Point to EMCDDA*. Drugscope, London.

MCM Research Limited (2004) *WTAG Binge-drinking Research*. MCM Research Limited, Oxford.

National Treatment Agency (2002) *Models of Care for Substance Misuse Services Part 1 & 2*. NTA, London.

Pates, R., McBride, A. & Arnold, K. (2005) *Injecting Illicit Drugs*, p. xiii. Blackwell Publishing, Oxford.

Plant, M. (1987) *Drugs in Perspective*, pp. 13–14. Hodder and Stoughton, London.

Rassool, G.H. (1998). *Substance Use and Misuse: Nature, Context and Clinical Interventions*. Blackwell Science, Oxford.

Rassool, G.H. (2002) Substance Use and Dual Diagnosis: Concepts, Theories and Models. In: *Dual Diagnosis: Substance Misuse and Psychiatric Disorders* (Rassool G.H., ed.). Blackwell Publishing, Oxford.

Royal College of Psychiatrists (1987) *Drug Scenes. A Report on Drugs and Drug Dependence*. The Royal College of Psychiatrists, Gaskell, London.

Royal College of Psychiatrists and Royal College of Physicians Working Party (2000) *Drugs: Dilemmas and Choices*. Gaskell, London.

Statistical Bulletin (1999) *Alcohol: 1976 Onwards*. Department of Health, London.

Westermeyer, R. (2002) *Harm Reduction And Illicit Drug Use*. http://www.habitsmart.com/index.html

World Health Organization (1981) *Nomenclature and classification of drug- and alcohol-related problems: A WHO Memorandum*. Bulletin of the World Health Organization, 59, 225–42.

4 Psychoactive Substances and their Effects

G.H. Rassool & J. Winnington

The drug experience: pharmacology, personality, environment

It is acknowledged that the effect a psychoactive substance or 'drug experience' will have on a given individual will depend on several other factors beside the pharmacological properties of the drug. The gamut of 'drug experience' involves interrelated sets of non-pharmacological and pharmacological factors. These include pharmacological factors, personality of the individual and the context or setting (Ghodse, 1995). The pharmacological factors include the chemical properties or type of drug used.

Different drugs have different modes of action on the body due to their pharmacological properties, the drug dosage and the route of administration. In addition, the effects or actions of a psychoactive drug are influenced by the personal characteristics of the drug user. These characteristics include factors such as the person's biological make-up, personality, gender, age and drug tolerance. In addition, the knowledge, attitude and expectations (psychological set) about a drug will have an influence on the 'drug experience'. For example, if an individual believes or expects (as a self-fulfilling prophecy) that a particular substance will produce a certain effect, the desired effect may be experienced. The last set of factors is the setting or context in which a drug is used. This includes the physical environment where the drug is used, the cultural influences of the community where the drug is consumed, the laws related to drug use and the context in which a drug is used. All the interrelated factors, pharmacological properties, individual differences and context of use influence the individual experiences of drug taking.

Specific drugs and their effects

This section focuses on the nature and effects of psychoactive substances. Each classification of substances will be examined including alcohol, hypno-sedatives, stimulants, hallucinogens, cannabis, tranquillisers and steroids. Names, legal status, sought after effects and adverse effects will also be presented.

Alcohol

Alcohol is taken orally as a drink and is our most commonly used social lubricant. Alcoholic drinks are measured in 'units'; a unit equates to one regular sized glass of wine, half a pint of beer or one measure/shot of spirits, but these only apply to normal strength drinks. Beer ranges from around 3.5% to over 12% alcohol by volume. Strong lagers such as Tenants Super and Kestral Super have around five units of alcohol per can. The maximum recommended intake per week for males is 21 units and for females it is 14 units, but spread over the week rather than drunk in one session. Alternative Department of Health guidance suggests sensible limits of no greater than 3–4 units per day for men and 2–3 units per day for women. Alcohol rapidly enters the bloodstream from the stomach and intestines. It takes about 30–90 minutes to have maximum alcohol blood concentration. Factors such as the strength of the drink, the presence of carbon dioxide and bicarbonate, decrease in body temperature, presence of food and tolerance of the individual will influence the effect of alcohol.

Legal status

Alcohol can be bought by adults (aged 18 years and over).

Sought after effects

In low to moderate doses, alcohol loweres inhibitions, increases confidence and sociability and produces a mild euphoric feeling. Safe drinking levels have been shown to protect against coronary heart disease in men over the age of 40 or women past the menopause.

Adverse effects

The effects are influenced by the amount, frequency and duration of use and the tolerance of the user. High doses of alcohol can have a range of effects, from slurred speech, ataxia, blurred vision and diminishing consciousness, depression of the central nervous system, to shock, coma and death. Alcohol also affects coordination, reaction time and judgement; it makes users particularly prone to accidents and trauma.

Large amounts of alcohol over a period of time can lead to hypothermia, inflammation of the stomach lining, ulcers, oesophageal varices and birth defects. A physical dependency can result from alcohol consumption and this can lead to marked physical withdrawal symptoms on cessation. These include nausea, tremors, cramps, vomiting, sweating, high temperature, hypertension, anxiety, restlessness and transitory hallucinations, stomach pains and even seizures or delirium tremens, called DTs. Toxicity usually results in vomiting, thus preventing fatal overdoses. However, inhaling vomit is responsible for a number of deaths every year. Alcohol is associated with violent incidents and suicide, with the risk of self-harm in heavy drinkers being much higher than in the general population.

Amyl, butyl and isobutyl nitrite

Amyl, butyl and isobutyl nitrites, known collectively as alkyl nitrites ('poppers', rush, locker room, hard core) are chemically related to nitrous oxide or laughing gas. They are clear, yellow, volatile and inflammable liquids with a sweet smell when fresh. When stale, the drug degenerates to a smell often described as 'smelly socks'. To users, the alkyl nitrites are known as 'poppers'.

Therapeutic use

Medically, amyl nitrite has been used in the treatment of angina and as an antidote to cyanide poisoning. Butyl nitrite has no therapeutic medical uses.

Illicit use

In the UK, drugs such as butyl nitrite are on sale in sex shops, pubs, bars and clubs. As a street drug, butyl nitrite comes in small bottles with screw or plug tops. It is sold mainly, but not exclusively, to the gay community. The drug is widely used for the 'rush' of blood to the brain and an initial rush is followed by light-headed feelings. It is used to facilitate sex (often among the gay community).

Legal status

Butyl nitrite is not classified as a drug and has no restrictions on its availability under current medicine or drug legislation. However, other laws such as the Offences Against the Persons Act 1861 may be used to restrict distribution of these substances.

Sought after effects

They are popular on the dance scene and in clubs and the effects are short-lived. Once inhaled, the effects are virtually instantaneous and last for 2–5 minutes. The blood vessels dilate, there is an increase in heart rate and the blood rushes to the brain. Those using the drug to enhance sexual pleasure report a slow sense of time, prolonged sensation of orgasm and the prevention of premature ejaculation. Alkyl nitrites are also used for the relaxation of the anal sphincter, easing anal intercourse. Sniffing of nitrites could cause a reduction in blood pressure and contribute to unconsciousness. Anyone with cardiovascular problems, glaucoma and anaemia should avoid using nitrites. The users often experience weakness, headache, facial flushing and nausea and vomiting. There appears to be no serious long-term effect of the drug as it is excreted rapidly from the body in healthy individuals.

Adverse effects

Tolerance to the drug develops within two to three weeks of regular use, but after a few days of abstinence, this tolerance is lost. There are no reports of withdrawal symptoms or psychological dependence. The substance causes a fall in blood pressure and rise in heart rate, which can lead to fainting and loss of balance, headache and nausea. Swallowing the liquid can be fatal, but this is rare.

Anabolic steroids

Steroids are hormones that occur naturally in the body and control the development and functioning of the reproductive system. The term anabolic means to chemically build up. Synthetic anabolic steroids, in particular the modified male sex hormone, testosterone, form the main market supplies.

Therapeutic use

Only two anabolic steroids are available on prescription in the UK. These are nandrolone (Durabolin) and stanozolol (Stromba). Anabolic steroids have an effect on muscle building and are medically used in the treatment of thrombosis, anaemia and muscle wasting.

Illicit use

Illicit anabolic steroids are used mainly by athletes and bodybuilders. The idea behind the use of these steroids is that because they build muscle bulk they will also increase strength. The drug can be taken in tablet form or by injection.

Legal status

Anabolic steroids are not controlled under the Misuse of Drugs Act 1971. They are, however, prescription only drugs and intent to supply can be an offence under the Medicines Act.

Sought after effects

Anabolic steroids increase the retention of nitrogen by the body, allowing this to be used to build muscle and body strength. Steroids also aid in the production of red blood cells, which has led to the belief that they might be helpful in increasing endurance. There is, however, no empirical evidence to support this.

Adverse effects

Although the substances may look like diverted pharmaceuticals, they are often illegally manufactured counterfeits. If the substance is injected, the usual risks apply. As anabolic steroids are modelled chemically on male hormones they can have a masculinising effect. Women may have an increase in body hair, a deepened voice, enlargement of the clitoris and decrease in breast size. Men may suffer from a decrease in sperm production and testes size and development of breast tissue. Some of these effects may be permanent and therefore irreversible. The increase in aggression is welcomed by athletes but sometimes the associated steroid mania has been blamed for violent crimes. Other physical problems are linked to steroid use, such as acne, coronary heart disease, raised blood pressure and possible liver and kidney damage. Physical dependence does not seem to be a problem but users have reported hypomania, mania, depression, anger and lethargy after stopping their use.

Cannabis

Cannabis (dope, draw, blow, resin, grass, skunk) is derived from a bushy plant, *Cannabis sativa*, which is easily cultivated in the UK. It is used as a relaxant or mild intoxicant. The active ingredients are concentrated in the resin at the top of the plant. 'Skunk' is a stronger breed. Hash or hashish is resin that is scraped from the plant and then compressed into blocks. Herbal cannabis, also known as marijuana, is a weaker preparation of dried plant material. The strongest preparation, cannabis oil, prepared from the resin is less common in the UK. Usually, these substances are mixed with tobacco and smoked. Sometimes they are smoked in a pipe, brewed in a drink or mixed with food. Smoking allows the user to regulate the dose because the effect is very rapid when used in this way. Cannabis is usually retailed in ounces (twenty-eight grams) or fractions of ounces, quarter of an ounce (seven grams), half an ounce (fourteen grams). Generally about half a gram of resin is used to make a couple of joints. The retail price varies depending on whether it is sold in herbal (grass) or resin form.

Therapeutic use

Compared with all other drugs controlled under the Misuse of Drugs Act, cannabis has the greatest non-medical usage. However, cannabis is indicated for the treatment of anorexia associated with weight loss in patients with AIDS, and to treat mild to moderate nausea and vomiting associated with cancer chemotherapy.

Legal status

Cannabis is controlled under the Misuse of Drugs Act (Class C), making it illegal to cultivate, produce, supply or possess the drug, unless a Home Office licence has been issued for research use or other special purposes. It is an offence to allow any premises to be used for cultivating, producing, supplying, storing or smoking of cannabis.

Sought after effects

Short-term use

The effects derived depend to a large extent on expectations, motivation and mood of the user. The effects of cannabis usually start just a few minutes after smoking and last from about one hour to several hours depending on how much is consumed. Some users experience an intense feeling of relaxation. The following are common effects: talkativeness, bouts of hilarity, relaxation and greater sensitivity to sound and colour. There is no hangover of the type associated with alcohol use. Whilst under the influence of cannabis, concentration and mental and manual dexterity are impaired, making tasks such as driving or any procedure requiring accuracy or precision both difficult and dangerous.

Long-term use

Opinion varies about the effects of long-term cannabis use. This may be partly because slowly developing and infrequent effects need large longitudinal samples to arrive at conclusive results, and these studies are rare. Like tobacco, frequently and chronically inhaled cannabis probably causes bronchitis and other respiratory problems and may also contribute to the development of lung cancer. Generally, people who smoke cannabis are more likely to use other drugs, and people who smoke tobacco and drink are also more likely to try cannabis. However, there is no evidence that the use of one drug actually causes people to use another (escalation theory). Whilst there is little evidence that cannabis can produce a physical dependence, regular use can produce a psychological need for the drug and some individuals may come to rely on it as a 'social lubricant'.

Perceptual distortion may also occur, especially with heavy use. If the drug is used whilst an individual is anxious or depressed, these feelings may be accentuated, leading to a feeling of panic. People chronically intoxicated on cannabis appear apathetic, sluggish, and they neglect their appearance. There may be particular risks for people with respiratory or heart disorders. Heavy use, particularly if strong varieties such as some forms of skunk are used regularly, can lead to psychosis. Heavy users of cannabis with personality disturbance or psychiatric problems may precipitate a temporary exacerbation of symptoms.

Ecstasy (MDMA)

Ecstasy (E, Adam, XTC, doves, 'Dennis the Menace', 'rhubarb and custard', 'New Yorkers', 'love doves', 'disco burgers', or 'phase 4') is often categorised as a hallucinogen, as in some respects it resembles LSD, leading to changes in states of consciousness, but it does not actually produce a hallucinogenic effect and does not usually lead to disturbances in a person's grasp of reality. It is manufactured from the components of methylamphetamine and safrole (a nutmeg derivative). It usually comes in tablet form, powder or in capsules with different shapes and colours.

Therapeutic use

Ecstasy was first manufactured in Germany in 1914 as an appetite suppressant, although it was never actually marketed for this purpose. It has been used in a limited way as an adjunct to various types of psychotherapy in order to facilitate the therapeutic process. In addition, the drug has also been used to some extent with terminally ill patients in order to help them come to terms with their situation and to communicate their feelings more easily.

Illicit use

The main use of ecstasy has been as a 'dance' or 'rave' drug. In the late 1980s it was given much publicity in the media, supposedly emphasising the dangers of the drug. A strong youth culture developed involving ecstasy, 'house music' and all night 'raves'.

Legal status

Ecstasy is a Class A drug.

Sought after effects

The effects start after about 20 minutes and can last for several hours. It is described as having a calming effect, with an enhanced perception of colours and sound. The user experiences euphoric feelings, and feelings of empathy, relaxation and meaningfulness.

Adverse effects

The adverse effects of ecstasy include tiredness, confusion, anxiety and depression. With higher doses the user can feel anxious and confused, and coordination can be impaired, making driving or similar activity very dangerous. If ecstasy is taken regularly over a period of a few days, the user can experience panic attacks, temporary paranoia or insomnia. Dependence is possible if it is taken frequently. Although ecstasy is not physically addictive, tolerance to the effects of the drug does build up. The use of this particular drug may be more hazardous for individuals with heart conditions, hypertension, a history of seizures or any type of psychiatric disorder. Sudden death through overheating and dehydration, or drinking too much water has led to collapse, convulsions or renal failure. Because of these ill effects, it is advised that wearing light, loose clothing, drinking plenty of non-alcoholic fluids as well as stopping dancing when feeling exhausted, could help reduce the possible complications of the drug. There is always a danger of the drug being contaminated by other substances, such as amphetamine mixtures, LSD and ketamine.

GHB

GHB (gammahydroxybutrate) is also known as (liquid ecstasy, GBL, BDO, GBH, blue nitro, midnight blue, renew trient, Reviarent, SomatoPro, serenity, enliven). It is a colourless liquid, with a slightly salty taste. The drug is usually sold in small 30 ml plastic containers (approximately £15) and consumed in capfuls. It is sometimes sold as 'liquid ecstasy', but is not related to ecstasy. In the past few years, GHB has become popular on the club scene, with users enjoying an alcohol-like high with potent positive sexual effects. It is also used by body-builders. The drug can take anything from ten minutes to an hour to take effect.

Legal status

Since 30 June 2003, GHB has been categorised as a Class C drug in the UK, with dealers facing up to five years in jail and possession punishable by up to two years in prison.

Sought after effects

GHB affects the release of dopamine in the brain, causing effects ranging from relaxation to sleep, at low doses. A small capful can make you feel uninhibited, exhilarated, relaxed and feeling good, with the effects lasting as long as a day, although it is difficult to give a clear 'safe' dose, as the concentration of the liquid will vary.

Adverse effects

As the dosage increases this can lead to disorientation, nausea, confusion, a numbing of the muscles or muscle spasms and vomiting. At high doses, convulsions, coma and respiratory collapse can occur. The drug also lowers blood pressure and in some cases people find breathing difficult. Overdosing can lead to a loss of consciousness and coma. It is not recommended that asthmatics or those with any form of respiratory or low blood pressure disorders take this drug. Because of its disabling effects, the exposure to the threat of sexual assault is high. There have been reports of the drug being used as a 'date rape' drug (like Rohypnol), with victims being slipped the drug via alcohol, or in coffee, tea or hot chocolate (it is almost tasteless).

Khat

Khat (also spelled quat, qat and kat) acts as a social lubricant mostly in Muslim countries, with links to (especially) the Yemen, Ethiopia or Somalia. It is an evergreen shrub (*Catha edulis*) that grows in parts of East Africa and the Middle East. It is transported to the UK by air and is generally preferred fresh as the leaves from the plant are most powerful when fresh. The user usually chews about two ounces of leaves or stems for a number of hours, swallowing the juice. Dryness of the mouth is caused by the juice so large amounts of liquid are also drunk. Effects start about a quarter of an hour into chewing and finish up to two hours after stopping. The main active substances in khat are cathine and cathinone, and these are closely related to amphetamines but are less potent.

Legal status

The khat plant is legal, but its active ingredients cathinone and cathine are Class C.

Sought after effects

Khat generally produces talkativeness, mild euphoria and hallucinations. In many countries it has social and cultural significance and it is mostly used as a social stimulant on festive occasions.

Adverse effects

Effects start after approximately 30 minutes, with stimulation and talkativeness. This is followed by a relaxed and introspective state that can last for up to five hours, often with insomnia. This is then followed by periods of lethargy, irritability and general hangover. Dependence can develop and heavy use can be problematic. Nausea, vomiting, mouth ulcers, abdominal pain, headache, palpitations, increased aggression and hallucinations can occur. Continued use can lead to cycles of sleeplessness and irritability and can, in the longer term, lead to psychiatric problems such as paranoia and possibly psychosis. Digestive problems such as constipation and stomach ulcers have frequently been reported to affect regular users. Khat is also often used with tobacco and hypno-sedatives such as benzodiazepines, which brings additional associated risks.

Hypno-sedatives

The hypno-sedatives include both hypnotics and minor tranquillisers. The barbiturates are: tuinal, membutal, sodium amytal, phenobarbital, and minor tranquillisers (benzodiazepines), diazepam (Valium), chlordiazepoxide (Librium), lorazepam (Ativan), nitrazepam (Mogadon), temazepam. Others include clomethiazole (Heminevrin) and chloral hydrate. The street names are downers, temazzies, eggs, jellies, mogadon, moggies, barbs and tranx.

Therapeutic use

Barbiturates have been used medically in anaesthesia and in the treatment of epilepsy, and rarely nowadays, insomnia. Minor tranquillisers are often prescribed for the relief of anxiety and stress.

Illegal use

Hypno-sedatives are drugs of misuse not only among the illicit drug population but also in the population in general. Benzodiazepines are usually taken by mouth but are sometimes ground up and injected. Temazepam was a serious problem, as a substitute for opiates, in the 1980s with users injecting the contents of oral temazepam capsules. This was greatly reduced when the formulations were banned from National Health Service prescription and additional controls were introduced.

Legal status

Benzodiazepines and barbiturates are prescription only medicines and are Class C and B controlled drugs respectively. It is illegal to supply these psychoactive substances and to possess them without a prescription.

Sought after effects

Barbiturates are depressant drugs and their effects are similar to alcohol intoxication. They include slurred speech, stumbling, confusion, reduction of inhibition, lowering of anxiety and tension, and impairment of concentration, judgement and performance.

Adverse effects

In the short term, users may experience tiredness, depression of respiration and sometimes dizziness and unsteady movement. In case of overdose, respiratory failure and death may result if these drugs are mixed with alcohol or with each other. Injecting these drugs is particularly hazardous, with increased risk of overdose, gangrene and abscesses. Barbiturates and minor tranquillisers are highly addictive and withdrawal symptoms include anxiety, insomnia, tension, headaches, cramps in the abdomen, pains in the limbs and even epileptic fits. Dependency on benzodiazepines or barbiturates is dangerous. Stopping use abruptly if dependent (usually after taking for three weeks or more) should be avoided and medical advice sought.

LSD and other hallucinogens

This section deals with a group of substances known as hallucinogens or hallucinogenic drugs. Lysergic acid diethylamide, known as LSD, is derived from a synthetic alkaloid (ergot). LSD is taken by mouth in extremely small doses (50–150 micrograms), which are usually on small paper squares. The effects tend to start about half an hour after taking it and last up to 12 hours or sometimes even longer, depending on the dosage. LSD is also known as acid, tabs or trips. Other hallucinogens include psilocybin (liberty cap mushrooms), *Amanita muscaria* (fly agaric mushrooms) and mescaline, which is derived from the peyote cactus. Mushrooms are also known as magic mushrooms. It usually takes about 30–50 mushrooms to produce a hallucinogenic experience similar to that experienced with LSD.

PCP, an animal tranquilliser, causes mind–body dissociation and a sensory deprived state. Ketamine ('special K', green, super K, vitamin K), a powerful anaesthetic, is becoming more popular and has the potential to cause hallucinations and other 'psychotic' outcomes. Ketamine is now a significant player in the UK drugs market. The drug first became popular within the gay clubbing scene but now has widened its appeal to a larger group of partygoers, edging its way onto the list of major drugs on sale in most areas (Druglink, 2005). It is usually a tablet or a white crystalline powder, which is snorted, but can also be in liquid form in small phials, which can be injected.

Therapeutic use

In ancient cultures the plants and the extracts have been used during religious rituals, witchcraft and employed as intoxicants in medicine. In recent times, LSD has been used occasionally in psychotherapy. Ketamine is a powerful anaesthetic used in animals and humans.

Illegal use

The widespread experimentation with LSD and other hallucinogens in the subculture of the 1960s resurfaced in the late 1980s. Experimentation with the drug in recent times has been associated with the advent of the club scene. In its pure form, LSD is a white powder, but is often supplied as an impregnated square of paper or as a drop on a piece of blotting paper and nearly always taken orally. LSD is also used in combination with amphetamines and ecstasy to enhance the perceptual experiences. The effect starts after about half an hour, and intensifies over a period of two to six hours. The effect may last up to 12 hours, depending on the dosage. The mushrooms, mentioned above, are sometimes eaten raw, cooked or brewed into a tea.

Legal status

LSD is a Class A controlled drug. Psilocybin or psilocybin-containing mushrooms are legal in their freshly picked state, but preparing them or growing or possessing them with intent to supply is illegal and restricted by the Misuse of Drugs Act 1971. Ketamine is not controlled under the Misuse of Drugs Act, but is controlled under the Medicines Act. Possession is not illegal, but people can be prosecuted for unauthorised manufacture or supply. Ketamine is currently under consideration by the Home Office to be made a Class C drug.

Sought after effects

The effects of the drug are dependent on the user's prior experience, mood, expectations and setting. It is much stronger in effect than psychedelic mushrooms or mescaline. A moderate dose will produce profound alteration in mood, sensation and consciousness, intensified sensory experiences and perceptual distortions. Confusion of time, space, body image and boundaries can occur with what have been called the blending of sight and sound. The user may 'see' sounds and 'hear' colours. Mushrooms are similar to LSD, but the trip is often milder and shorter.

Adverse effects

There is no physical dependence or withdrawal symptom associated with recreational use of LSD. The side effects and toxicity of the drug may cause panic, confusion, impulsive behaviour and unpleasant illusions (a bad trip), flashbacks and may precipitate psychotic reactions. Cases of accidental death due to impaired judgement have occurred but this is extremely rare. The negative and unpleasant effects are much more likely to arise if the user is in a negative mood or situation, or mixes hallucinogens with other drugs or alcohol.

Fly agaric mushrooms often cause nausea and stomach pain. However, the greatest danger with hallucinogenic mushrooms is that the user may take a similar looking poisonous species by mistake. Tolerance builds up with LSD and mushrooms in so far as the user needs to space out 'trips' to get the desired effects.

Ketamine may impair memory and aggravate existing psychosis, anxiety or depression. Prolonged use may cause disorientation and gradual detachment from the world. A few deaths have occurred through overdose, heart or respiratory failure. With large or repeat doses hallucinations occur, for example loss of sense of time, feeling disconnected from the body, near-death experiences. Large doses can lead to loss of consciousness.

Opiates and opioids

The term opiate refers to any psychoactive substance either natural or synthetic in origin that has an effect similar to morphine. Opiates are derived from the opium poppy although there are a number of psychoactive synthetic substitutes. The drug opium is obtained from scarifying the seed of the poppy. Morphine and codeine are extracted from opium, and heroin is manufactured chemically from morphine. Some of the commoner opiate drugs are: codeine, heroin, pethidine, methadone, morphine and dipipanone hydrochloride (Diconal). The street names for heroin are smack, junk, gear, scag, H, scat, tiger, chi, elephant, harry, dragon. Methadone is also known as doll, red rock, juice or 'script'.

Therapeutic uses

The medical applications of opiates include effective relief of pain, treatment for diarrhoea and vomiting, and as a cough suppressant. Morphine, for instance, is widely used for short-term acute pain resulting from fractures, burns and the later stages of terminal illnesses. Methadone is often prescribed to heroin addicts for maintenance or withdrawal purposes. Some of the opiates such as pethidine, morphine, dihydrocodeine and methadone are highly addictive.

Illicit use

The most popular opiate as an illicit drug of misuse is heroin. The drug is swallowed, smoked (chasing the dragon – heated on silver paper and the smoke inhaled), sniffed or injected (either subcutaneously or intravenously). Diverted pharmaceutical opiates and opioids may be formulated for injection, oral use, or occasionally as suppositories. Tablets are sometimes crushed and injected. If heroin powder is injected it is generally mixed with water or lemon juice. It is sold illicitly as a powder and is usually brown, but can be white. Habitual users of heroin may generally consume half a gram to over one gram per day.

Legal status

Heroin, pethidine, morphine, dihydrocodeine and methadone are Class A controlled drugs. Codeine and dihydrocodeine are Class B but Class A if prepared for injection. Distalgesic, dextropropoxyphene and buprenorphine (Temgesic) are Class C.

Sought after effects

In moderate doses, opiates produce a range of generally mild physical effects apart from the analgesic effect. It induces euphoria, which may wear off, but users continue to use the drug to avoid withdrawal symptoms. Heroin users report the ability of the drug to induce a relaxed detachment from pain and anxiety. The depressant effects reduce the activity of the nervous system including reflex functions such as coughing, respiration and heart rate. They also dilate the blood vessels, thus giving a feeling of warmth. Opiates such as heroin provide powerful relief from physical pain (for which they are used medically) and also of psychological pain. Methadone effects are similar to heroin and may be prescribed to prevent opiate withdrawal symptoms. Methadone tincture cannot be injected, thus reducing the risks associated with injecting behaviours.

Adverse effects

Heroin dependence develops after repeated use over several weeks and sudden withdrawal leads to anxiety, nausea, muscle pains, sweating, diarrhoea and gooseflesh. Tolerance develops quickly so that larger amounts of the same drug are needed to produce the same effect. During a period of abstinence (in treatment or prison), tolerance diminishes quickly so that individuals can easily overdose by taking their usual dose. Overdose occurs as a result of depression of the respiratory centre in the brain, which leads to respiratory and cardiac arrest and death unless immediate medical attention is received. Though stupor, coma and death can occur from overdoses, there is generally little effect on the motor skills and sensation. The user of opiates may appear detached or withdrawn with contraction of the pupils.

However, most complications arise from unsterile injections and adulterated street drugs. Heroin taken by injection is also a risk factor in contracting hepatitis B and C, HIV and septicaemia. If the supplies of the drug are cut off, symptoms may become apparent 8 to 24 hours after the last dose. The drug must have been used daily for at least two to three weeks for physical withdrawal symptoms to occur. The withdrawal symptoms include anxiety, insomnia, diarrhoea, aches, tremor, sweating, muscular spasms, sneezing and yawning. The severity of withdrawal symptoms will depend on the extent of an individual's dependence. Methadone is also addictive and can cause overdose within an hour of administration or after two or three days, as the drug builds up in the body. It causes constipation and irregular menstrual periods, though conception is still possible.

Stimulants

Stimulants are synthetic powders available in a variety of tablets and capsules, sometimes in combination with other drugs. In the 1950s and 1960s they were widely prescribed for symptoms of depression and as appetite suppressants. The main recommended use now is in the treatment of pathological sleepiness and paradoxically, in some cases, for treatment of hyperactivity in children. These drugs may be taken orally or sniffed in powder form, smoked or dissolved in water and injected. Methylphenidate (Ritalin) and diethylpropion (Tenuate, Apisate) have a similar effect to amphetamines, but are less potent. Amphetamines, known as speed, whizz, sulph, uppers, are swallowed, sniffed, smoked or injected (by crushing the tablets).

Cocaine (charlie, coke, snow, foot, lady, C) is a drug with powerfully stimulant properties. It is a white powder derived from the leaves of the Andean coca shrub. It is expensive, and until recently was seen as a rich man's drug. A small amount of the drug is usually 'sniffed' or 'snorted' up the nose through a tube and absorbed through the nasal membranes, although sometimes the substance is injected. Freebasing consists of smoking cocaine base (or crack). Crack cocaine (rocks, ready wash, ice, base) is whitish in colour and looks like irregular lumps of sugar. This is a more potent way of administration than snorting and produces a 'rush' similar to the experience of injecting cocaine.

Most 'street stimulants' are illicitly manufactured amphetamine sulphate powder. The production process is relatively simple and large quantities are available on the illicit market. Illicit amphetamine, heavily diluted with adulterants (often to 15% purity), is easily available and sells at £20–30 (GBP) per gram. An occasional user may take a few weeks to consume half a gram, while a heavy user might consume up to six grams per day of relatively impure substance. Many cocaine and crack users also take other drugs, including heroin. A highly dangerous practice is injecting a mixture of heroin and cocaine (known as snowballing or speedballing). Alcohol is often mixed with cocaine to produce coca-ethylene, which is toxic.

Legal status

All amphetamines and similar stimulants are 'prescription' only drugs under the Medicines Act. Most are also controlled under the Misuse of Drugs Act, with the exception of some mild stimulants. Amphetamine, dex- and methyl-amphetamine, phenmetrazine and methylphenidate are in Class B, but if prepared for injection the increased penalties of Class A apply. Diethylpropion and other amphetamine like stimulants are in Class C. Cocaine, its derivative salts and the leaves of the coca plant come under Class A of the Misuse of Drugs Act. As in the case of some opiates, a doctor must be licensed by the Home Office before prescribing cocaine. Such prescribing is, however, very uncommon.

Sought after effects

Amphetamines create arousal and activate the user in a manner similar to adrenalin, which the body produces naturally. Heart and respiratory rate are speeded up and pupils widen and appetite lessens. The user feels more energetic, confident and cheerful. The experience of these effects creates the possibility of psychological dependence. As the individual's energy is depleted the predominant feelings may be anxiety, irritability and restlessness. The short-term effects of cocaine are similar to those of amphetamines. When sniffed, the psychological effects peak after 15–30 minutes, leading to the dose being repeated approximately every 20 minutes in order to maintain the effect. When cocaine is smoked the effects are more immediate.

Adverse effects

Amphetamines

High and repeated doses of amphetamines can produce delirium, panic, hallucinations and feelings of persecution. The effects of a single dose last about three to four hours, leaving the user feeling tired and depleted. It can take a couple of days for the body to recover fully. Amphetamines and other stimulants merely postpone fatigue and hunger without satisfying the need for rest and nourishment. Heavy prolonged use also exposes the individual to the risk of cardiovascular problems. This applies particularly to people with hypertension and anyone who does strenuous exercise whilst taking the drug (for example athletes).

Cocaine

Several quickly repeated doses can lead to extreme agitation, anxiety, paranoia and sometimes hallucination. Excessive doses can lead to death from respiratory or heart failure. In order to maintain the desired effects the regular user has to take increasingly large doses, often several times the normal level. On cessation, the individual is likely to feel deeply depressed, lethargic and very hungry. Regular and high dose use can lead to delusions, hallucinations and paranoia. These symptoms may develop into a psychotic state and it can then take the person several months to recover fully. Heavy long-term use can cause debilitation due to lack of sleep and food, leading to lowered resistance to illness generally. In the case of cocaine, with heavy frequent use, increasingly unpleasant symptoms develop. Instead of euphoria there is uncomfortable restlessness, extreme excitability, nausea, insomnia and weight loss. This can lead to a state similar to paranoid psychosis. Repeated sniffing can also damage the nasal septum.

Volatile substances

More than a hundred commercially available products are now used to get high. Some organic based substances produce effects similar to alcohol or anaesthetics when their vapours are inhaled. Some of these are used as solvents in glue, paint/nail varnish removers, rubber, cement, Tippex™, dry cleaning fluids, degreasing compounds and thinning fluids. Others are used as propellant gases in aerosols and fire extinguishers or as fuels such as petrol, cigarette lighter gas and magic markers. Sniffers of volatile substances heighten the desired effect by increasing the concentration of the vapour and excluding air, for example, by sniffing from a bag or by placing a plastic bag over the head while inhalation takes place.

Solvent abuse seems to occur in very localised areas, for example in a housing estate, school or particular group. The age group 12–15 years is mainly involved and some of these children continue to sniff glue for several years. Glue and other volatile substances are easily available in shops. The Government has produced guidelines for retailers to ensure that these products are stocked out of the reach of children and to restrict the sales to adults.

Legal status

The Intoxicating Substances Supply Act, passed in 1985, makes it an offence to supply a young person under 18 years with a substance that the supplier knows or has reason to believe will be used 'to achieve intoxication'. The law is mainly directed to shopkeepers but could also be applied to anyone who sells or gives a young person a sniffable product.

Sought after effects

Inhaled solvent vapours are absorbed quickly through the lungs and rapidly reach the brain. Part of the effect is the reduction in oxygen intake. Respiratory rate and heart rate are depressed, and repeated or deep inhalation can result in an 'overdose', causing disorientation, loss of control and unconsciousness. The experience is similar to being drunk, and experienced sniffers try to achieve a dream-like state. There is an immediate euphoria with confusion, unsteadiness and lack of coordination. Distorted perceptions and hallucinations can also occur. The effects appear quickly and disappear within a few minutes to half an hour of sniffing being stopped. There may be a hangover effect with headache and poor concentration for about a day.

Adverse effects

There is considerable risk of accidental injury or death if the individual becomes intoxicated in a hazardous environment. During vomiting, there is the risk of choking if the sniffer has been intoxicated to the point of unconsciousness. If a plastic bag has been placed over the head in order to assist inhalation of the substance, suffocation becomes a real risk. Some volatile substances such as aerosol gases and cleaning fluids can sensitise the heart, causing heart failure, especially if exertion takes place at the same time. Some gases squirted directly into the mouth can cause death from suffocation. Sniffing from small bags held to the mouth or nose has caused fewer deaths than the practice of inhaling butane and similar gases with plastic bags placed over the head.

Long-term heavy solvent abuse can result in moderate and lasting impairment of brain function, particularly affecting the control of movement. Chronic misuse of aerosols and cleaning fluids can cause renal and hepatic damage. The practice of sniffing leaded petrol can cause lead poisoning. Chronic misuse can affect general performance, along with evidence of weight loss, depression and tremor. These symptoms usually clear when sniffing ceases. Tolerance can develop, but physical dependence does not constitute a significant problem. Psychological dependence occurs in susceptible youngsters with concomitant family or personality problems. These individuals are also more prone to becoming 'lone sniffers' instead of the usual pattern of sniffing in groups.

References

Druglink (2005) *Ketamine*. September/October. Drugscope, London.

Drugscope. Information leaflets on drugs. Drugs Material in English and Other Languages. http://www.drugscope.org.uk

Ghodse, A.H. (1995) *Drugs and Addictive Behaviour*. Blackwell Science, Oxford.

Rassool, G.H. (1998) *Substance Use and Misuse. Nature, Contexts and Clinical Interventions*. Blackwell Science, Oxford.

5 Mental Health: an Introduction

G.H. Rassool & J. Winnington

Introduction

Mental and behavioural disorders are universal public health problems and about 450 million people suffer from mental disorders. One person in four will develop one or more mental or behavioural disorders during their lifetime and about 873 000 people die by suicide every year (World Health Organization, 2001). Five of the ten leading causes of disability worldwide are psychiatric conditions, including depression, alcohol use, schizophrenia and compulsive disorder (Murray & Lopez, 1996). In the European Union, around 58 000 people die each year as a result of suicide or self-inflicted injury and most suicide deaths are linked to mental illness, in particular depression (Kerkoff *et al.*, 1994). Of the ten countries with the highest rates of suicide in the world, nine are in the European region.

Mental health problems represent not only an immense psychological, social and economic burden to society, but also increase the risk of physical illnesses. Mental disorders affect and are affected by chronic conditions such as cancer, heart and cardiovascular diseases, diabetes and HIV/AIDS. Individuals with mental disorders are often subjected to social isolation, poor quality of life and increased mortality. Untreated, mental disorders bring about unhealthy behaviour, non-compliance with prescribed medical regimens, diminished immune functioning and poor prognosis. These disorders are the cause of staggering economic and social costs. The *World Health Report 2001* (WHO, 2001) outlines a new understanding and provides new hope and a comprehensive review of what is known about the burden of mental disorders and the principal contributing factors. It examines the scope of prevention and the availability of, and obstacles to, treatment. It provides a critical review of service provision and planning and concludes with a set of far-reaching recommendations that can be adapted by every country according to its resources and needs.

In England, mental ill health is so common that at any one time around one in six people of working age have a mental health problem, most often anxiety or depression. One person in 250 will have a psychotic illness, such as schizophrenia or bipolar affective disorder (manic depression) (Department of Health, 1999). In 2000, the Office for National Statistics (ONS) carried out a survey of psychiatric morbidity of people aged 16 to 74 years living in private households in Great Britain, and found that about one in six adults aged between 16 and 74 living in private households had a neurotic disorder (depression, anxiety, mixed anxiety and depression disorder, phobia, obsessive-compulsive disorder or panic disorder). A new report *The Neglected Majority* (Sainsbury Centre for Mental Health, 2005) indicated that one fifth of individuals who have depression in England need help that their general practitioners cannot give. The report calls for a new type of intermediate mental health care for this group. Intermediate mental health care is a way of bridging the gap between primary and specialist services.

The *National Service Framework* (Department of Health, 1999) focuses on the mental health needs of working age adults up to 65. This *National Service Framework* sets out standards in five areas; each standard is supported by the evidence and knowledge base, by service models, and by examples of good practice.

- Standard 1 addresses mental health promotion and combats the discrimination and social exclusion associated with mental health problems.
- Standards 2 and 3 cover primary care and access to services for anyone who may have a mental health problem.
- Standards 4 and 5 encompass the care of people with severe mental illness.
- Standard 6 relates to individuals who care for people with mental health problems.
- Standard 7 draws together the action necessary to achieve the target to reduce suicides.

These standards will be challenging for all mental health services and those delivering service provision in primary care and specialist settings to individuals with dual diagnosis. About 90% of mental health care is provided solely by primary care, making mental health consultations second only to those for respiratory infections (Goldberg & Huxley 1992; Murray & Lopez, 1996). The importance of primary care in addressing mental health problems and the delivery of primary care mental and neurological health services is addressed in Standard 2 of the *National Service Framework for Mental Health* (Department of Health, 1999).

Mental disorders

The following section gives a brief overview of the common mental disorders. It is worth noting that many substance misusers have experienced mental health problems. More than 50% of those seeking help for substance misuse have had a mental disorder in the previous six months. It is reported that around 30% of those seeking help for mental health problems have current substance misuse problems (Department of Health, 1998).

Anxiety

Anxiety disorders are serious medical disorders that affect approximately 5% of the population at any one time, affecting more women than men. Anxiety disorders often start in the twenties but may begin earlier and may cause people a number of different physical and psychological problems. According to the WHO's *Guide to Mental Health in Primary Care* (WHO, 2000), anxiety disorders are generalised anxiety, panic attacks, phobias, obsessive-compulsive disorders and post-traumatic stress disorders. Each anxiety disorder has its own distinct features but they all have a common theme of excessive, irrational fear and dread.

Generalised anxiety

Some individuals suffer from anxiety and have exaggerated worry and tension about health, money, family or work even though there is little or nothing to provoke it. Generalised anxiety is much more than the normal anxiety people experience day to day. Having this disorder means it is difficult to get through the day, and individuals always anticipate disaster. The features of generalised anxiety are dizziness, sweating, fatigue, headaches, muscle tension, muscle aches, difficulty swallowing, trembling, twitching, irritability, hot flushes, poor concentration and insomnia.

Individuals with generalised anxiety seem unable to relax and they may startle more easily than other people. Unlike individuals with several other anxiety disorders, those suffering from generalised anxiety do not avoid certain situations as a result of their disorder and are able to function in social settings or in their the job. Generalised anxiety may be triggered by stress factors and rarely occurs alone; it is usually accompanied by another anxiety disorder, such as depression or substance misuse. Individuals who suffer from anxiety usually smoke more, and may drink more alcohol too, increasing their risk of physical ill health (Department of Health, 1999).

Panic attacks

For individuals suffering from panic attacks, the symptoms of anxiety develop suddenly and increase in intensity over a few minutes. Individuals characteristically believe that they will lose control and often have fears of collapsing, imminent heart attack, going mad or other personal or social disaster. Panic attacks are characterised by palpitations, chest pain, choking feelings, churning of the stomach, dizziness, feeling of unreality or fear of impending doom. Panic attacks tend to subside within a short period of time and individuals may develop intense anxiety between episodes. However, panic attacks may lead to avoidance of a situation or location where a previous attack occurred. But not every individual who experiences panic attacks will develop panic disorder, for example many people have one attack but never have another. Panic disorder is often accompanied by other serious conditions such as depression and drug or alcohol misuse. Panic disorder is one of the most treatable of the anxiety disorders, responding in most cases to medications or carefully targeted psychotherapy.

Phobias

Another sort of anxiety disorder is called a phobia, in which people have problems in certain situations. Phobias are irrational fears of people, places, things and events. Some individuals with phobias have such restricted lives that they avoid normal, everyday activities such as shopping, driving or even going to work. The three most common phobias are simple phobia, agoraphobia and social phobia. Many individuals have minor phobias, particularly of animals or insects, but their lives do not become restricted and they are able to carry on their social functioning. Agoraphobia is a severe form of phobia and it involves fear of crowded shopping places, lifts, public transport or even open spaces. If this avoidance is carried to extreme lengths it can be disabling. Social phobias are twice as common in women as in men and involve an intense fear of doing something embarrassing or humiliating in public. For example, a fear of answering the telephone or eating in the public arena are common situations encountered by individuals with social phobias.

Obsessive-compulsive disorder

Obsessive-compulsive disorder involves anxious thoughts or rituals that lead to repetitive behaviour. Individuals with this disorder are overwhelmed by persistent, unwelcome thoughts or images, or by the urgent need to engage in certain rituals. The occurrence of obsessional thoughts is characteristically associated with an increase in anxiety leading to rituals and compulsions such as excessive cleaning or hand washing. Most individuals with this condition recognise that what they're doing is senseless, but they are unable to cease it. Attempts to resist the thoughts and compulsions result in extreme tension and anxiety, which can only be relieved by carrying out the rituals or compulsions. But for individuals with obsessive-compulsive disorder the activities are time-consuming, very distressing and interfere with daily life. Depression, other anxiety disorders or eating disorders may accompany obsessional-compulsive disorder.

Post-traumatic stress disorder

Post-traumatic stress disorder (PTSD) is a debilitating psychological condition that can develop following an extremely distressing or terrifying event. Often, individuals with PTSD have persistent frightening thoughts and memories of their ordeal and feel emotionally numb, especially with people they were once close to. PTSD can result from any number of traumatic incidents such as mugging, rape or torture; being kidnapped or held captive; child abuse; serious accidents such as car or train crashes; and natural disasters such as floods or earthquakes. The event that triggers PTSD may be something that threatened the person's life or the life of someone close to them. Or it could be something witnessed, such as massive death and destruction after a building is bombed or a plane crashes.

It is characterised by repeated flashbacks in the form of nightmares and disturbing recollections during the day. Individuals with PTSD may also experience other sleep problems, feel detached or numb, lose interest in things they used to enjoy and have trouble feeling affectionate. They may feel irritable, more aggressive than before or even violent. Things that remind them of the trauma may be very distressing, which could lead them to avoid certain places or situations that bring back those memories. Anniversaries of the traumatic event are often very difficult. PTSD is diagnosed only if the symptoms last more than a month and, occasionally, the illness doesn't show up until years after the traumatic event. The disorder is often accompanied by depression, substance misuse or one or more other anxiety disorders.

Relationship of anxiety disorders with substance misuse

Evidence from research studies has shown substantial co-occurrence between anxiety disorders and alcohol problems and indicates that alcohol misusers are at two to three times the risk of suffering from an anxiety disorder (Ross *et al.*, 1988). The self-medication hypothesis has been popular, and in many studies patients describe using alcohol to control their phobic fears and anxiety (Bibb & Chambless, 1986). It is reported that alcohol can increase clinical anxiety, especially after prolonged drinking and during withdrawal, and thus anxiety disorders such as panic disorder and generalised anxiety disorder (GAD) may be related to these situations rather than be a primary psychiatric disorder in these individuals (Harrison & Abou Saleh, 2002). Anxiety disorders may be a risk factor for the development of substance misuse, and anxiety symptoms are likely to be present during chronic intoxication and withdrawal. In a study examining the relationship between social phobia and cocaine dependence Myrick & Brady (1997) found a lifetime prevalence of social phobia in these cocaine dependant individuals to be 13.9%. They also found that the social phobic individuals were more likely to have additional psychopathology, use multiple psychoactive substances and were more likely to develop alcohol misuse at an earlier age. Research has shown a high level of substance use disorders with individuals who have PTSD. There is evidence to suggest that many substance misusers have been exposed to traumatic events at an early age. Studies have found that 64% of cocaine misusers had been exposed to a range of types of trauma and that 68% of admissions to a substance abuse treatment centre reported histories of physical and sexual abuse (Wasserman *et al.*, 1992; Ellason *et al.*, 1996). PTSD symptoms can be altered by substance use. Cocaine tends to worsen PTSD symptoms whereas opiates, alcohol and cannabis showed an improvement in PTSD symptoms (Bremner *et al.*, 1996).

Depression

Depression is the most common mental disorder, and each year one woman in every fifteen and one man in every thirty will be affected by depression (Meltzer *et al.*, 1994). Most of the 4000 suicides committed each year in England are attributed to depression. A recent review of the literature concluded that depression could be a major risk factor both for the development of cardiovascular disease and for death after a myocardial infarction (Musselman *et al.*, 1998). A depressive disorder is an illness that involves the body, mood and thoughts, and affects lifestyle and behaviour. It affects the way an individual eats and sleeps, the way one feels about oneself, and the way one thinks about things. It is reported that depression in people from black and ethnic minority groups, refugees and asylum seekers is frequently overlooked, although the rate has been found to be 60% higher than in the white population, with the difference being twice as great for men (Nazroo, 1997). Depressive disorders come in different forms: major depression, bipolar or unipolar depression, dysthymia, post-natal depression, seasonal affective disorder and chronic fatigue syndrome. However, within these types there are variations in the number of symptoms, their severity and persistence.

Major depression is manifested by a combination of symptoms that interfere with normal daily activities and result in the inability to work, study, sleep, eat and enjoy once pleasurable activities. The signs and symptoms of depression are (adapted from WHO, 2000):

- Low or sad mood
- Loss of interest or pleasure

- Insomnia, early morning awakening, or oversleeping
- Disturbed appetite and/or weight loss or overeating and weight gain
- Feelings of hopelessness, pessimism
- Feelings of guilt, worthlessness, helplessness
- Loss of interest or pleasure in hobbies and activities
- Decreased libido
- Decreased energy, fatigue, being 'slowed down'
- Difficulty concentrating, remembering, making decisions
- Suicidal thoughts and acts
- Restlessness, irritability

Some physical illnesses such as Parkinsonism, multiple sclerosis and hypothyroidism and some drugs (beta-blockers, oral contraceptives, corticosteroids) produce depressive symptoms and these conditions should be excluded before a diagnosis of depression is made.

Dysthymia

A less severe type of depression, dysthymia involves long-term, chronic symptoms that lower the mood but do not disable. Many individuals with dysthymia continue to function but interpersonal relationships may be affected. Individuals suffering from this condition may also experience major depressive episodes at some time in their lives.

Bipolar disorder

Bipolar depression, also known as manic-depressive illness, involves cyclical mood swings between severe depression and high elation. Sometimes the mood switches are dramatic and rapid, but most often they are gradual. When in the depressed cycle, an individual can have any or all of the symptoms of a depressive disorder. When in the manic cycle, the individual may be overactive, over-talkative and have a great deal of energy. Mania often affects thinking, judgement and social behaviour in ways that cause serious problems and embarrassment. Some of the symptoms of mania are:

- Abnormal or excessive elation
- Irritability
- Decreased need for sleep
- Grandiose notions
- Increased talking
- Racing thoughts
- Increased sexual desire
- Markedly increased energy
- Poor judgement
- Inappropriate social behaviour

Unipolar depression is depression without the accompanying cyclical mood swings.

Post-natal depression

Many women are particularly vulnerable after the birth of a baby. The hormonal and physical changes, as well as the added responsibility of caring for the newborn can be factors that lead to post-natal depression in some women. Post-natal depression is identical to depression and the majority of onsets occur during the first one to three months following childbirth. Some women will also develop psychotic illness within four weeks of childbirth and this disorder is characterised by symptoms such as hallucinations, delusions and gross impairment and functioning. The onset is rapid and requires emergency hospitalisation. Severely depressed mothers may resort to suicide, which is the second most common form of maternal death in the year after birth (Confidential Enquiry into Maternal Deaths in the UK, 1998).

Seasonal affective disorder (SAD)

Seasonal affective disorder, or SAD, is an affective or depressive disorder. Most SAD sufferers experience normal mental health throughout most of the year, but experience depressive symptoms in the winter. Symptoms may start emerging between September and November and continue until March, April or even May. Around 20% of cases are fairly mild, and are known as the 'winter blues', or sub-syndromal SAD, occurring mainly during December, January and February. But between 2 and 5% of cases have severe SAD and can't function in winter without continuous treatment (MIND, 2004). The symptoms are many and varied, and people can experience any of the following common effects (MIND, 2004):

- Lethargy or fatigue: lacking in energy and being unable to carry out normal daily routine
- Sleep problems: oversleeping, finding it hard to stay awake during the day, sometimes having disturbed nights and early morning waking
- Depression (including post-natal depression): feeling sad, low, weepy, guilty, a failure; sometimes hopeless and despairing, sometimes apathetic and feeling nothing
- Mood changes: in some people, bursts of overactivity and cheerfulness (hypomania) in spring and autumn
- Overeating: craving carbohydrates and putting on weight (which may increase negative feelings)
- Bulimia: eating large amounts of food and then vomiting
- Social problems: irritability and not wanting to see people
- Abusive behaviour
- Concentration problems: difficulty 'thinking straight', making decisions or concentrating
- Anxiety: tenseness and inability to cope with everyday stresses, panic attacks
- Loss of libido: not being interested in sex or physical contact
- Alcohol and drug misuse
- Get constant colds, infections and other illnesses
- Period problems

Various aetiologies have been suggested in the causation of SAD. One possibility is that SAD is related to a lack of serotonin and that exposure to full-spectrum artificial light may improve the condition by stimulating serotonin production, although this has been disputed. Another theory is that melatonin produced in the pineal gland is the primary cause. Another possibility is a problem affecting the nerve pathways in the brain and disrupting the body clock (Johansson *et al.*, 2001; 2003; MIND, 2004). SAD is rare, if existent at all, in the tropics, but is measurably present in higher latitudes. SAD is a more serious disorder, sometimes triggering dysthymia or clinical depression.

Relationship of mood disorders with substance misuse

Depression is considered to be important in the development of alcohol problems and dependence. Studies have shown that effective treatment for the mood disorder has a positive impact on the outcome of alcohol related disorders. Cocaine is associated with high rates of mood symptoms and disorders (Weiss *et al.*, 1986), both in major depression and bipolar disorder. Opiate use can produce or exacerbate depressive symptoms, and opiate users appear to have difficulty managing dysphoric mood states, suggesting that dysphoria may be a primary determinant of opiate drug use (Harrison & Abou Saleh, 2002). Alcohol can cause many mood symptoms, both due to chronic use and acute withdrawals, or may be used to self-medicate primary mood disorders. It is recognised that there is an association between alcohol misuse and mood disorders and studies have shown a higher than expected rate of bipolar disorder and major depression. Strakowski *et al.* (1992) studied age of onset and co-morbidity for first presentation of bipolar disorder and found that 24% had a co-morbid diagnosis of alcohol dependence, and that the onset of substance misuse preceded the presentation of bipolar disorder by a year in the majority of patients. Sex differences in the relative frequencies of primary alcoholism and primary depression have been identified. Males tend to have higher rates of alcoholism with secondary depression whereas females tend to have higher rates of primary depression with secondary alcoholism (Schuckit, 1983; Hesselbrock *et al.*, 1985). In a study of 204 patients with bipolar affective disorder, past substance misuse was evident in 34% (Goldberg *et al.*, 1999). This was most often alcohol (82%), cocaine (30%), marijuana (29%), sedative-hypnotic or amphetamine (21%) and opiate (13%) abuse. Those with a substance misuse were more likely to be male, divorced, separated or widowed. In addition, they were significantly more likely to have histories of medication non-compliance and suicidal ideation at the time of the manic episode.

Schizophrenia

Schizophrenia is the most common psychotic disorder and is characterised by apprehension, confusion, perceptual abnormalities, abnormal thought processing and expression, strange beliefs and fears, and hallucinations. The disorder can be divided into acute and chronic features. In the acute phase of the disorder, psychotic symptoms (such as hallucinations and delusions) usually emerge in men in their late teens and early twenties and in women in their mid-twenties to early thirties. Hallucinations are of common occurrence. Individuals with schizophrenia may hear voices other people don't hear or believe that others are reading their minds, controlling their thoughts or plotting to harm them. These experiences are terrifying and can cause fearfulness, withdrawal or extreme agitation. Delusional beliefs are also very common, particularly those with ideas of persecution. For example, the individuals may believe that they are being poisoned by others, receiving messages from radio or television or being watched and observed. Cognitive impairments often interfere with the patient's ability to lead a normal life and earn a living, and can cause great emotional distress.

The symptoms of schizophrenia fall into three broad categories:

- Positive symptoms: hallucinations, delusions, thought disorder and disorders of movement (clumsy and uncoordinated).
- Negative symptoms: flat affect (immobile facial expression, monotonous voice), lack of pleasure in everyday life, diminished ability to initiate and sustain planned activity, and speaking infrequently, even when forced to interact.
- Cognitive symptoms (or cognitive deficits): poor executive functioning (the ability to absorb and interpret information and make decisions based on that information), inability to sustain attention, and problems with working memory (the ability to keep recently learned information in mind and use it right away).

Individuals with schizophrenia are not especially prone to violence, but aggression is more likely in conjunction with acute disorder and may be associated with drug or alcohol misuse. Substance misuse always increases violent behaviour, whether or not the individual has schizophrenia. Violent behaviour is often directed at family members if the individual has paranoid schizophrenia. The chronic symptoms of schizophrenia include affective blunting, apathy, poverty of thought and speech, social withdrawal and self-neglect. Since many people with schizophrenia have difficulty holding a job or caring for themselves, the burden on their families and society is significant as well.

Relationship of schizophrenia with substance misuse

Some individuals who misuse drugs show symptoms similar to those of schizophrenia, and people with schizophrenia may be mistaken for people who are high on drugs. However, substance use may exacerbate schizophrenic symptoms and produce psychotic symptoms in their own right, with the impact of the substance use varying depending on the class of drug used, the quantity consumed, the route of administration and the state of use (Harrison & Abou Saleh, 2002). People with schizophrenia are three times more likely to abuse alcohol and six times more likely to abuse drugs. There is evidence to suggest that up to 50% of patients suffering from schizophrenia have either drug or alcohol problems (Andreasson *et al.*, 1987).

Patients suffering from schizophrenia seem to have a preference for activating drugs such as amphetamines, cocaine, cannabis and hallucinogens (Baigent *et al.*, 1995; Ries *et al.*, 2000). Symptoms such as mania, psychosis, depression, anxiety and personality disorder may be present. Stimulants may exacerbate psychotic symptoms, increase mood lability and interfere with sleep. Cannabis use has been reported to increase delusions, hallucinations, depression and anxiety. Schizophrenic patients who misuse alcohol may be more likely to exhibit hostile behaviour, paranoid thoughts and depression than non-alcohol using patients (Harrison & Abou Saleh, 2002). Substance misuse can also reduce the effectiveness of treatment for schizophrenia, making it more likely that individuals will not follow their treatment programme. The most common form of substance misuse in individuals with schizophrenia is an addiction to nicotine. Quitting smoking may be especially difficult for people with schizophrenia, since nicotine withdrawal may cause their psychotic symptoms to get worse temporarily.

The role of medication in mental illness

Medication is essential to control severe and enduring mental health problems because of the neuro-pharmacological imbalances underlying these conditions. Medications used in mental health services are categorised as antipsychotic medications, antidepressants, anxiolytics and mood stabilisers.

Antipsychotic medication

Antipsychotic medications are mainly used to control the active psychotic symptoms of schizophrenia, schizo-affective disorders, mania and depression. In low dosage, they are sometimes prescribed for those individuals with severe anxiety disorders or personality disorders. In the community, the medications are given as depot injections at intervals of weeks where compliance is uncertain. The common side effects are sedation, tremors and disorders of muscular movements. The newer compounds, 'atypical' antipsychotics, are better at treating the negative symptoms of psychotic illnesses and are less likely to induce disorders of muscular movements. The side effects reported include weight gain, sexual problems and diabetes.

Antidepressant medication

Antidepressants are mainly used to treat depression and the depressive phase of manic-depressive psychosis. These generally take three to six weeks for the medication to be effective. Their main function is to improve or elevate mood. The older tricyclic antidepressants tend to have more side effects than the newer types such as the selective serotonin reuptake inhibitors (SSRIs). The older tricyclic drugs are also more dangerous in overdose. Common side effects are a dry mouth, drowsiness, nausea, weight gain and sexual problems.

Anxiolytic medication

Anxiolytic medications are mainly used to relieve anxiety and help induce sleep. Benzodiazepines are typical of this group and tolerance and dependence are problematic. They should generally only be prescribed for short periods of time because of their high addictive potential.

Mood stabilisers

Mood stabilisers are prescribed to individuals with bipolar disorders, severe depression and in some cases of personality disorders. Lithium carbonate is a potentially toxic drug and regular blood tests are performed to ensure the blood levels remain in the therapeutic range. In addition, there are potential risks to the thyroid and the kidney in the long term, so it is often prescribed to individuals who have relapsed. Drugs used in epilepsy, such as carbamazepine and sodium valproate are also sometimes used as mood stabilisers.

Conclusion

Individuals with recurrent or severe and enduring mental illness (disabled for two or more years by impaired social behaviour) and co-morbidity with substance misuse have complex needs, which may require the continuing care of specialist mental health services and substance misuse services. It has been reported that around 30% of those seeking help for mental health problems have current substance misuse problems, and of individuals seeking help for substance misuse, more than half have had a mental disorder in the previous six months (Department of Health, 1998). Individuals with substance misuse and psychiatric disorders find it hard to engage with appropriate services and suicide is a high risk factor amongst this group (Appleby, 1999). Assessments of individuals with mental health problems, whether in primary or specialist care, should consider the potential role of substance misuse and how to access appropriate specialist input. The *Dual Diagnosis Good Practice Guide* (Department of Health, 2002) provides a framework within which staff can strengthen services so that they have the skills and organisation to tackle this demanding area of work. The authors' key message is that substance misuse is already part of mainstream mental health services and this is the right place for skills and services to be. Mental health services must also work closely with specialist substance misuse services to ensure that care is well coordinated.

References

Andreasson, S., Engstrom, A., Allebeck, P. & Rydeberg, U. (1987) Cannabis and schizophrenia: a longitudinal study of Swedish conscripts. *The Lancet*, 1483–6.

Appleby, L. (1999) *Safer Services: National Confidential Inquiry into Suicide and Homicide by People with Mental Illness*. Department of Health, London.

Baigent, B., Holme, G. & Hafner, R.J. (1995) Self reports of the interaction between substance abuse and schizophrenia. *Australia and New Zealand Journal of Psychiatry*, 29, 69–74.

Bibb, D.L. & Chambless, D.L. (1986) Alcohol use and abuse amongst diagnosed agoraphobics. *Behaviour Research Therapy*, 24, 49–58.

Bremner, J.D., Southwick, S.M., Darnell, A. *et al.* (1996) Chronic PTSD in Vietnam combat veterans: course of illness and substance abuse. *American Journal of Psychiatry*, 153, 369–75.

Confidential Enquiry into Maternal Deaths in the UK (1998) Why mothers die: Report on Confidential Enquiries into Maternal Deaths in the United Kingdom 1994–1996. HMSO, London.

Department of Health (1998) *Expert Seminar on Dual Diagnosis and the Management of Complex Needs*. Department of Health, London.

Department of Health (1999) *National Service Framework for Mental Health: Modern Standards and Service Models*. Department of Health, London.

Department of Health (2002) *Dual Diagnosis Good Practice Guide*. HMSO, London.

Ellason, J.W., Ross, C.A., Sainton, K. & Mayran, L.W. (1996) Axis I and II co-morbidity and childhood trauma history in chemical dependency. *Bull Menninger Clinical*, 60, 39–51.

Goldberg, D. & Huxley, P. (1992) *Common Mental Disorders: a Biosocial Model*. Routledge, London.

Goldberg, J.F., Garno, J.L., Leon, A.C. *et al.* (1999) A history of substance abuse complicates remission from acute mania in bipolar disorder. *Journal of Clinical Psychiatry*, 60, 733–40.

Harrison, C.A. & Abou Saleh, M.T. (2002) Psychiatric disorders and substance misuse: psychopathology. In: *Dual Diagnosis: Substance Misuse and Psychiatric Disorders* (Rassool G.H., ed.). Blackwell Publishing, Oxford.

Hesselbrock, M.N., Meyer, R.E. & Keener, J.J. (1985) Psychopathology in hospitalised alcoholics. *Archives of General Psychiatry*, 42, 1050–5.

Johansson, C., Smedh, C., Partonen, T. *et al.* (2001) Seasonal affective disorder and serotonin-related polymorphisms. *Neurobiology Disease*, April, 8 (2), 351–7.

Johansson, C., Willeit, M., Levitan, R. *et al.* (2003) The serotonin transporter promoter repeat length polymorphism, seasonal affective disorder and seasonality. *Psychological Medicine*, 33 (5), 785–92.

Kerkhof, A.J.F.M., Schmidtke, A., Bille-Brahe, U., Deleo, D. & Lönnqvist, J. (1994) *Attempted Suicide in Europe. Findings from the Multicentre Study on Parasuicide by the WHO Regional Office for Europe DWSO Press*. Leiden University, The Netherlands.

Meltzer, H., Gill, B., Petticrew, M. & Hinds, K. (1994) *OPCS Survey of Psychiatric Morbidity in Great Britain*. Bulletin No. 1. HMSO, London.

MIND (National Association for Mental Health) (2004) *Understanding Seasonal Affective Disorder*. Mind Publications, London.

Murray, C.J.L. & Lopez, A.D. (1996) *The Global Burden of Disease: a Comprehensive Assessment of Mortality and Disability from Diseases, Injury and Risk Factors in 1990 Projected to 2020*. Geneva, World Bank, Word Health Organization and Harvard School of Public Health.

Musselman, D.L., Evans, D.L. & Nemeroff, C.B. (1998) The relationship of depression to cardiovascular disease. *Archives of General Psychiatry*, 55, 580–92.

Myrick, H. & Brady, K. (1997) *Co-morbid Social Phobia and Cocaine Dependence*. American Psychiatric Association New Research Abstracts, Washington, DC.

Nazroo, J.Y. (1997) *Ethnicity and Mental Health: Findings from a National Community Survey*. Policy Studies Institute, London.

Office of National Statistics (2000) *The Prevalence of Psychiatric Morbidity among Adults aged 16–64 Living in Private Households in Great Britain*. HMSO, London.

Ries, R.K., Russo, J., Wingerson, D. *et al.* (2000) Shorter hospital stays and more rapid improvement among patients with schizophrenia and substance use disorders. *Psychiatric Services*, 51, 210–15.

Ross, H.E., Glaser, F.B. & Germanson, T. (1988) The prevalence of psychiatric disorders in patients with alcohol and other drug problems. *Archives of General Psychiatry*, 45, 1023–32.

Sainsbury Centre for Mental Health (2005) *The Neglected Majority*. Sainsbury Centre for Mental Health, London. www.scmh.org.uk

Schuckit, M.A. (1983) Alcoholic patients with secondary depression. *American Journal of Psychiatry*, 140, 711–14.

Strakowski, S.M., Tohen, M., Stoll, A.L. *et al.* (1992) Comorbidity in mania at first hospitalisation. *American Journal of Psychiatry*, 149, 554–6.

Wasserman, D.A., Havassy, B.E. & Boles, S.M. (1992) Traumatic events and post-traumatic stress disorder in cocaine users entering private treatment. Presented at the College on Problems of Drug Dependence Annual Meeting.

Weiss, R., Mirin, S.M. & Micheal, J.L. (1986) Psychopathology in chronic cocaine abusers. *American Journal of Drug Alcohol Abuse*, 12, 17–29.

WHO (2000) *WHO Guide to Mental Health in Primary Care* (UK Version). Royal Society of Medicine, London. www.whoguidemhpcuk.org

WHO (2001) *The World Health Report 2001: Mental Health: New Understanding, New Hope*. World Health Organization, Geneva.

6 Alcohol and Dual Diagnosis

K. Moore

Introduction

Alcohol use is a socially approved behaviour that has 'an important role within our society' (Epke, 2003). It is actively promoted in many cultural, social and religious circumstances, and assists in supporting national economies through taxation (Prime Minister's Strategy Unit, 2004). Groups from all walks of life and ages celebrate intoxication as a rite of passage applauded by their peers, whilst at the same time the effects of intoxication are negatively moralised and marginalised (Room, 2005). Yet some of the most well known jazz artists who have had serious mental illnesses and alcohol problems have lead successful and productive lives (Royal College of Psychiatrists, 2003). As health providers, we have known for many years the negative impact of alcohol on physical, social, financial and mental well-being. Indeed, there is a bewildering amount of research and commentary related to the wide spectrum of effects of alcohol, from promoting alcohol use as beneficial to health, to precipitating violence and significant physical or mental health consequences.

Nursing is undergoing rapid changes in social and political arenas, presenting clinicians with challenges in expanding professional roles and responsibilities. The inclusion of dual diagnosis as a mainstream mental health responsibility and particularly that of mental health and alcohol is one area where clinical responsibility remains at times contentious. It is now widely acknowledged that dual diagnosis patients using alcohol are commonplace in primary care and mental health settings. Formal recognition of this is outlined in the *National Service Framework for Mental Health* (Department of Health, 1999), *Models of Care* for drug misuse treatment (Health Advisory Service, 2001; National Treatment Agency, 2002), which clearly state that where co-morbidity of mental health and substance misuse (dual diagnosis) issues occur, this is the remit of mental health clinicians.

For nurses, the management of alcohol problems in all settings continues to be difficult and fraught with high levels of violence and aggression towards staff (Royal College of Psychiatrists, 2000; Tucker, 2002; Cole, 2005). The ongoing concerns 'are expressed by both staff and patients alike' on the impact alcohol has on safety, when featuring in acute mental health episodes (Williams, 2000). Yet nurses, in particular, have specialist skills in communication and the management of high expressed psychological need and altered perceptual states, making them ideal clinicians to working with dual diagnosis patients who use alcohol.

Relationship of alcohol and mental health

Common links with alcohol and mental health include depression, suicidal behaviour, anxiety, obsessive-compulsive disorders, bipolar disorders, schizophrenia and personality disorders (Institute of Alcohol Studies, 2004). Nursing care and management of the mental health patient with alcohol problems must incorporate three broad factors: physical health, mental health (including risk) and social functioning. The links between alcohol and mental health can be extremely complex. However, there are four broad characteristics used in dual diagnosis to explain relationships (Abdulrahim, 2001):

(1) Alcohol is used to medicate psychological distress/symptoms (self-medication)
(2) Alcohol use causes psychological distress/symptoms (side effect)
(3) Alcohol use that has no causal or preventative mechanism for psychological distress or symptoms
(4) Underlying trauma resulting in alcohol use and mood disorders

The *Alcohol Harm Reduction Strategy for England* (Prime Minister's Strategy Unit, 2004) clearly states that mental health and alcohol problems are of high concern, particularly in relation to suicide, vulnerability and mental well-being. This is linked with social situations such as homelessness and physical health consequences for the individual. Whilst the alcohol strategy serves to broadly define social tasks and responsibility within mental health, the responsibility for changing alcohol consumption does not necessarily lie with the individual if they are 'genuinely unable to exercise that choice' (Prime Minister's Strategy Unit, 2004).

Mental health patients who use alcohol can express overwhelming needs that, as clinicians, we feel unprepared for and overly challenged by (McCaffery *et al.*, 2002). However, Barnes *et al.* (2002) emphasise the need for basic training in addictions for mental health staff, acknowledging the need for mental health and alcohol services to work in close collaboration. From experience, we know that by increasing basic alcohol knowledge and using existing skills, nurses can form warm, empathic relationships and develop an organised approach to anticipating care, achieving positive outcomes in alcohol management (Soden & Murray, 1993; NDARC, 2003).

What are the key concerns for mental health?

One of the first issues we must look at when working with dual diagnosis patients using alcohol is the belief system that we use in relation to alcohol use. Mental health service users are no exception to the social norms of alcohol use. In some cases we consider some to be more vulnerable to the effects of alcohol being used in maladaptive ways or medicating distressing symptoms, and view others as making a life choice. Traditionally, for mental health patients, this meant that many were excluded from accessing treatment on the basis of one of these problems. Because of this, stigma and stereotyping is experienced, which is significantly increased when treatment is offered reluctantly, and as a result of a crisis only.

New developments in psychiatry and substance misuse are driven by public opinion in the wake of high profile, high risk events (Ward & Applin, 1998). Such events, whilst engendering public outrage, also precipitate change. Public events can and do influence our thoughts and practice in relation to when and how we intervene (Walker *et al.*, 1998; Drucker, 2003–4). The Royal College of Psychiatrists clearly recommends that behaviour, rather than the individual, should be stigmatised (Royal College of Psychiatrists, 2001). Yet in practice this can be difficult when faced with managing aggression, violence and self-harm as a consequence of alcohol consumption, given that alcohol use can be the direct cause of such behaviours. Clearly, there are associations between all levels of alcohol use and lowering of inhibitions, anger thresholds and aggressive outbursts, which nurses are constantly managing as front-line staff.

One key driver in developing mental health care is risk management. Many initiatives are developed with the sole aim of reducing harm to self and others. Mental health nurses have an advantage over their substance misuse colleagues as assessment of risk is a basic component of all interactions within mental health. Substance misuse services have now begun to address such issues. However, with alcohol problems this is significantly complicated by physical consequences, social situations and resultant mental health needs.

Using a models of care framework for alcohol management in dual diagnosis

Models of Care (National Treatment Agency, 2002) is a Government initiative which sets out to describe a national framework of commissioning and treatment for substance misuse services, promoting evidence based practice and good practice guidelines. The model promotes a single point of access, integrated treatment pathways focusing on screening and assessment, levels of treatment interventions, care planning and coordination of care. Importantly, Models of Care is based on the mental health community programme approach.

Models of care relationship to mental health and the care programme approach

Broadly, the models parallel each other, and the levels of care are similar in nature. However, Models of Care in relation to alcohol views in-patient treatment of mental health and alcohol as a highly specialist treatment in mental health settings, whilst mental health services see this as specialist substance misuse work. Fundamentally, views on the management of alcohol problems remain diametrically opposed for the dual diagnosis patient. Dual diagnosis patients may be engaged in different levels of treatment, with different services at the same time, and do not necessarily follow a linear pattern, with the levels of care not necessarily being mutually exclusive. Table 6.1 presents the Models of Care relationship to mental health and the care programme approach (CPA).

Where to start – triage

As a starting point it is worth noting that, generally, mental health patients do not respond well to confrontational approaches or abstinence based

Table 6.1 Models of care relationship to mental health and CPA.

Tier/CPA Level	Alcohol service level of interventions	Mental health service level of interventions
Tier 1	Relates to primary care services, such as GP, social services, housing, A & E departments, voluntary advice/self-help agencies, education and vocational services	Relates to primary care services such as GP, social services, housing, A & E departments, voluntary advice/ self-help agencies, education and vocational services No CPA required
Tier 2 or Standard CPA	Alcohol-related advice or drop-in service Outreach service Low threshold or GP clinics Liaison with other general medical sectors All service users would be triaged	Mental health drop-in, open access or advice agencies GP referral for assessment Standard CPA Liaison with other general medical sectors All service users would be triaged
Tier 3 or Enhanced CPA Structured community and specialist services	Structured community treatment with a named population Day programmes for substance misuse Community prescribing Specialist subgroup work with criminal justice, treatment and testing orders Liaison with other specialist and general agencies, including joint working practices	Community treatment with a named population Day programmes for mental health Community clinics Specialist subgroup work with home treatment, outreach and crisis teams Liaison with other specialist and general agencies, including joint working practices Enhanced CPA
Tier 4a Residential services	In-patient detoxification services In-patient rehabilitation services Residential dual diagnosis services	
Tier 4b Highly specialist non-substance misuse services	Treatment at specialist general medical services such as liver and HIV units	In-patient admission to acute psychiatric service, elders' service, adolescent or regional specialty service In-patient admission to forensic services Treatment at specialist general medical services such as liver and HIV units

treatment models. This may make the situation more difficult, emphasising a sense of shame, guilt, stigma and blame on the individual, meaning that they do not seek early treatment and remain engaged. Confrontational or abstinence models may precipitate or enhance feelings of anger and suspicion and heighten paranoia, raising the potential for aggression and non-engagement. As nurses we must achieve a balance between creating doubt or dissonance in engaging, whilst provoking or promoting change.

As skilled communicators nurses learn to ask questions on some of the most sensitive aspects of life, in a manner that is both empathic and supportive. Asking questions about alcohol is no different. At first, sensitive topics feel uncomfortable, but the more practice we have, the more comfortable and sure we feel; this is true of asking about alcohol in non-judgemental ways. At all levels of nursing, regardless of the place and nature of the presentation, specific basic questions need to be asked when assessing alcohol and its impact:

- The amount of alcohol consumed (number of cans, pints or bottles when the individual is unsure)
- The type of alcohol used (beer, spirits, cider); where possible get the name of the drink, such as super strength ciders or normal strength beers

Both these questions will help calculate the number of units (percentage of alcohol in the drink) the person has consumed. It is, however, important not to leave it just there, you also need to ask:

- The time of day drinking started (or the usual start time for the first alcoholic drink)
- Number of days per week alcohol is consumed or the usual drinking pattern over a day, week or month

These two questions will help establish the nature of drinking in the spectrum of social drinking to problem drinking or dependency.

- Finally, you need to ask whether they experience any changes or problems the day after drinking, as this will help to establish any physical or psychological impact (for example tremor, sweats, shakes, blackouts, panic attacks)

In dual diagnosis, the use of screening tools has been tested in different settings, advocating basic questionnaires such as CAGE (Mayfield *et al.*, 1974) in primary care practice, and the AUDIT (Meltzer, 2003) is recommended for dual diagnosis in all settings (Piccinelli *et al.*, 1997; NDARC, 2003; Abou-Saleh, 2004). Additional physical testing by breath alcohol testing, routine blood testing (for main corpuscular volume) and gamma glutamyl transferase (GGT) are also useful, as when raised these can indicate alcohol use. It is important for nurses at any stage of assessment or intervention to be aware of the local resources in relation to either alcohol or mental health use, and to seek advice, support or referral on to these services if needed.

Working with non-problematic alcohol use

At this level, intervention is usually opportunistic, occurring as situational contacts or brief interventions; completing a basic alcohol triage should be considered at every opportunity. In a one-to-one situation, nurses should consider the reason for presentation, and as standard practice ask all patients about their alcohol use (Freeman, 2002). In relation to mental health needs, key cues for targeted questioning would relate to presentations that include stress, tension, anxiety, low mood and psychological distress (Royal College of Psychiatrists, 2005). Interventions by nurses can often be completed in one session using a minimal intervention, such as ensuring patients have access to the information they need to make informed choices, information on sensible drinking limits, clear and safe advice on alcohol reduction, advice on completion of simple alcohol diaries and mental health distress assessment. A follow-up appointment is useful but not essential. If appropriate, additional appointments composed of 5–6 face-to-face sessions can be provided, focusing on concise information on alcohol use and reduction. Assessment building on minimal triage would consider the level of dependence by use of simple alcohol diaries that are retrospective. It is important to include exploring motivation of the individual to change; relapse assessment and cues for relapse would be included in the follow-up sessions (NDARC, 2003).

Working with intoxication

Situational crises often precipitate treatment; nurses in GPs' surgeries, A & E departments, psychiatric liaison teams or crisis/home treatment teams would be more likely to have contact with this patient group presenting with acute distress or mental illness with intoxication. Presentations include individuals with alcohol and panic attacks, suicidal features/self-harm behaviour, depression with suicidal features, domestic violence, homicidal thoughts, psychotic symptoms, personality disorders and social phobias. Indeed, there is a well documented relationship between alcohol and aggression, where alcohol is thought to 'focus attention onto salient cues in threatening circumstances' (Zeichner *et al.*, 1994).

The presenting mental health need may not meet the criteria for referral to a mental health clinic or team; however, meaningful interventions can be offered. The assessment of alcohol and mental health would be more specific with a focused assessment to define alcohol or mental health need (Rassool, 2002). At this stage one issue may be a more hidden problem. Nurses would need to consider completing a basic alcohol assessment and assessment of any withdrawal symptoms. Importantly, a risk assessment related to psychiatric symptoms, increased levels of risk, historical risk patterns or crisis presentations needs to be completed. For some individuals this may be their first presentation to services, and interventions offered can be both assessment and treatment.

Intervention strategies predominantly rely on the level of risk presented by the individual. For nurses, presentations that involve feelings and thoughts of suicide are often the most difficult to manage and these are the situations with perhaps the fewest protocols to support decision making (McCaffery *et al.*, 2002). It can be easy to feel that the patient presenting in an intoxicated state, expressing suicidal thoughts and plans, is attention seeking and acting out (Sidley & Renton, 1996). A generally held belief is that intoxicated patients cannot be assessed. This presents a conundrum, as the tragedy of not assessing due to intoxication is that the use of alcohol is one of the key factors in 80% of individuals who complete suicide (McCaffery *et al.*, 2002). However, when intoxication and suicidal thoughts are present, the immediate actions are tied to the duty of care (NMC, 2004).

Alcohol users, like their general psychiatric counterparts, have similar features in relation to depression and feelings of hopelessness. They do, however, express more feelings/episodes of aggression, impulsive behaviour, lower self-esteem and poor problem solving skills (Hawton *et al.*, 2003). At this stage it is recommended that treatment of the risk and intoxication occur at the same time. This can mean that assessment and reassessment is necessary over time, as the level of intoxication may influence the level of the immediate risk (Mann *et al.*, 1999). Initially, the task for nurses is safety and, second, enhancing the level of motivation to address the issues, supporting the desire to change.

Building motivation is one of the basic principles in working with someone who does not acknowledge that they have a problem (Prochaska & DiClemete, 1986). This style of communication relies on active listening and reflection to support and 'nudge' a decision balance in favour of admitting a problem and/or receiving treatment. However, this can involve multiple crisis presentations before an individual can achieve motivation to act. An empathic, non-confrontational communication style is recommended, as scare tactics increase feelings of frustration, lack of control and poor self-esteem.

Strategies supporting motivation for change include education on associations between alcohol and the presenting psychological/psychiatric problem, use of objective written information such as retrospective alcohol diaries, liver function testing and balance sheets listing the pros and cons of continuing without change and the perceived effects of change. If there is time available or where there is the facility for repeat sessions, conversations around barriers to change can be explored, using reframing techniques to emphasise either the alcohol or mental health element to promote change. Finally, some individuals may also need the introduction or alteration of medication for more integrated treatment of either the alcohol or the mental health issues. This needs to be completed in partnership with medical colleagues (Department of Health, 2002; Crome & Myton, 2004).

Nursing staff need to consider two practice elements; first, whether they can work in partnership with the individual on either the psychiatric or the alcohol element of the presentation and, second, whether the patient would want or need more specialist services to assess and manage the level of need and risk. If in doubt, contact your local community mental health team (CMHT) or alcohol service for advice and/or onward referral. Longer-term strategies may involve more focused interventions by referring to an alcohol or mental health agency, and could involve combination treatments, face-to-face interventions and support across multiple agencies, in a coordinated fashion for intensive treatment.

Working with problem drinking and dependent drinking

Where risk drives interventions with intoxication, the same is true for mental health patients who have problematic binge or dependent drinking patterns. For patients with a serious and enduring mental illness (SMI) the use of a standard or enhanced CPA can act as the pivot for treatment pathways. The Department of Health (2002) recommends that dual diagnosis issues at this level require care coordination in order to manage integrated treatment across multiple agencies. Mental health nurses are often at the forefront of being both coordinators of care and providers of care in in-patient and community settings.

Acute admissions of dual diagnosis patients with alcohol problems, as voluntary patients or under section of the Mental Health Act, places mental health nurses in conflicting dilemmas. First, personal views can be challenged or reinforced by aggressive behaviours; second, professionally they need to present themselves as empathic and supportive; and finally, they need to control and maintain an alcohol free and safe environment (Department of Health, 2002). This can lead to difficult ward dynamics, conflicts and ward subcultures developing, in part sustained and enforced by use of the Mental Health Act and leave/discharge status (Freeman, 2002). In the growing body of literature, evidence suggests that supporting restrictions for the supply/consumption of alcohol in the absence of any other intervention is 'almost certainly doomed to failure' (Williams, 2000). Thus mental health nurses are often in a no-win position. Similarly, the dilemma for community staff is the need to maintain alcohol free areas by either banning or ignoring attendance for treatment while intoxicated, or risking a home visit to an address that may have associations with alcohol related violence.

It is possible to take a proactive role in completing a comprehensive assessment and intervening with mental health patients who use alcohol. However, rather than a single event, assessment is an ongoing process and can take days, weeks or months to complete, depending on the mental health of the person at the time of contact. Short-term or quick resolutions are less likely, as both the mental health and substance misuse elements need to be fully understood. Outpatient work with mental health patients who have alcohol problems and/or dependency can take between 6 and 12 months, with regular weekly appointments, and sometimes longer.

The comprehensive alcohol assessment builds on the basic alcohol assessment and includes patterns of use, withdrawal symptoms, psychological history, self-harm, levels of risk for both mental health and alcohol use and history of trauma. Exploration of any physical problems experienced, social issues related to childcare, relationships, domestic violence, housing, employment and finances need to be included. Patients should also be asked about their history with forensic services, legal problems, arrests, fines, charges or any outstanding warrants, as these are often the social consequences of alcohol use. Each element helps the assessor to develop an understanding of links between biological, social and psychological factors/triggers for the patient, related to their dual diagnosis over time.

In planning care, the degree of immediate risk is used to determine how, when and where psychiatric services intervene. This can be outpatient community mental health services where immediate risk is low but mental health needs are high, or emergency reception centres/crisis teams or in-patient units where immediate risk is high and mental health needs are high or even under section of the Mental Health Act. Based on assessment, individualised care plans reflecting mental health and alcohol use are developed, covering the initial presentation, with a step-wise approach to individualised treatment, considering risk and strategies that address psychosocial functioning.

Where alcohol causes physical withdrawal syndromes, detoxification is a treatment intervention that complements the skills of nursing and mental health nursing. Whilst detoxification can be a very physical process (Trevisan *et al.*, 1998), there are a number of psychological elements that mental health nurses are skilled at observing and managing, including hallucinations, delirium, altered mental states, hyper-vigilance, anxiety, paranoia, depression, tactile hallucinations and levels of risk. The principles of patient care in alcohol detoxification in dual diagnosis are similar to alcohol detoxification alone: monitoring of dehydration, blood pressure, dietary intake, orientation to time, place and person, and sleep are basic aspects of mental health observations, and where needed, in-patient treatment should be secured for more complex presentations (Myrick & Anton, 1998; Watts, 2001).

Patients need a non-stimulating, non-threatening environment. Staff need to use a steady, consistent approach, which is the same for mental health patients in an over stimulated or paranoid state. It is important to explain all actions clearly and in a manner that outlines your intentions; the approach is completed in a friendly, supportive manner with good use of eye contact. Low lighting at night will help reduce perceptual disturbances and, in combination with appropriate medications, maximise opportunities for a positive outcome and the ability for both the patient and mental health staff to move into a proactive stage of intervention.

The role for nurses

Nurses have the skills to work with this complex group, and do so on a daily basis, using transferable skills from many aspects of nursing care. From assessment and planning, to the delivery of care, mental health nurses use core interventions such as communication and listening, developing trust, encouraging change and accepting resistance. They have key roles in facilitating combinations of interventions using regular individual time for counselling, motivational interviewing, relapse prevention, assertiveness training, social behaviour therapies, cognitive behavioural approaches, outreach approaches and family interventions. Using a model of care for patients using alcohol, or a care programme approach, nurses are well placed to facilitate jointly coordinated agency approaches that are negotiated with the patient, and, where appropriate, facilitate medication management for the mental health or detoxification in home, outpatient or hospital settings, depending on need. These skills make nurses ideal clinicians in treatment provision and review of care for mental health patients using alcohol.

Short, medium or long-term treatment for mental health patients using alcohol requires clear and consistent approaches across multiple agencies, with realistic timeframes for interventions to work. Many individuals can and do successfully engage in treatment that leads to positive change over time. That is not to say that nurses or mental health nurses carry this responsibility alone, a partnership approach to working with alcohol problems in acute mental health settings is needed. Certainly, primary care nurses, GPs, social workers, medical colleagues, probation, alcohol teams, housing and forensic teams have equal roles to play in successfully identifying and intervening with this complex group.

References

Abdulrahim, D. (2001) *Substance Misuse and Mental Health Co-morbidity (Dual Diagnosis)*. The Health Advisory Service, London.

Abou-Saleh, M. (2004) Dual diagnosis: management within a psychosocial context. *Advances in Psychiatric Treatment*, 10, 352–60.

Barnes, A., Murray, M., Ritchie, F. & Jones, M. (2002) Dual diagnosis: developing the skills base. *Mental Health Practice*, 5 (7), 16–19.

Cole, A. (2005) Four in five nurses on mental health wards face violence. *British Medical Journal*, 330, 1227.

Crome, I. & Myton, T. (2004) Pharmacotherapy in dual diagnosis. *Advances in Psychiatric treatment*, 10, 413–24.

Department of Health (1999) *National Service Framework for Mental Health*. The Stationery Office, London.

Department of Health (2002) *Dual Diagnosis Good Practice Guide. Mental Health Implementation Policy Guide*. HMSO, London.

Drucker, E. (2003–4) Where is the addiction field headed? The future of treatment in a drug crazed world requires attitude shift. *Cross Currents*, (Winter edition). Centre for Addiction and Mental Health, Canada.

Epke, H. (2003) Preventing alcohol abuse – a community strategy. *Journal of Community Nursing*, 17 (2), 16–19.

Freeman, J. (2002) Dealing with drugs in acute psychiatry: knowing the score. *Mental Health Practice*, 5 (8), 18–22.

Hawton, K., Houston, K., Haw, C. & Townsend, E. (2003) Co-morbidity of axis I and axis II disorders in patients who attempt suicide. *American Journal of Psychiatry*, 160, 1494–500.

Health Advisory Service (2001) *The Substance Misuse Advisory Service: Commissioning Standards: Drug and Alcohol Treatment and Care*. Health Advisory Service, London.

Institute of Alcohol Studies (2004) *Alcohol and Mental Health*. Institute of Alcohol Studies, Cambridgeshire.

Levy, A. & Scott-Clark, C. (2004) Under the Influence. *Society Guardian*, November.

McCaffery, R., Lee, A., Pramod, J. & Scott, J. (2002) A survey of opinions on the management of individuals who express suicidal ideation while intoxicated with alcohol. *Psychiatric Bulletin*, 26, 332–4.

Mann, J., Waternaux, C., Haas, G. & Malone, K. (1999) Toward a clinical model of suicidal behavior in psychiatric patients. *American Journal of Psychiatry*, 156, 181–9.

Mayfield, D., McLeod, G. & Hall, P. (1974) The CAGE questionnaire: validation of a new alcoholism screening instrument. *American Journal of Psychiatry*, 131, 1121–3.

Meltzer, H. (2003) Developing a common instrument for mental health. In: *EUROHIS: Developing Common Instruments for Health Surveys* (Nosikov, A. & Gudex, C., eds). World Health Organization, IOS Press.

Myrick, H. & Anton, R. (1998) Treatment of alcohol withdrawal. *Alcohol Health & Research World*, 22 (1), 38–43.

NDARC (National Drug and Alcohol Research Centre) (2003) *Guidelines for the Treatment of Alcohol Problems*. National Alcohol Strategy, Commonwealth of Australia, Canberra.

National Treatment Agency (2002) *Models of Care for Treatment of Adult Drug Misusers*. National Treatment Agency, London.

Nursing and Midwifery Council (2004) *The NMC Code of Professional Conduct: Standards for Conduct, Performance and Ethics*. Nursing and Midwifery Council, London.

Piccinelli, M., Tessari, E., Bortolomasi, M. *et al.* (1997) Efficacy of alcohol use disorders identification test as a screening tool for hazardous alcohol intake and related disorders in primary care: a validity study. *British Medical Journal*, 314–420.

Prime Minister's Strategy Unit (2004) *Alcohol Harm Reduction Strategy for England*. Cabinet Office, London.

Prochaska, J. & DiClemete, C. (1986) Towards a comprehensive model of change. In *Treating Addictive Behaviours: Process of Change* (Miller, W. & Heather, N., eds). Plenum Press, New York.

Rassool, G.H. (2002) Substance misuse and mental health: an overview. *Nursing Standard*, 16 (50), 47–53.

Room, R. (2005) Stigma, social inequality and alcohol and drug use. *Drug and Alcohol Review*, 1 (24), 143–55.

Royal College of Psychiatrists (2000) *Drug and Alcohol Abuse 'Rife' on Psychiatric Wards*. Annual Meeting, Royal College of Psychiatrists, Edinburgh.

Royal College of Psychiatrists (2001) *Changing Minds Campaign. Drugs and Alcohol – Whose Problem is it Anyway? Who Cares?* Royal College of Psychiatrists, London.

Royal College of Psychiatrists (2003) *Creative Artists and Psychiatric Disorder*. Press release, Royal College of Psychiatrists, London.

Royal College of Psychiatrists (2005) *Alcohol: Our Favourite Drug*. Fact Sheet. Royal College of Psychiatrists, London.

Sidley, G. & Renton, J. (1996) General nurses' attitudes to patients who self harm. *Nursing Standard*, 1 (10), No. 30.

Soden, T. & Murray, R. (1993) Motivational interviewing techniques. In: *Alcohol and Drug Problems: A Practical Guide for Counsellors* (Howard, B., Harrison, S., Carver, V. & Lightfoot, L., eds). Addiction Research Foundation, Toronto, Canada.

Tucker, R. (2002) The enigma of violence: developing a therapeutic response. *Mental Health Practice*, 5 (5), 4–6.

Trevisan, L., Boutros, N., Petrakis, I. & Krystal, J. (1998) Complications of alcohol withdrawal. Pathophysiological insights. *Alcohol Health & Research World*, 22 (1).

Walker, L., Jackson, S. & Barker, P. (1998) Perceptions of the psychiatric nurse's role: a pilot study. *Nursing Standard*, 12 (16), 35–8.

Ward, M. & Applin, C. (1998) *The Unlearned Lesson*. Wynne Howard Books, London.

Watson, H. (2000) Problem drinkers among acute care patients. *Nursing Standard*, 14 (40), 32–5.

Watts, M. (2001) The significance of drinking context for home detoxification. *Nursing Standard*, 15 (8), 33–7.

Williams, R. (2000) Substance use and misuse in psychiatric wards: a model task for clinical governance. *Psychiatric Bulletin*, 24, 43–6.

Zeichner, A., Allen, J., Gianocola, P. & Lating, J. (1994) Alcohol and aggression: effects of personal threat on human aggression and affective arousal. *Alcoholism, Clinical and Experimental Research*, 18 (3), 657–63.

7 Eating Disorders and Dual Diagnosis

M. Abuel-Ealeh & R. Barrett

Introduction

Although recent times have witnessed an increased interest in eating disorders, these major mental health problems have existed and were known for hundreds of years before. Definitions, explanations and fashions have evolved over time, but the challenge, indeed enigma (Bruch, 1978), of understanding why people, the vast majority of whom are young women, but with a notable increase amongst young men too, continue to torture themselves almost to death through determined starvation or excessive bingeing followed by vomiting, purging and starvation, remains largely unresolved. In our society there are greater pressures on women to control their weight, together with a tendency for thinness to be increasingly valued as social status rises (Evans, 2003).

The aims of the chapter are to examine the relationship of eating disorders with mental health and substance misuse and to present an overview of the various ranges of service approaches and strategies used in the care and treatment of people with eating disorders.

Anorexia nervosa

Anorexia nervosa is seen as an illness, which has undergone major change, especially over the past 40 years. This is seen by Russell (1995) to be congruent with societal attitudes, which attribute great importance to thinness in women. In addition, it appears that the incidence of anorexia nervosa has increased over the past 50 years and this may be due to changing socio-cultural factors. Crisp's (1992) view is that the central psychopathology of anorexia nervosa is rooted in the biological and psychological experiences accompanying the attainment of the adult weight. He saw anorexia nervosa as an attempt to cope with fears and conflicts associated with psychobiological maturity, and emphasised the meaning of sub-pubertal weight in developmental terms (Crisp, 1992).

According to Crisp (1992), the prevalence rate of anorexia nervosa is 86 per 100 000 females. He calculated that the number of 'hard core' anorexics in the UK amounted to 215 per 500 000 population. This calculation is equivalent to 23 650 anorexia sufferers in the UK in any given period of time. Even though the vast majority of sufferers of anorexia nervosa are young females, it is not unknown amongst males. There is a fair degree of agreement that the ratio of male to female sufferers is around 1:10. The mortality rate of anorexia nervosa is 20% of all sufferers after a mean duration of 20 years of the illness (Crisp, 1992). A major cause of death in relation to co-morbidity is suicide, owing to depression being the most likely psychiatric disorder to accompany both anorexia nervosa

Table 7.1 Diagnostic criteria for anorexia nervosa (DSM-IV).

(1) Refusal to maintain body weight at or above a minimally normal weight for age and height, (for example weight loss leading to maintenance of body weight less than 85% of that expected or failure to make expected weight gain during period of growth, leading to body weight less than 85% of that expected).
(2) Intense fear of gaining weight or becoming fat, even though underweight.
(3) Disturbance in the way in which one's body weight or shape is experienced, undue influence of body shape and weight on self-evaluation, or denial of the seriousness of current low body weight.
(4) In post-menarchal females, amenorrhoea, that is the absence of at least three consecutive menstrual cycles (a woman is considered to have amenorrhoea if her periods occur only following hormone administration, for example oestrogen).

Anorexia nervosa is further classified into two types: *restrictive type* when the sufferer does not regularly engage in binge eating or purging behaviour (that is self-induced vomiting or the misuse of laxatives or diuretics); *purging type* when the sufferer regularly engages in binge eating or purging behaviour (that is self-induced vomiting or the misuse of laxatives or diuretics).

and bulimia nervosa. Table 7.1 presents the DSM-IV (APA, 1994) diagnostic criteria of anorexia nervosa and Table 7.2 presents the commonly occurring features observed in people suffering from anorexia nervosa.

Table 7.2 Commonly occurring features observed in people suffering from anorexia nervosa.

Anorexia nervosa
Severe weight loss
Distorted body image, misconception about body weight and size
Lack of concern about low body weight
Excessive exercising
Self-induced vomiting and purging
Fatigue and decreased energy
Sleep disturbance, difficulty in sleeping
Feeling cold, intolerance of cold, low body temperature
Headaches
Abdominal pain, constipation
Amenorrhoea
Bradycardia
Low blood pressure
Brittle nails
Yellow skin, especially palms
Growth of soft downy hair all over the body, known as lanugo
Irritability and anxious energy
Depression
Isolation and loss of friends
Personality changes
Perfectionism

Bulimia

Whilst anorexia nervosa has a long history, bulimia nervosa, in contrast, is of recent origin. It was as recently as the 1970s when the syndrome of bulimia nervosa was first described (Russell, 1979). According to Lacey (1992), the prevalence rate of bulimia nervosa is 3% of females aged 15–40 years. As may be noted, this is significantly higher than the prevalence rate of anorexia nervosa.

Bulimia nervosa shares various similarities with anorexia nervosa but it also has very distinct features. In both eating disorders there is a fear of fatness with an accompanying urge to lose weight, what Bruch (1978) in her classic account of anorexia nervosa refers to as 'the relentless pursuit of thinness'. This constant pursuit of thinness is no less evident in people with bulimia nervosa, yet there is much less likelihood of weight loss; indeed, many individuals with bulimia nervosa are of normal weight. The best way to explain the absence of severe weight loss in bulimia nervosa is by pointing to its distinguishing feature, namely bingeing. Such eating patterns are representative of this severe disorder and constitute a classification that has its own distinguishing features that are at odds with the classic disorder anorexia nervosa. Anorexia nervosa, unlike other eating disorders, in its most severe form is easily discernible, to the point of not being easily mistaken for any other mental health problem. Those with bulimia nervosa, in contrast, may go undetected for a long time, due largely to the marked likelihood of the disorder being concealed by sufferers, who are typically very secretive.

The roots of bulimia nervosa are again quite distinct from those of anorexia nervosa. In terms of family dynamics alone, the 'golden girl', described by Bruch (1978), prior to the onset of the anorexia nervosa is compliant, obedient and fits the idealised picture of the model daughter. As Gordon (1999) indicates, a differential pattern is apparent in people with bulimia nervosa. The daughter who goes on to develop bulimia nervosa is, according to Gordon, likely to have resented her mother. She is likely to have viewed her mother as weak, and despised her accordingly, whilst typically identifying closely with her father, whom she perceives as a strong figure whom she respects and wants to emulate. This girl's experience of bulimia nervosa is likely to have involved poor emotional regulation, along with marked ambivalence and a chaotic lifestyle. Bulimia nervosa may even manifest as a proneness to being driven by impulses that cannot be controlled (Lacey & Evans, 1986). This characterisation itself offers early notice of what will be described below in terms of co-morbidity and bulimia nervosa. The extreme version represents the antithesis of the 'golden girl', the 'reckless rebel' who is yet vulnerable, with a tendency towards an accompanying mood disorder, and less frequently, personality disorder (Godt, 2002). The person with bulimia nervosa presents in a way far removed from the person with anorexia nervosa, but whilst not likely to markedly lose weight, she is no less in need of support than the person with severe emaciation. Tables 7.3 and 7.4 present the DSM-IV (APA, 1994) diagnostic criteria of bulimia nervosa and the characteristics observed in people suffering from bulimia nervosa.

Table 7.3 Diagnostic criteria for bulimia nervosa (DSM-IV).

(1) Recurrent episodes of binge eating. An episode of binge eating is characterised by both eating, in a discrete period of time (for example in any two-hour period), an amount of food that is definitely larger than most people would eat in a similar period of time (taking into account time since last meal and social context in which eating occurred; and a sense of lack of control over eating during the episodes (for example a feeling that one can't stop or control what or how much one is eating).
(2) Recurrent use of inappropriate compensatory behaviour to avoid weight gain, self-induced vomiting.
(3) A minimum average of two episodes of binge eating and two inappropriate compensatory behaviours a week for at least three months.
(4) Self-evaluation is unduly influenced by body shape and weight.
(5) The disturbance does not occur exclusively during episodes of anorexia nervosa.

Bulimia nervosa is further classified into two types: *purging type* when the sufferer regularly purges after binge eating via self-induced vomiting or the abuse of laxatives; *non-purging* type when the sufferer does not engage in self-induced vomiting or laxative abuse. Some may use compensatory methods of dieting or exercising.

Source: American Psychiatric Association (1994).

Table 7.4 Commonly occurring features observed in people suffering from bulimia nervosa.

Bulimia nervosa
Binge eating large amounts of food
Self-induced vomiting and/or purging
Secretive, devious and deceptive behaviour
Frequent visits to the lavatory after meals to get rid of food eaten
Menstrual disturbances
Sore throat and erosion of dental enamel due to frequent vomiting
Dehydration and poor skin condition
Parotid gland swelling
Russell's sign, the presence of bruises, calluses on the thumb or hand, secondary to trauma from self-induced vomiting
Absent gag reflex
Peripheral oedema, swelling of hands and feet
Healthy appearance
Fatigue, decreased energy and lethargy
Headaches
Abdominal pain, bloating, heartburn and constipation
Feeling out of control, helpless and lonely
Depression and mood swings

Differences between anorexia and bulimia

Apart from the actual medical complications of bulimia nervosa, there are cardinal signs, which can act as distinguishing features of bulimia nervosa, alerting health care professionals and lay people alike. The swollen parotid glands are one telltale abnormality, producing a so-called 'hamster' appearance. 'Russell's sign' involves calluses or abrasions on the knuckles of the hand, caused by using the hand to stimulate the gag reflex. Erosion of dental enamel on the teeth is likely to be present in people with bulimia nervosa who have been vomiting for four years or more (Mitchell, 1995). Though having fewer serious untoward medical complications than those evident in anorexia nervosa, which is somewhat surprising given the extremes of behaviour evident in bulimia nervosa, symptomatology of the organ systems of the body has to be monitored, and may on rare occasions prove to have very serious consequences indeed.

Electrolyte imbalance, characterised by water retention, swelling and abdominal bloating may well be evident. Large amounts of potassium are lost in the urine and due to vomiting, chloride is lost. This can lead to marked weakness and cardiac arrhythmias. Metabolic acidosis also occurs, brought on by the abuse of laxatives. Many people with bulimia nervosa brush their teeth after vomiting but this promotes the loss of enamel. Gastrointestinal complications are associated with problems in swallowing. This raises concern because of repeated assaults on the oesophagus from forced vomiting. Gastric dilation poses the danger of gastric rupture, and may be the most common cause of mortality; several dozen cases have been reported. Rupture of the oesophagus is rare but not unknown. It is thought that pressure changes in the gut are evident, resulting in the patient being unable to vomit. Dehydration and laxative misuse can result in reflex constipation. The rectal walls may on occasion become so weakened that they protrude through the anus and require surgery. Finally, cardiomyopathy and other types of myopathy resulting from the misuse of emetics can occur.

The mortality rate of bulimia nervosa is seven times higher than that of the general population (Nielsen, 2001) (the mortality rate of anorexia nervosa is 20 times the rate of the general population). Nielsen (2001) reports that 3% of bulimia nervosa sufferers die. Simon (2002) reports that the mortality rate of patients with bulimia nervosa undergoing therapy after six years was 1%.

Aetiology of eating disorders

The aetiology of eating disorders remains contentious and controversial. Much remains uncertain and perhaps unknown. There is, however, a high level of agreement on the idea that the causation of eating disorders is multifactorial. Family characteristics such as enmeshment, rigidity, over protectiveness, intense family atmosphere, lack of privacy within the family, lack of conflict resolution and involvement of the anorectic child in unresolved family conflicts have been seen as possible contributory factors (Minuchin *et al.*, 1978). Other family related stress factors include a family move to new neighbourhood, a period of time the child spent away from home, family history of eating problems and disorders, unusual familial interest in food, weight and shape, and parents working in the food or fashion industry.

Kay (1999) suggested that anorexia nervosa and bulimia nervosa might be seen as familial disorders with biological correlates. He highlighted family and genetic influences. For example, family studies showing 7–10 times higher prevalence rates of eating disorders amongst relatives of people with eating disorders when compared with controls, and higher concordance levels amongst monozygotic relative to dizygotic twins. Palmer (1995) put forward a 'general hypothesis' that postulates that premature, unwanted and coercive sexual experience in early life may lead to impaired personal development, problems with self-esteem and relationships, which in turn may contribute to the causation of any adult psychological disorder. The proposition that childhood sexual abuse has a greater link with eating disorders was called by Palmer the 'specific hypothesis'. Vandereycken & Hartley (1996) subscribe to the idea that various socio-cultural factors contribute to the causation of eating disorders. This view is supported by Palmer (2000), who suggests that eating disorders have some relationship to culture, but this remains controversial.

Included under this rather large umbrella are factors such as culture, race, class, media, ethnicity, religion, gender, housing and education. The idea that anorexia nervosa, for example, is seen as an illness of Westernised cultures remains fairly popular but it has been challenged in more recent times. According to McCourt & Waller (1996), eating disorders and disturbed eating attitudes have been found in a wide variety of cultures; these may be linked to acculturation to 'Western' ideals, but eating disorders amongst young Asian women living in the UK may be the product of culture clash rather than acculturation.

Contextualising eating disorders with dual diagnosis

This extreme form of bulimia nervosa is closely associated with co-morbidity. It must be emphasised that this group of sufferers is at the extreme end of the continuum of bulimia nervosa, representing no more than 10% of the total of people with bulimia nervosa. Activities such as self-harm, substance misuse, even offending and sexual promiscuity are statistically associated with each other and are far from being random activities. In Lacey's (1992) sample 40% of sufferers exhibited co-morbidity, and 8 to 10% had a severe personality disorder.

The relationships of women with multi-impulsive bulimia nervosa are interesting. In a study of the sexual partners of women with normal weight bulimia nervosa (Lacey, 1992), out of a sample of 112 patients, 73 (65%) reported having a sexual partner at first assessment, with only nineteen married and living with their husbands. Such relationships tended to be abusive or with a 'safe' man; the latter category is defined as a meaningless relationship, the patients saw no future in it and were not in love. Patients are more likely to have an alcohol misusing partner. Indeed, it is common for partners to drink alcohol to excess. Forty percent of partners reported drinking over 36 units of alcohol per week, with marked depressive features as part of the picture, as are a tendency to have weight problems, be overweight or, in a few instances, have a history of clinical obesity. Finally, women with multi-impulsive bulimia nervosa are likely to report having been sexually abused. Lack of control and impulsivity in bulimia nervosa are closely associated with personality disorder. Hostility and impulsive anger are both aspects of borderline personality disorder (BPD). Patients with such characteristics are likely to be associated with multi-impulsive personality disorder. Another aspect of co-morbidity in regard to bulimia nervosa is personality disorder. Prevalence rates of personality disorder in samples of people with bulimia nervosa range from 21 to 77% (Wonderlich, 1995).

Suicidal thoughts and suicide itself are associated with anorexia nervosa, bulimia nervosa and depression. Cooper (1995) indicates that about half of people with eating disorders have a lifetime history of affective disorders. The tendency is towards bulimia nervosa and, less often, the purging subtype of anorexia nervosa. Studies have shown that 8 to 33% of people with bulimia nervosa also have obsessive compulsive disorder. Cooper (1995) argues, however, that there could be a closer link between obsessive compulsive disorder and depression than with eating disorders.

Eating disorders and substance misuse

Certain commonalities are evident in the way people experience both eating disorders and substance misuse. In binge eating, for example, there is a commonly held notion of urges or 'cravings' to consume food. The notion of craving is consistent with the World Health Organization's (1969) definition of drug dependence as including 'a compulsion to take the drug on a continuous or periodic basis in order to experience its physical effects'. As Rassool (2002) comments, there is a consensus over this definition, and it has been widely adopted. Loss of control is another common feature. Denial and secrecy are again features found in both disorders. In eating disorders, for example, binge eating is viewed as an addiction. It is notable, for example, that Overeaters Anonymous has a 12-step approach adapted from Alcoholics Anonymous. In this paradigm, treatment is associated with total abstinence.

However, there are difficulties in viewing eating disorders as analogous with substance misuse. Wilson (1995) argues that the physical dependence, withdrawal, craving and loss of control found in addictive disorders are not characteristic of binge eating. Moreover, there is no evidence of craving in bulimia nervosa from any kind of chemical disturbance. In a study conducted by Turner *et al.* (1991) bulimia nervosa patients and controls consumed a 500 ml drink of 1200 kcal or an inactive placebo mixture. Results showed little carbohydrate specific response in either group. Findings did not concur with the idea that binge eating is mediated by carbohydrate craving. In fact, the ratings for 'good mood' were lower in the patients following carbohydrate consumption. The loss of control thesis in eating disorders doesn't fit as comfortably with the principle of craving for a given substance as it does in regards to substance misuse. Thus the notion of 'one drink away from a drunk' has little credence in relation to eating disorders. The equivalent in bulimia nervosa, for example 'one bite away from a binge', whilst premised on the notion of loss of control akin to its counterpart in substance misuse, has little meaning in that the craving for a specific food is not evident. People with bulimia nervosa differ in another way from those with substance misuse in that the focus in bulimia nervosa is on the amount eaten, not the actual constituents of the food. There is very little evidence that bulimia nervosa involves bingeing on a high sugar/high fat food.

Higher co-morbidity exists in relation to eating disorders and substance misuse than can be expected in the general population. Evidence suggests that patients with anorexia nervosa and bulimia nervosa have significantly higher rates of past and present substance misuse than is observed generally (Wilson, 1995). One study by Higuchi *et al.* (1993), involving over 2000 female twins, showed a significant lifetime association between bulimia nervosa and alcoholism. In bulimia nervosa, substance misuse is best viewed as a coping mechanism, in other words the self-medication hypothesis of dual diagnosis theory (Rassool, 2002).

Approaches to the care and treatment of people with eating disorders

Evolution and change in emphasis over time has influenced not only how eating disorders are perceived and explained but also the general approach to care and treatment. Whereas previously care and treatment were imposed upon the patient, there is now a greater emphasis on engaging the client and persuading them to seek and accept the help on offer. The severe weight loss in anorexia nervosa demands that the sufferer is offered the help they need even if this is sometimes delivered against their will. Forcing anorexia nervosa sufferers to receive help under section of the Mental Health Act remains highly politically incorrect, so much so that some in-patient treatment centres often sweep this under the carpet, and declaim that such strategies are against their professional practice.

Commonly used approaches to treatment of people with eating disorders utilise psychodynamic psychotherapy, cognitive behavioural therapy, family therapy, motivational interviewing and interpersonal psychotherapy. The whole spectrum of professional workers is engaged in working with this client group with medical and nursing staff, nutritionists, clinical psychologists and family therapists making a major contribution. Self-help groups and other voluntary services continue to make an important contribution. In a typical voluntary sector setting, it is likely that the main focus is on feelings rather than food. For example, the person with bulimia nervosa, rather than being educated on accepted weight management principles, is at one such centre likely to be offered anything from aromatherapy, through to reflexology and shiatsu massage, and not all these interventions are commonly found in the more traditional settings. The Eating Disorders Association is a charitable trust that, within its remit, has focused on the promotion of self-help interventions with the use of accompanying manuals. Self-help programmes are to be found in the leading specialist centres in the NHS (Treasure *et al.*, 1996; Treasure, 1997). Sequential treatment for bulimia nervosa incorporating a self-care manual is but one example of self-help services available in the statutory sector.

Nursing care of people with eating disorders

The care of people with eating disorders is increasingly a multidisciplinary undertaking. However, whilst due recognition must be given to the respective roles of all members of the eating disorders team, this is not the remit of this section. Such a focus has already been provided in existing literature such as Hindmarch (2000). There has, to date, been little in the way of published work on the nurse's role in service delivery, be that in specialist or non-specialist settings. This issue relates to shortcomings in the treatment of people with eating disorders in acute mental health care, leading the National Institute for Clinical Excellence to issue for consultation its draft guidelines on clinical practice on eating disorders (NICE, 2003). Nurses, as key players in the delivery of care, are clearly implicated and will be found in the front line in further development of services. The nurse's role as coordinator of the multidisciplinary team cannot be underestimated.

The therapeutic relationship is considered to be the cornerstone of the care of people with eating disorders and mental health nursing in general. It is applicable at any stage in the stepped care model in eating disorders services (Robinson, 1998), ranging from community care at one end of the spectrum to in-patient acute mental health and specialist unit care at the other extreme. The in-patient setting represents the traditional model of the nurse, who is a key figure in both engagement with the client and as the strict supervisor in re-feeding, and this context forms the focus of the overview of nursing approaches. Halek (1997) highlights the prerequisites for effective nursing interventions. The key position of nurses, particularly in re-feeding, brings such prerequisites into sharp focus.

First of all, consistency is essential. All team members must work within the same rules and practice strict adherence to such principles, not least because some clients may be adept at exploiting divisions within the team and create a 'splitting' effect. Reliability is also an important component in the care of people with bulimia nervosa. These clients are educated to establish more structure and order in their lives, and if an arrangement or appointment is not kept with the client, all attempts to establish trust may be lost. Reliability is therefore essential if such clients are to be helped to share their inner turmoil, something that they normally shroud in secrecy.

The issue of boundaries may also be a central tenet in the nursing approach to people with eating disorders. Nurses may be engaged in their very own adolescent struggles, or through the weight restoration process may have come to closely identify with the client. Such an instance underscores the need for regular clinical supervision, due to the fact that if boundaries are transgressed, the entire concept of consistency may be thrown into disarray. Nurses must develop self-awareness, such that they are constantly on the alert to any potential undermining of team solidarity. The fact that the nursing approach is a team activity only serves to highlight the need for careful management of boundaries (Halek, 1997).

Halek (1997) also makes reference to managing anxiety. Decisions ought not to be made in a climate of crisis management. Due to the severe emaciation of people with severe anorexia nervosa and, moreover, its high mortality rate, it is perhaps understandable that management of such a client may be underwritten by panic. Such a reaction in the nursing team, in particular, is compounded by the fact that, as experienced nurses in this specialism often report, it is the nursing team that is often held responsible for the client's lack of weight gain in the re-feeding programme. This view, which is a corollary of the nurse's proximity to the client, must be challenged within the multidisciplinary milieu. Such responsibility must be diffused across the whole spectrum of care and not be centred solely on nurses.

Authenticity is another important aspect of the nurse's role. Openness and genuineness are an essential part of the equation, notably in relationships with nurse managers and supervisors. Safety is paramount. Above all, the nurse should be reflexive and open to self-exploration. An example of this is in terms of the strict regime imposed in the re-feeding programme for anorexia nervosa, in which the client defies logic, appearing fully committed to a state of self-starvation. Feelings and thoughts are likely to come into sharp focus, and it might appear to the inexperienced practitioner that the approach is tantamount to bullying. The re-feeding process is necessary because it can literally save lives, not overlooking the fact that for many nurses it is an unpleasant intervention. What might seem an affront on basic human rights comes to be seen as a necessary therapeutic endeavour. It presents the greatest challenge in the care of people with eating disorders, due to the fact that it manifests, to all intents and purposes, as coercion.

However, as Davidson (2000) documents, the fulcrum of re-feeding is meal supervision, which cannot fail to arouse strong emotions in nurses who, as is their duty, must seek to ensure that the client eats the meal, even though this may take an interminable time. In this kind of scenario, it is to be expected that the nurse will sometimes be drawn to question the meaning of it all and, essentially, to be open to feelings. Being truthful to the client, according to Halek (1997), is important, yet this doesn't mean sharing every element of one's doubts and criticisms regarding the approach. Understanding clients is irrevocably linked with how one is responding to a client, and in turn how the nurse appears to people in their care.

It cannot be emphasised enough that communication skills are at the heart of the nursing approach, not just in terms of the parenting style interaction at the initial stages of weight restoration in severe anorexia nervosa. It is hoped that there will be a shift towards more mutuality in the therapeutic alliance in which nurse and client function as partners in the care process. What is notable is that no sufferer of an eating disorder has retrospectively complained of being coerced into eating. Rather, on recovery there is often, conversely, an appreciation of the support given through such a very difficult time. To date, no client has appealed against coercive treatment under the terms of the Human Rights Act 1999. This is significant in itself.

Listening is important. Ideally, the nurse should be attentive to the person communicating inner thoughts and feelings, and needs to be sufficiently skilled to understand that the exchange between them is but a rare opportunity for a meaningful therapeutic intervention. There may not be many opportunities for such reciprocal verbal exchange until the road to recovery is reached. Eating disorders can often be found in people who do not reveal feelings or who actively avoid doing so. The nurse has a pivotal role in helping clients verbalise their thoughts and emotions.

One forum for communication is therapeutic group work, albeit in terms of the nurse acting as facilitator. The idea is that effective management of people with eating disorders can be achieved by fostering group dynamics and enabling members to apply group pressure as a therapeutic medium. Davidson (2000) is very critical of this process, arguing that the purpose of it is kept very vague, yet there is much to be said for a therapeutic group providing solace for an individual with bulimia nervosa, for example highlighting to them that they are not alone in their suffering.

Another important skill in nursing and management of people with both anorexia nervosa and bulimia nervosa is the capacity to deal with silence. It is a good idea to put open questions to the person who is very reticent in sharing anything. If the client takes a long time to answer questions, one strategy is to ask why (Prestwood, 2001). A little window of insight into the world of eating disorders may be provided if the person reports having to work out the nurse's response, in addition to having to prepare a further answer to that response. Such 'second-guessing' can be seen as indicative of a desperate search for control over one's situation, to such an extent that it has progressed to the severely debilitating state of anorexia nervosa. Tables 7.5 and 7.6 present the key elements of helping people suffering from anorexia nervosa and bulimia nervosa.

Preventative aspects

Increasingly, there is concern about the effects of widespread dieting, particularly amongst schoolgirls. Currently, the huge popularity of the 'Doctor Atkins' diet has served to compound such worries, but it has been reported that almost half of 14-year-old schoolgirls may be dieting at any one time. Success in young women has come to be associated with slimness, such that their self-esteem may be irrevocably linked not solely with educational or occupational achievement, but with a quest for the perfect body. Such striving for self-control may be bought at a high price. Whilst dieting does not directly cause eating disorders, there is a connection, and measures have to be taken to educate a target population most predisposed to developing eating disorders.

The current authors established a programme of prevention in local secondary schools in 2000. This involved conducting a survey in all secondary schools in the local catchment area (Abuel-Ealeh *et al.*, 2001). Forty per cent of the total number of secondary schools surveyed agreed to a one-hour presentation being delivered by the project team, which included eating disorder practitioners drawn from the local range of mental health services. A teacher in each school agreed to act as the liaison person. Some members of the prevention team had undertaken the Care and Understanding of People with Eating Disorders programme run by the current authors at Anglia Ruskin University. The groups were made up of both boys and girls wherever possible and utilised a comprehensive prevention of eating disorders educational package, which included a video featuring young people

Table 7.5 Key elements of helping people suffering from anorexia nervosa.

(1) The safety of sufferers is of prime importance. They should be kept in the best possible physical condition, challenging though this is.

(2) Despite the strong resistance to food, which is likely to be present, all attempts need to be made in order to meet minimum nutritional needs and to maintain electrolyte balance. The intention in the longer term is weight restoration and establishing healthy eating habits.

(3) If care is being provided in in-patient settings, then it may be necessary to provide one-to-one support and supervision during and after meals. This is one of the hardest tasks a nurse may have to undertake since the sufferer will see it as impinging on their privacy as well as on any attempt at establishing a therapeutic nurse–patient relationship.

(4) Weight monitoring is often a necessary part of any given programme of care of people with anorexia nervosa. If the client is in an in-patient unit, weighing may take place up to twice a week. This would normally be carried out on the same day, at the same time, using the same clothes. In such situations, the nurse needs to ensure that clients are not using tactics such as drinking large amounts of water before weighing or loading up their pockets with objects that will increase the reading of the scales.

(5) Depression is common among sufferers of anorexia nervosa so it is essential to judiciously monitor the potential for suicide and to provide repeated assurance and support as appropriate.

(6) Encouraging clients to explore and talk about their feelings may be helpful. The focus should be on exploring healthier behaviours and more effective strategies in coping with anxiety.

(7) A good degree of understanding of key psychotherapeutic approaches to care and treatment, for example cognitive behaviour therapy, may be helpful in enabling the nurse to work with sufferers and to explain some of the cognitive processes associated with anorexia nervosa, such as overgeneralisation. Proficiency in the principles of problem solving may be helpful in enabling sufferers to prioritise their problems in order to tackle these gradually.

(8) Education of both the sufferer and their family is essential. The focus may be in enabling them to understand the nature of anorexia nervosa, to provide different explanations and ways of helping.

Table 7.6 Key elements of helping people suffering from bulimia nervosa.

(1) In rare instances, in-patient care may be necessary. In the event of medical complications such as ruptured oesophagus, collapsed rectum or serious electrolyte imbalance, medical care will be indicated.

(2) Co-morbidity is often evident in bulimia nervosa, with associated substance misuse or mood disorder; if this is accompanied by severe suicidal ideation or the person is actively suicidal, in-patient care will be required.

(3) A therapeutic alliance is essential, in which the nurse can demonstrate an understanding of the distress encountered in bulimia nervosa. Only by gaining the person's trust will the nurse be in a position to promote the expression of inner feelings without shame and by so doing help the person seek treatment and, ultimately, a full recovery.

(4) In light of the fact that dietary restraint underpins binge eating, it is important to help the person with bulimia nervosa to understand that resisting the commitment to dieting will in turn help eliminate bingeing. Equally, education on the adverse effects of binge eating, self-induced vomiting and the abuse of diuretics and laxatives is necessary.

(5) Guidance in modifying distorted thinking is important. Explain the cognitive view of the development of bulimia nervosa, so as to outline how concerns about body shape and weight link with low self-esteem and in turn inappropriate behaviour. Intervention is aimed at helping to break the binge-purge cycle.

(6) Establish a structured and systematic approach to meals. An ordered regime is important in that it introduces an element of stability to the person with bulimia nervosa, thereby challenging the disrupted eating patterns that are characteristic of this disorder.

(7) The teaching of self-help strategies is an important component of this approach, in that it helps the person not only identify the negative thoughts, emotions and interpersonal stressors encountered in bulimia nervosa, but primarily promotes the adoption of a problem solving approach with consequent regulation of one's own behaviour and higher self-esteem.

(8) Encourage clients to record distorted thought and emotions accompanying incidents of binge eating and purging. This will help them learn to identify triggers of the binge-purge cycle, with a view to alleviating the emotional instability in the disorder.

who had recovered from eating disorders. The prevention package itself, along with educational leaflets, was left with the liaison teacher and every effort was made to maintain contact and provide support. It was emphasised, however, prior to the presentation and afterwards that the project team were to provide education but not therapeutic interventions or counselling. On evaluation, schools reported that no prevalence of eating disorders was apparent but everybody, pupils and staff alike, were more informed about the detection of eating disorders, the features of eating disorders and ways to get help if required.

Conclusion

The above initiative was taken in the absence of any conclusive evidence that prevention programmes are effective. Successive authors have commented on prevention of eating disorders programmes in general or have evaluated specific initiatives (Fairburn, 1995; Vandereycken & Noordenbos, 1998). The central tenet of scepticism regarding prevention of eating disorders in young people is the marked difficulty in identifying at-risk individuals. Moreover, no evidence base exists to demonstrate the efficacy of such prevention initiatives, any more than anti-smoking campaigns, which tend to be on a much larger scale and have swallowed up vast amounts of funding. The current authors contend that, even in the absence of clear evidence that prevention actually has any effect in reducing prevalence in general, or succeeds in stopping the relentless progression of an eating disorder in just one individual, it is not an option to give up and not try to tackle this devastating problem. If nothing else, the greater understanding and awareness of eating disorders, developed in the population as a whole, will have made the undertaking worthwhile.

References

Abuel-Ealeh, M., Ashbey, R. & Barrett, R. (2001) Survey of students from an eating disorders programme, *Nursing Standard*, 15 (47), 3–39.

American Psychiatric Association (1994) *Diagnostic and Statistical Manual of Mental Disorders*, 4th edn (DSM-IV). APA, Washington, DC.

Bruch, H. (1978) *The Golden Cage: The Enigma of Anorexia Nervosa*, Vintage, New York.

Cooper, P.J. (1995) Eating disorders and their relationship to mood and anxiety disorders. In: *Eating Disorders and Obesity. A Comprehensive Handbook* (Brownell, K.D. & Fairburn, C.G., eds), pp. 159–64. Guilford Press, New York.

Crisp, A. (1992) Anorexia Nervosa: Diagnostic issues; physical complications; prevalence, models of psychopathology. Conference proceedings, Eating disorders and their treatment – anorexia nervosa and bulimia nervosa, a two-day multidisciplinary conference (25 and 26 November 1992). St. George's Hospital Medical School, London.

Davidson, B. (2000) Psychiatric nursing: The no-man's land between patient and therapist. In: *Eating disorders. The Multiprofessional Approach* (Hindmarch, D., ed.) Whurr, London.

Evans, P.C. (2003) 'If only I were thin like her, maybe I could be happy like her'. The self-implications of associating a thin female ideal with life success. *Psychology of Women Quarterly*, 27 (3), 209–14.

Fairburn, C.G. (1995) The Prevention of Eating Disorders. In: *Eating Disorders and Obesity. A Comprehensive Handbook* (Brownell, K.D. & Fairburn, C.G., eds), pp. 289–93. Guilford Press, New York.

Fairburn, C.G., Cooper, Z., Doll, H. & Welch, S. (1999) Risk factors for anorexia nervosa: three integrated case-control comparisons. *Archives of General Psychiatry*, 56, 468–76.

Godt, K. (2002) Personality disorders and eating disorders: the prevalence of personality disorders in 176 female outpatients with eating disorders. *European Eating Disorders Review*, 10, 103–9.

Gordon, R.A. (1999) *Eating Disorders: Anatomy of a Social Epidemic*. Blackwell, London.

Halek, C. (1997) Eating disorders. The role of the nurse. *Nursing Times*, 93 (28), 9–15 July, 63–6.

Higuchi, S., Suzuki, K., Yamada, K., Parish, K. & Kono, H. (1993) Alcoholics with eating disorders: prevalence and clinical course. *British Journal of Psychiatry*, 162, 403–6.

Hindmarch, D. (ed.) (2000) *Eating Disorders. A Multiprofessional Approach*. Whurr, London.

Kay, W.H. (1999) The new biology of anorexia and bulimia nervosa: implications for advances in treatment. *European Eating Disorders Review*, 7, 157–61.

Lacey, J.H. (1992) Homogamy: the relationships and sexual partners of normal-weight bulimic women. *British Journal of Psychiatry*, 161, 638–42.

Lacey, J.H. & Evans, C. (1986) The impulsivist: a multi-impulsive personality disorder. *British Journal of Addiction*, 81, 715–23.

Lewis, V.J. & Blair, A. (1991) In: *Psychology and Social Issues: a Tutorial Text* (Cochrane, R. & Caroll, D., eds). The Falmer Press, London.

McCourt, J. & Waller, G. (1996) The influence of sociocultural factors on the eating psychopathology of young Asian women in British society. *European Eating Disorders Review*, 4 (2), 73–83.

Minuchin, S., Rosman, B.L. & Baker, L. (1978) *Psychosomatic Families: Anorexia Nervosa in Context*. Harvard University Press, Cambridge, Mass.

Mitchell, J.C. (1995) Medical Complications of Bulimia Nervosa. In: *Eating Disorders and Obesity. A Comprehensive Handbook* (Brownell, K.D. & Fairburn, C.G., eds). Guilford Press, New York.

National Institute for Clinical Excellence (2003) The National Institute for Clinical Excellence issues for consultation its guidelines on clinical practice on eating disorders.
http://www.NICE%20EDs files\ NICE%20EDs.htm

Nielsen, S. (2001) Epidemiology and mortality of eating disorders. *Psychiatric Clinics of North America*, 24 (2), 201–14.

Palmer, R. (1995) Childhood sexual abuse and eating disorders. The proceedings of the third St. George's Hospital eating disorders conference – engaging the patient (6–7 March 1995).

Palmer, R. (2000) *Helping People with Eating Disorders. A Clinical Guide to Assessment and Treatment*. J. Wiley & Sons, Chichester.

Prestwood, C. (2001) The role and function of the psychiatric nurse in the treatment of eating disorders. Personal Communication.

Rassool, G. Hussein (2002) Substance use and dual diagnosis: concepts, theories and models. In: *Dual Diagnosis: Substance Misuse and Psychiatric Disorders* (Rassool, G.H., ed.). Blackwell Publishing, Oxford.

Robinson, P.H. (1998) Community treatment of eating disorders. Paper presented at the winter meeting of the Royal College of Psychiatrists, London, 20–23 January.

Russell, G.F.M. (1979) Bulimia nervosa. An ominous variant of anorexia nervosa. *Psychological Medicine*, 9, 429–48.

Russell, G. (1995) Anorexia nervosa through time, In: *Handbook of Eating Disorders – Theory, Treatment and Research* (Szmukler, G., Dare, C. & Treasure, J., eds). Wiley, Chichester.

Simon, H. (2002) *How Serious is Bulimia Nervosa Without Serious Weight Loss (Anorexia)?*
http://www.ucdmc.ucdavis.edu

Treasure, J.L. (1997) *Anorexia Nervosa: a Survival Guide for Sufferers and Those Caring for Someone with an Eating Disorder*. Psychology Press, Hove.

Treasure, J.L., Schmidt, U.H., Troop, N.A., Tiller, J.M., Todd, G. & Turnbull, S. (1996) A randomised controlled trial of sequential treatment for bulimia nervosa incorporating a self-care manual. *British Journal of Psychiatry*, 168, 94–8.

Turner, M. St J., Foggo, M., Bennie, J., Carroll, S., Dick, H. & Goodwin, G.M. (1991) Psychological, hormonal and biochemical changes following carbohydrate bingeing: a placebo controlled study in bulimia nervosa and matched controls. *Psychological Medicine*, 21, 123–33.

Vandereycken, W. & Hartley, P. (1996) Socio-cultural aspects of eating disorders. Editorial in *European Eating Disorders Review*, 4 (2), 71–2.

Vandereycken, W. & Noordenbos, G. (1998) *The Prevention of Eating Disorders*. Athlone Press, London.

Wallcraft, J. (1997) *Healing Minds*. Mental Health Foundation, London.

Wilson, G.T. (1995) Eating Disorders and Addictive Disorders. In: *Eating Disorders and Obesity. A Comprehensive Handbook* (Brownell, K.D. & Fairburn, C.G., eds). Guilford Press, New York.

Wonderlich, S.A. (1995) Personality Disorders and Eating Disorders. In: *Eating Disorders and Obesity. A Comprehensive Handbook* (Brownell, K.D. & Fairburn, C.G., eds). Guilford, New York.

World Health Organization (1969) *Sixteenth report of WHO Expert Committee on Drug Dependence. Technical Report Series, 407*. WHO, Geneva.

Yellowlees, A. (2000) *Working with Eating Disorders* (Health Awareness). Heinemann Educational, Oxford.

8 Problem Drug Use and Personality Disorders

P. Phillips

Personality disorders

The aetiology, diagnosis, treatment and legal status of personality disorders are currently attracting the interest of mental health professionals and law makers in a significant way (Welch, 2002; National Institute for Mental Health in England, 2003). This interest, and the subsequent clinical research activity being undertaken, was substantially aided by the introduction in the DSM-IV of a special axis (axis II) for the classification of personality disorders. Millon (1981) comments that: 'the long drought is over and a revival of the rich heritage of the forties and fifties is underway'. Despite this, personality disorder diagnoses and labels are routinely used in a pejorative way in British mental health practice. It is commonly accepted that personality disorders and drug use are often associated with each other in clinical practice and theory (Daley *et al.*, 1993) and this supposed relationship is summarised by Nace *et al.* (1990) who suggest: 'the pharmacological effects of alcohol and drugs induce personality regression with a weakening of ego function'. Personality disorders are marked by a wide range of reported features including difficulty recognising and dealing with painful emotional states and regulating behaviour, impaired personal relationships, poor frustration tolerance, need for immediate gratification, poor response to stress and poor interpersonal skills.

The relationship between personality disorder and illicit drug use

However, the relationship between personality disorder and problematic drug use is frequently very complex and thought by many commentators to be not fully understood. The clinical characteristics and criteria for a diagnosis of personality disorder are thought to be commonly found in drug users (Dackis & Gold, 1992). The validity of this argument, however, needs to be examined in light of the largely behavioural criteria established for the diagnosis of personality disorder, which can be seen to assign pathological personality labels to individuals who are experiencing temporary episodes of mental health/personality difficulties, rather than to those who have experienced these symptoms in a pattern that might suggest more than a transient association. Blume (1989) demonstrates this argument well in a US study of two hundred opiate 'addicts' diagnosed with antisocial personality disorder, finding that at two-year follow-up over half of the subjects no longer met the criteria for the diagnosis. Further to this Sievewright & Daly (1997) suggest that the validity of personality disorder diagnoses may be unreliable in people with problematic drug use, in that criminal activities (a common diagnostic criterion for personality disorders) may be entirely related to behaviours secondary to problematic drug use (that is acquisitive crime that funds continued drug use and prevents withdrawal features).

The Epidemiological Catchment Area Survey (ECAS) (Regier *et al.*, 1990), which formed part of the US National Institute of Mental Health epidemiological catchment area programme, found a 'severe substance misuse' rate of 83.6% in persons diagnosed with antisocial personality disorder. Regier *et al.* (1990) suggest that finding this statistically significant association between the two disorders (personality disorder and 'substance misuse') constitutes evidence that one disorder may have an aetiological role in the other, and that an underlying biological vulnerability to these disorders exists in affected individuals. This 'vulnerability' hypothesis has gained support elsewhere. Campbell *et al.* (1993) suggest that the presence of a personality disorder increases vulnerability to problem drug/alcohol use and complicates the pattern of drug using behaviour.

Other commentators indicate that the method of assessment of both drug use and personality is highly correlated to reported prevalence rates of problem drug use amongst those with personality disorders. This is particularly pertinent where the Millon clinical multi-axial inventory (Millon, 1983) was used to diagnose personality disorder, as opposed to clinical interview based instruments such as the personality disorders examination (Loranger, 1988). A comprehensive Dutch study, conducted in Amsterdam (DeJong *et al.*, 1993), examined the prevalence of personality disorders in hospitalised alcohol patients and 'polydrug addicts'. This study found high rates of personality disorder, along with a study by Craig (1987). In this survey 263 subjects were recruited to the study (178 alcohol patients and 86 'drug addicts'), who entered the same therapeutic community concurrently. Diagnoses were assigned according to the DSM-III-R, and subjects were assessed for personality pathology using the structured interview for DSM-III personality disorders. The alcohol patients were found to have a personality disorder rate of 78%, the average number of disorders per patient being 1.8. The most common disorder types in this group were histrionic (34%), dependent (29%), avoidant (19%), compulsive (19%) and borderline (17%). The 'polydrug addicts', however, had a prevalence rate of 91%, the average number of personality disorders being 4.0 per patient. The most common disorder types in this group being borderline (65%), histrionic (64%), passive-aggressive (49%), antisocial (48%) and dependent (35%). In comparing the results of the groups in this study DeJong *et al.* (1993) found a significantly higher prevalence of certain personality disorders in the 'polydrug addicts' group. These groups were the paranoid, schizotype, histrionic, antisocial, borderline and passive aggressive disorders.

Perhaps the personality disorder most commonly associated with drug use is antisocial personality disorder. The DeJong study (DeJong *et al.*, 1993) found a prevalence of only 5% for this group in the above sample. This is known to be significantly lower than found in other studies. However, DeJong explains this by suggesting that the age of onset of drug use was proportionately higher, with a subsequent shorter 'addiction' history, thereby leading to lower rates of antisocial 'behaviour'. A further variable factor to be taken into account when examining the DeJong study is the judicial and involuntary placement of many of the subjects in the 'polydrug addicts' sample group. The findings of this study lead DeJong *et al.* (1993) to critically question the validity and clinical usefulness of classifying 'drug addiction' separately from personality disorder. This was the case in earlier versions of the American DSM, for instance in DSM-I. 'Alcoholism' and 'drug addiction' were classified as personality disorders and regarded by the psychiatric establishment to be sub-types of sociopathic personality disturbance.

However, with this in mind, because much (but not all) illicit drug use is by its nature illegal, an assumption that using the drug in the first place constitutes antisocial or sociopathic behaviour is made, thereby legitimising the relationship between drug use and personality disorder.

Shared characteristics: substance misuse and personality disorders

It is suggested that there are a number of shared characteristics between substance misuse and personality disorder. These are lowered self-esteem, self-confidence, self-satisfaction, social confidence, assertiveness, personal control and self-efficacy. Dusenbury & Botvin (1992) also add external locus of control to this list of shared personality characteristics, whilst generalising that drug users 'tend' to have a number of shared negative patterns of behaviour in common with people with personality disorder. These are higher anxiety levels, impulsivity, rebelliousness and need for approval. Dusenbury & Botvin (1992) suggest that these groups are more pessimistic, and are more alienated from 'appropriate' cultural and social values. Campbell *et al.* (1993) also suggest that persons with the combination of problem drug use and personality disorder are often self-centred, vulnerable to psychosis, are unable to endure periods of low mood and have extreme difficulty with the sense of self-identity.

These findings are echoed by DeJong *et al.* (1993) who suggest that once an opioid dependence is established the user's life is largely concerned with the procurement and use of the drug, which is characterised by marked behavioural patterns. This pattern, described by Noorlander (1985), is referred to as 'junkie syndrome', and includes lying, criminal acts, manipulation, lack of responsibility, egocentricity, feelings of superiority, exaggeration in the expression of emotions, lack of real emotionality, and rapid shifting of emotional states. DeJong *et al.* (1993) go further to suggest that these behavioural patterns are so similar to those of personality disorders that it is impossible to separate them from pre-existing personality disorders. This argument, however, does not consider the notion that the criminal status of much drug use is central to the behaviours described above, and reinforces the stereotypes concerning drug users and the commonality with the diagnostic criteria and professional attitudes towards personality disorders. Lindesmith (1940) describes these stereotypes in his paper 'Dope fiend mythology': the drug addict as a violent criminal, the drug addict as a moral degenerate and the drug addict as emotionally inferior.

The personality disorders most commonly associated with drug use are antisocial (psychopathic) and borderline (Nace *et al.*, 1983; Koenigsberg *et al.*, 1985). However, here the diagnostic criteria can contradict itself: the *Diagnostic and Statistical Manual* (version IV) states that the features of a personality disorder must have been present for a considerable length of time, having commenced in childhood, or early adulthood, but then goes on to list 'substance misuse' as a diagnostic criterion in borderline personality disorder, and discusses its relevance to antisocial personality disorder. Robins & Przybeck (1985) go further in suggesting that 'substance misuse' in adolescents under the age of 15 positively contributes to the development of psychopathology, specifically including personality disorder. These views often seem to represent the current psychiatric thinking about the relationship between personality and drug use, as illustrated in this case study.

Case study

Helen is a 27-year-old woman, currently maintained on an injectable script of methadone. She has been in treatment with the drug dependence unit for 18 months, during which time she has had numerous psychiatric and medical admissions. Helen's history is lengthy since she started to use drugs and alcohol 12 years ago. During this time Helen suffered ongoing sexual assault by an older family member, and an older stranger to the family. Helen presented to the mental health services on a number of occasions during her childhood with symptoms of depression, eating disorder and self-harm. She has been resident in children's homes for much of her early adulthood. Helen's presence in the drug unit causes tremendous staff anxiety, as there have often been difficulties in the management of Helen's behaviour in the past. Helen's ability to establish and maintain interpersonal relationships has been severely damaged by her early experiences of sexual abuse, and she regularly engages in self-harming behaviour, including cutting, overdosing and jumping from buildings.

Helen entered treatment using heroin, methadone, cocaine, amphetamines and benzodiazepines, mostly by injection, and alcohol. During the period of her treatment Helen has made significant progress in the way in which she uses drugs; she now uses her script of injectable methadone, which she has reduced by one third in the past year, and 'treats' herself to other drugs (cocaine, amphetamines and benzodiazepines) when she can afford to do so, usually on a weekly basis. Helen's psychiatric diagnosis is that of borderline personality disorder, and consequently her relationship with the local mental health services is somewhat difficult.

Helen regularly sees the mental health worker attached to the drug unit, who works with Helen around the management of both her drug use and her mental health problems. This relationship has been established using trust, respect and advocacy as main principles. Through the relationship Helen is able to separate out what she uses to self-medicate her symptoms of emotional distress and what she enjoys using. This understanding is a key to enabling Helen to develop more adaptive ways of coping, whilst accepting that drug use may not be the most harmful behaviour Helen may engage in during times of crisis. This management strategy is fiercely disapproved of by mental health services.

Helen is now denied any access to mental health services in her locality, as each time she has been in hospital she has not been able to continue her prescription of injectable methadone, and her access to in-patient facilities has been stopped completely after rumours that she was supplying other patients on the ward with illicit drugs. The local psychiatrist states that as the patient is not ready to consider abstinence there is nothing mental health services can do to help her. Helen continues to experience mini-psychotic episodes in the community periodically, but continues to do well.

Implications for practice

There are many implications for practice raised by the case study. A key notion in addressing them is accepting personality disorder and problematic drug use as a dual diagnosis, in attempting to understand the relationship between the drug use and the mental health problems experienced by the client. This is of paramount importance in mental health settings, as accepted British medical definitions of dual diagnosis often exclude those with non-psychotic mental health problems, thereby missing valuable opportunities presented by clients to address their drug use and its relationship to their current difficulties. This is seen in much of the prominent US literature regarding the differences in treating the 'mentally ill chemical abusers and addicted' (MICAAs) as opposed to the 'chemically abusing mentally ill' (CAMIs).

Sciacca (1990) suggests that integrated treatment models developed in the USA (Minkoff, 1989) are inappropriate for those who are not *primarily mentally ill* because of the 'manipulative aspects of their coexisting character pathology'. This presents many difficulties in attempting to define and provide appropriate care and treatment for those with a dual diagnosis of personality disorder and problematic drug use for a number of reasons (Phillips, 1998):

- It promotes a culture of 'non disclosure' for clients with personality disorder and problematic/harmful drug use.
- It does not consider drug use as effective self-medication in a harm reduction continuum.
- It fails to acknowledge the ethos and phenomenology of the drug taking experience, and the opportunities it can afford people with mental health problems.

Little research evidence is available that describes effective interventions for dually diagnosed clients with personality disorder and problem drug use. Beck *et al.* (1993) suggest that cognitive behavioural approaches to this combination appear promising, but require further evaluation. Cognitive behavioural work with clients with personality disorder and problem drug use commences with a thorough and comprehensive assessment of both problems, and their relationship to each other. An element of flexibility is essential for 'appointment' type work with drug users because of the difficulties faced with this often 'hard to reach' group. In practice this may mean that a number of appointments may have to be offered before the client attends to be seen.

To identify a personality disorder in a drug user always necessitates a careful evaluation of the client's drug free beliefs and behaviours that are influenced by psychoactive drugs. It is likely that a high degree of similarity between drug free and drug using beliefs and behaviours indicates a high probability of personality disorder. A marked divergence of beliefs and behaviours between drug free and drug using periods can often indicate that the personality aspects are related to drug using behaviours.

The assessment process should include:

- Why did the client start using drugs, and in what setting?

- How did using drugs lead to problem drug use? (What was the psychological and emotional landscape at the time?)
- How did the client function before using drugs, and how do they function currently?
- What personality traits were present during the time before the client started using drugs?
- What personality traits are/were present when the client is/was abstinent (whether enforced or chosen abstinence)?

It is important to get collateral information from as many reliable sources as possible in formulating/assessing the client. This can include reviewing clinical notes from drug services, mental health services and other agencies involved in the care of the client. It is important to review past treatment experiences with the client when embarking on cognitive behavioural work, and reflect on changes in drug use and personality over time (for instance many drug users report that cocaine use effects significant personality changes). It is equally important to hear and understand the experience of drug using from the client in answering the basic assessment questions. Beck *et al.* (1993) suggest that using provocative imagery techniques are helpful in assisting clients to remember and contact their emotions, for example asking clients to close their eyes and imagine the environment in which they use, or buy or sell.

Goal setting as treatment

Beck *et al.* (1993) suggest that there are two standard goals of treatment, which are to reduce 'drug dependency', and to assist clients to learn more adaptive ways of coping with problems. It is, however, crucial to work with clients' own goals in therapeutic work. It may be that some clients seek a drug free lifestyle, and others wish to continue using drugs/alcohol. As health workers, an appropriate response to this desire is to engage with the client using harm minimisation approaches. In this way an acceptance that the client does use drugs helps the client feel accepted as a person, rather than 'just a drug user'. Using harm reduction approaches can also help the client to remain in control of the direction and pace of the therapeutic work.

Management issues

Alongside the therapeutic approaches described above, there are a number of other key elements in working with those with a dual diagnosis of personality disorder and problem drug use, which concern the attitudes of staff who treat and care for them. The language we use as professional health care workers, such as 'addiction' and 'substance abuse/misuse', derive from a culturally shaped and defined understanding of drug use, which immediately pathologises and alienates clients. This language forms part of the commonly held belief amongst mental health workers that clients suffering from personality disorder do not respond to treatment, and that resources are more effectively utilised elsewhere in mental health services. This does not aid in the establishment of a therapeutic alliance with clients. It is therefore highly important to adopt a willingness to be open, non-punitive and non-judgemental about drug use with clients, which should include discussing the benefits using has for the client, alongside the negative effects of drug use in the client's life. Adoption of these basic attitudinal principles may help to engage the client in a helpful dialogue in which behaviour is not personalised, but understood as part of the process of therapy. Clients with this combination of problems also often require help of a more practical nature: help with current legal problems, housing and accessing 24-hour support, and this is an important factor in establishing a relationship that is responsive and in which change can be monitored.

References

Beck, A.T., Wright, F.D., Newman, C.F. & Liese, B.S. (1993) *Cognitive Therapy of Substance Abuse*. The Guilford Press, New York.

Blume, S.B. (1989) Dual diagnosis: psychoactive substance abuse and the personality disorders. *Journal of Psychoactive Drugs*, 21, 139–44.

Campbell, M., Gonzalez, N.M., Ernst, M., Silva, R.R. & Werry, J. (1993) Antipsychotics (neuroleptics). In: *Practitioner's Guide to Psychoactive Drugs for Children and Adolescents*. (Werry, J.S. & Aman, M.G., eds). Plenum, New York.

Craig, R.J. (1987) A psychometric study of the prevalence of DSM-III personality disorders among treated opiate addicts. *International Journal of Addiction*, 23, 115–24.

Dackis, C.A. & Gold, M.S. (1992) Psychiatric Hospitals for Treatment of Dual Diagnosis. In: *Substance Abuse: A Comprehensive Textbook*. (Lowinson, J.H., Riuz, P. & Millman, R.B., eds). Williams and Williams, Baltimore, Md.

Daley, D.C., Moss, H.B. & Campbell, M.S.N. (1993) *Dual Disorders: Counselling Clients with Chemical Dependency and Mental Illness*. Hazelden, Minn.

DeJong, C.A.J., Van den Brink, W., Harteveld, F.M. & Van den Wielden, E.G.M. (1993) Personality disorders in alcoholics and drug addicts. *Comprehensive Psychiatry*, 34 (2), 87–94.

Dusenbury, L. & Botvin, G.J. (1992) Applying the competency enhancement model to substance abuse prevention. In: *The Present and Future of Prevention* (Kessler, M., Goldston, S.E., eds), Primary Prevention of Psychopathology series, Vol. 15, pp. 182–95. Sage Publications Newbury Park, Calif.

Koenigsberg, H.W., Kaplan, R.D., Gilmore, M.M. & Cooper, A.M. (1985) The relationship between syndrome and personality in DSM-III: experience with 2462 patients. *American Journal of Psychiatry*, 142, 207–12.

Lindesmith, A. (1940) Dope fiend mythology. *Journal of Criminal Law and Criminology* (31), 199–208.

Loranger, A.W. (1988) *Personality Disorders Examination Manual*. DV Communications Inc., New York.

Millon, T. (1981) *Disorders of Personality, DSM-III*. Wiley, New York.

Millon, T. (1983) *Millon Multi-axial Inventory Manual*, 3rd edn. National Computer Systems, Minneapolis, MN.

Minkoff, K. (1989) An integrated treatment model for dual diagnosis of psychosis and addiction. *Hospital and Community Psychiatry*, 40, 1031–6.

Nace, E.P., Saxon, J.J. & Shore, N. (1983) A comparison of borderline and non-borderline alcoholic patients. *Archives of General Psychiatry*, 40, 54–6.

Nace, E.P., Davis, C.W. & Gaspari, J.P. (1990) Axis I co-morbidity in substance abusers. *American Journal of Psychiatry*, 148, 118–20.

National Institute for Mental Health in England (2003) *Personality Disorder: No Longer a Diagnosis of Exclusion*. NIMHE, London. http://www.dh.gov.wc/PublicationsandStatistics

Noorlander, E.A. (1985) Behaviour of heroin addicts: the so-called junkie syndrome. In: *Psychiatry and Addiction*. Dutch Society of Psychiatry, Amsterdam, The Netherlands.

Phillips, P. (1998) The mad, the bad and the dangerous – harm reduction in dual diagnosis. *International Journal of Drug Policy*, 9, 345–9.

Regier, D., Farmer, M.E., Rae, D. *et al.* (1990) Co-morbidity of mental disorders with alcohol and other drugs of abuse: results from the epidemiological catchment area. *Journal of the American Medical Association*, 264, 2511–18.

Robins, L.N. & Przybeck, T.R. (1985) Age of onset of drug use as a factor in drug and other disorders. In: *Etiology of Drug Use: Implications for Prevention* (Jones, C.L. & Battjes, R.J., eds). NIDA Research Monogram 56, DHHS, Washington, DC.

Sciacca, K. (1990) Introduction to program development for comprehensive services for mental illness, chemical abuse and addiction. Paper presented at the 34th Annual Conference of the American Association for Partial Hospitalisation. Philadelphia.

Sievewright, N. & Daly, C. (1997) Personality disorder and drug use: a review. *Drug and Alcohol Review*, 16, 235–50.

Welch, S. (2002) *Personality Disorders and Substance Misuse*. Department of Health Expert Papers Series. www.doh.gov.uk

Part 2

Special Populations

Chapter 9 Black and Ethnic Minority Communities: Substance Misuse and Mental Health: Whose Problems Anyway?

Chapter 10 Vulnerable Young People and Substance Misuse

Chapter 11 Meeting Multiple Needs: Pregnancy, Parenting and Dual Diagnosis

9 Black and Ethnic Minority Communities: Substance Misuse and Mental Health: Whose Problems Anyway?

G.H. Rassool

Introduction

Race, culture, ethnicity, mental health and substance misuse have always been contentious issues from the socio-political, economic and health perspectives. Historically, black and ethnic minority communities (BME) have been the victims of negative stereotypes, social exclusions, health inequalities, disparate treatment and racism, and these factors have continued to contribute to the epidemiological health care gap between black and ethnic minority communities and whites.

The UK is a multicultural society with approximately 7.9% of the total population (4.6 million people) representing black and ethnic minority communities (OPCS, 2001). In England people from ethnic minority groups made up 9% of the total population in 2001/02 compared with only 2% in both Scotland and Wales. Nearly half (48%) of the total ethnic minority population are established in metropolitan geographical areas and reside predominantly in the London region, where they comprise 29% of all residents, and in the West Midlands, West Yorkshire and Greater Manchester (Balarajan & Raleigh, 1992; OPCS, 2001). Indians were the largest minority group, followed by Pakistanis, those of mixed ethnic backgrounds, black Caribbeans, black Africans and Bangladeshis. The remaining ethnic minority groups each accounted for less than 0.5% but together accounted for a further 1.4% of the UK population.

It is apparent that black and ethnic minority groups in the UK are a heterogeneous group with varying values, attitudes, religious beliefs and customs that affect the patterns of mental health and substance misuse. This cultural diversity with a wide variation in lifestyle, health behaviour, religion and language has profound effects on their perception and recognition of health problems and ill health constructed within the paradigm of Western medicine and health care systems (Rassool, 1995). This growing diversity has strong implications for the provision of health care in both mental health and substance misuse services. Nurses and other health care professionals need to be aware of the existence of ethnic minorities within the community they serve. The practitioners should be able to assess the health care needs of the ethnic groups and develop services that take account of linguistic, religious and cultural differences (Department of Health, 1999a).

The aims of the chapter are to provide an overview of substance misuse and mental health and to examine the issues and problems faced by black and ethnic minority groups. The implications for the nursing interventions and cultural competence are also presented.

Policy initiatives: substance misuse and mental health

This section will focus on strategies and policies on substance misuse and mental health relevant to black and ethnic minority groups.

Substance misuse

It has been notable that recent national drug policies in the UK have failed to address the health status and health care needs of black and ethnic minority groups (Lord President of the Council, 1998). The task force reviewing services for drug misusers (1996) focused briefly on responding to the needs of black and ethnic minority groups and the inclusion of staff from these groups. According to the Advisory Council on the Misuse of Drugs (ACMD, 1998) 'Ethnic differences in patterns of drug misuse suggest that the needs of some minority ethnic groups are marginalised by existing services, which tend to focus on injecting rather than smoking'.

The current UK drug policy *Tackling Drugs to Build a Better Britain* (Department of Health, 1998a) and the updated drug strategy (Department of Health, 2002) recognised the failure of black and ethnic minority drug users to utilise the range of available treatment services and provided guidance for those involved in the purchasing and provision of drug services to tackle race equality, accessibility and practice. In addition, the strategy encouraged drug action teams (DATs) to undertake health care needs assessments and consider cultural diversity in service provision and delivery. The National Treatment Agency (2001) has identified diversity as one of its key strategic objectives, recognising the need to ensure equal access to service provision regardless of age, gender, sexuality, disability and ethnicity.

In *Models of Care* (NTA, 2002), a framework for the commissioning and delivery of drug services in the UK, the treatment needs of black and ethnic minority substance misusers are recognised throughout the document. In addition, there is a specific section on black and ethnic minority communities (pp. 130–8) focusing on service accessibility and service utilisation, the barriers to drug treatment services, service appropriateness, professional guidance and legal framework, care pathways, needs assessment and treatment. The document also reiterates that service provisions need to be sensitive to the needs of these groups, aware of legislation relating to race and racial discrimination, and to employ approaches in order to maximise treatment engagement and retention of these groups.

Mental health

There have been significant policy and service development initiatives within mainstream mental health services over the past five years. National initiatives such as the Government's plans for improving mental health services for working age adults are set out in the paper, *Modernising Mental Health Services: Safe, Sound and Supportive* (Department of Health, 1998b). *The National Service Framework for Mental Health* was launched in 1999 (Department of Health, 2000). This covers the mental health needs of working age adults and specifically addresses unacceptable variations in services across England. However, these policies do not adequately address the particular needs of black and ethnic minority groups and there is no specific standard set for ethnic minority mental health.

The Mental Health Policy Implementation Guide: Dual Diagnosis Good Practice Guide (Department of Health, 2002) summarises current policy and good practice in the provision of mental health services to people with severe mental health problems and problematic substance misuse. The guide contains a section on people from black and ethnic minority communities, claiming that although there are no definitive studies on the influence of culture and ethnicity upon individuals with a dual diagnosis, it is known that severe mental illness and substance misuse present differently across cultures and ethnic groups. The guide points out, for example, that ethnicity is associated with poor access to services and with different meanings and values attributed to drugs and alcohol. Service provision must therefore be congruent with, and sensitive to, the needs of each minority ethnic group.

Inside Outside: Improving Mental Health Services for Black and Minority Ethnic Communities in England (Sashidaran, 2002) sets out proposals for reforming the service experience and service outcome of people from black and ethnic minority groups who experience mental ill health and who come into contact with mental health services, as users or carers. The main focus for change is the pervasive ethnic inequality that currently exists within mental health services. The central objective of this initiative is to reduce and eventually eradicate such disparities and, by doing so, make mental health services appropriate for and relevant to a multicultural society. For the first time since the inception of the NHS, a national approach aimed at reducing and eliminating ethnic inequalities in health service experience and outcome is being advocated.

The latest document *Delivering Race Equality in Mental Health Care: an Action Plan for Reform Inside and Outside Services and the Government's Response to the Independent Inquiry into the Death of David Bennett* (Department of Health, 2005) combines a five-year action plan for reducing inequalities in black and ethnic minority patients' access to, experience of, and outcomes from mental health services; and the Government response to the recommendations made by the inquiry into the death of David Bennett. *Delivering Race Equality in Mental Health Care* is an action plan for achieving equality and tackling discrimination in mental health services in England for all people of black and ethnic minority status, including those of Irish or Mediterranean origin and east European migrants. The programme is based on three 'building blocks':

- More appropriate and responsive services: achieved through action to develop organisations and the workforce, to improve clinical services and to improve services for specific groups, such as older people, asylum seekers and refugees, and children.
- Community engagement: delivered through healthier communities and by action to engage communities in planning services, supported by 500 new community development workers.
- Better information: from improved monitoring of ethnicity, better dissemination of information and good practice, and improved knowledge about effective services. This will include a new regular census of mental health patients.

A summary of the long-term vision of the Government strategy in delivering race equality in mental health services is summarised in Table 9.1.

Table 9.1 Vision for delivering race equality in mental health service by 2010.

Service characterised by:
• Less fear of mental health services amongst BME communities and service users. • Increased satisfaction with services. • A reduction in the rate of admission and in the disproportionate rates of compulsory detention of BME to psychiatric in-patient units. • Fewer violent incidents that are secondary to inadequate treatment of mental illness. • A reduction in the use of seclusion in BME groups. • The prevention of deaths in mental health services following physical intervention; more BME service users reaching self-reported states of recovery. • A reduction in the ethnic disparities found in prison populations. • A more balanced range of effective therapies, such as peer support services and psychotherapeutic and counselling treatments, as well as pharmacological interventions that are culturally appropriate and effective. • A more active role for BME communities and BME service users in the training of professionals, in the development of mental health policy, and in the planning and provision of services. • A workforce and organisation capable of delivering appropriate and responsive mental health services to BME communities.

Source: Department of Health (2005).

Another piece of legislation that is relevant to the above policies and initiatives is the Race Relations (Amendment) Act 2000 (Home Office, 2000), which places a general duty on specified public authorities to work towards reducing institutional racism, the elimination of unlawful discrimination and to promote race equality of opportunity. In relation to mental health and substance misuse services, the Act requires the services not to discriminate on the grounds of race in employment, policies, service provision and delivery. The codes of practice are enforceable by the Commission for Racial Equality (Commission for Racial Equality, 2001).

Taken altogether, the implementation of policies and guidance in both mental health and substance misuse, with adequate monitoring, should enable the appropriate services to remedy their institutional failings in meeting the needs of black and ethnic minority groups.

Prevalence and patterns of mental health and substance misuse

This review will draw heavily on literature relating to the prevalence and pattern of substance misuse and mental health, dealing with these separately. There is limited data on the epidemiology and extent of dual diagnosis in black and ethnic minority service users.

Mental health

There is a dearth of research on the relative prevalence of mental health problems amongst different black and ethnic minority groups in the UK. A recent review commissioned by the Department of Health (Wright *et al.*, 2000) showed the absolute poverty of research in relation to ethnicity and mental health and, moreover, the relative lack of commitment to commission such work. There have been few population surveys of ethnic differences in the prevalence of mental illness, with most work focusing on rates of contact with services for those with psychotic disorders (Sproston & Nazroo, 2002). This is due to the difficulty of accessing large numbers of ethnic minority informants in general population surveys. Research studies based on contact with services provide information that is only the tip of the iceberg in terms of the true prevalence of mental disorders in black and ethnic minority groups. However, evidence based on clinical and epidemiological research, clinical observations, the testimonies of service users and carers points unequivocally to the racially discriminatory nature of current mental health services and significant discrepancies in service outcome between minority ethnic groups and the majority ethnic group (Iley & Nazroo, 2001; Jones, 2002; Bhui, 2002; Sainsbury Centre for Mental Health, 2002).

A recent study of the rates of mental disorders in black and ethnic minority communities (Sproston & Nazroo, 2002) represents probably the most comprehensive assessment to date of the prevalence of mental health problems amongst ethnic minority groups in England. The findings indicate that there are relatively modest differences in the rates of these disorders between individuals of white, Irish, black Caribbean, Bangladeshi, Indian and Pakistani ethnicity. There were small but statistically significant variations in the prevalence of mental health problems across ethnic groups. Compared with white informants of the same gender, Irish men and Pakistani women had significantly higher, and Bangladeshi women lower, rates of mental disorders. Amongst men, no statistically significant differences were found between ethnic groups when individual ICD-10 (World Health Organization, 2003) diagnoses were considered.

The findings also indicate a very low prevalence of anxiety disorders amongst the Indian group, whilst Irish men had the highest rate of anxiety disorders but the lowest rate of depressive episodes. Amongst women, the prevalence of all types of ICD-10 disorder was least common in the Bangladeshi group, whilst depressive episodes and anxiety disorders were most common amongst Indian and Pakistani women. There was evidence that somatic symptom scores were elevated amongst Bangladeshi men and South Asian women (especially those of Indian and Pakistani origin). A UK national survey of psychiatric morbidity amongst black and ethnic minority groups (Singleton *et al.*, 2001) found that South Asian adults (19.2%) and those in the group classified as 'other' (20.4%) appeared to have higher rates of prevalence for most neurotic disorders than their white counterparts (16.3%), whilst black adults appeared to have lower rates than both groups (14.1%), but the results were not statistically significant.

In contrast to studies on rates of contact with services, this national study of prevalence rates of psychosis indicated a two-fold higher rate for black Caribbean people compared with the white group, but this was only statistically significant for women. However, rates of psychosis were twice as high for black Caribbean women as for white women. It was not significant for men or the total black Caribbean population and was not significant at the level of estimated rates of psychosis. This finding is consistent with the only other national survey that has estimated the prevalence of psychotic illnesses amongst different ethnic groups (Nazroo, 1997). The findings also contradict the view that suggested that the onset of psychotic illnesses is particularly high amongst young black Caribbean men (Cochrane & Bal, 1989) as this study indicated that rates for the young black Caribbean people were not particularly elevated.

The estimated prevalence rate of psychotic illness

in Irish people was to similar to that for the white group, but the Indian and Pakistani groups had higher prevalence rates for psychosis than the white group, although none of these differences were statistically significant. In contrast, the Bangladeshi group had a lower rate than the white group but not significantly so. A UK national survey of psychiatric morbidity amongst black and ethnic minority groups (Singleton *et al.*, 2001) indicated that the prevalence of functional psychosis (mainly schizophrenia or bipolar disorder) appeared to be three times greater (0.6% and 1.8% respectively) for the black Caribbean population compared with the white population. It is worth pointing out that although more black Caribbean people are treated for psychosis, this may not indicate that they are more likely to have such illness. Rather, it is suggested that the way they express their symptoms may be interpreted in such a way (misdiagnosed) and that they are more likely than others to be prescribed treatment for these symptoms (Littlewood & Lipsedge, 1989; Fernando, 1989; Nazroo & King, 2002).

National data show that women born in India and East Africa have a 40% higher suicide rate than women born in England and Wales (Raleigh & Balarajan, 1992). The high-risk group for suicide is young women of South Asian origin without previous psychiatric history. It has been suggested that for the young South Asian people cultural conflict is seen as a precipitating factor in suicide and parasuicide (Raleigh *et al.*, 1990; Raleigh, 1996; Bhugra *et al.*, 1999a,c; Department of Health, 2001). However, it has been indicated that Indian/African, Asian and Pakistani groups who stated that they were depressed had similar rates of suicidal thoughts as the white group across gender and age groups. This is in contrast to other research studies that have found a high rate of suicide amongst young South Asian women (Sproston & Nazroo, 2002). Significantly, high rates of suicide amongst Irish-born people of both sexes, with particularly high rates amongst young women are also reported (Bracken *et al.*, 1998; Leavey, 1999), although a recent study suggests that these rates may in fact be an underestimate (Neeleman & Farrell, 1997). Young black women may be vulnerable to suicide, and social risk factors may precipitate serious mental disorders and possibly suicidal behaviour in African and African-Caribbean people (Raleigh, 1996; Whitley *et al.*, 1999; Department of Health, 2001).

Drug misuse

Historically, black and ethnic minority communities have been the victims of negative stereotypes in respect to substance misuse. The 1920s saw the 'birth of the British drug underground' and is associated with the popular myth that characterised 'the Chinese population as drug dealers and sexual deviants who preyed upon vulnerable young white women' (Kohn, 1992). More recently, the media presentation has resulted in the perception of particular ethnic minorities being susceptible to the misuse of psychoactive substances: Rastafarian, cannabis; Irish, alcohol; and in Africans, the transmission of HIV and AIDS (Rassool, 1997). Nevertheless, these beliefs and stereotypes, with racial undertones, have remained in the popular or collective consciousness of the nation and mask the full understanding of the state of knowledge regarding the patterns of use, perceptions and health beliefs of black and ethnic minority groups towards the use of psychoactive substances (Rassool, 1997). The social, psychological, environmental and economic positions of black and ethnic minority groups in the UK, especially the young, indicate that they face an increasing risk of drug and alcohol problems. A comprehensive literature review on drug use and related service provision is provided elsewhere (National Treatment Agency, 2003). It is reported that there is far more information on drug use amongst South Asian populations (Bangladeshis, Indians and Pakistanis) than amongst other black and minority groups especially from refugees and asylum seekers groups (National Treatment Agency, 2003).

Prevalence and patterns

A brief overview of the prevalence and patterns of drug and alcohol misuse by black and ethnic minority groups is presented in this section. Evidence from both quantitative and qualitative surveys strongly indicates that the rate of prevalence of drug misuse within the black and ethnic minority groups, particularly amongst South Asians, is lower than that of the white population, but with increasing trends (Ramsey & Spiller, 1997; Parker *et al.*, 1995, Ramsey *et al.*, 2001). However, there are clear indications that drug misuse is increasingly being reported amongst young black and ethnic minority women (National Treatment Agency, 2003). The substances misused by black and ethnic minority groups are not clearly different from those used by the white population, but there seem to be preferences for a certain class or classes of substances and mode of consumption by different ethnic groups, which are linked with the historical and cultural characteristics of each ethnic group (Oyefeso & Ghodse, 1993; Oyefeso *et al.*, 2000; Sangster *et al.*, 2002). It is argued that compulsory hospital admissions distort the statistics of problematic drug use amongst black Caribbean and African males, as a result of the use of 'stop and search' tactics and the diagnosis 'cannabis psychosis' (Harrison *et al.*, 1997).

Cannabis is the most widely used illicit drug amongst the younger members of black and ethnic minority communities, and presentations to drug services by black Caribbeans are more likely to focus on crack cocaine than other ethnic groups (including white groups) (Sangster *et al.*, 2002). Heroin is the drug of choice amongst young South Asians in some areas of England, particularly amongst Pakistani and Bangladeshi males. In some cases, heroin is also the first drug used (Gilman, 1993; Perera, 1996, 1998; Chaudry *et al.*, 1997; Sherlock *et al.*, 1997; Patel, 2000; Patel *et al.*, 2001; Sheikh *et al.*, 2001; Webster, 2001). Heroin was reported to be used by South Asian, Iranian, Vietnamese and Chinese people (Patel *et al.*, 1998; Whittington, 1999; Sangster *et al.*, 2002). Cocaine was reported as the main drug of use by black Caribbean, African and 'other' drug users than either South Asian or white drug users (Daniel, 1993; Perera *et al.*, 1993). Crack cocaine has been reported to be used by young Bangladeshis and Kashmiris (Sheikh *et al.*, 2001). These observations suggest that the widely held assumptions of the substance specific, cultural stereotypes that Asians do not use opiates and cocaine are gradually becoming less tenable.

There is also the contention that injecting drug use behaviour is uncommon amongst black and ethnic minority groups. Injecting by black and ethnic minority drug users is generally reported to be less prevalent than amongst white drug users, largely because of the lack of BME drug users presenting at needle exchanges (Sangster *et al.*, 2002). However, South Asians have been reported to be injecting heroin by Chaudry *et al.* (1997); Patel *et al.* (1998, 2001); Pearson & Patel (1998); Sheikh *et al.* (2001); Webster (2001); and Sangster *et al.* (2002). Studies have also reported that young South Asian males injecting steroids (Pearson & Patel, 1998; Ram, 2000; Sheikh *et al.*, 2001). Sangster *et al.* (2002) report injecting amongst black Caribbean heroin users in London, suggesting that this may be linked to the tendency for drug users to switch to heroin whilst in prison. Although there is generally a low uptake of needle exchanges by South Asian drug injectors, South Asian males have been shown to access injecting equipment via white friends or white girlfriends by Pearson & Patel (1998); Patel (2000); Patel *et al.* (1998); and Sheikh *et al.* (2001). There is great concern that dangerous injecting practices are occurring, particularly amongst South Asian female drug-injecting sex workers (Hall, 1999).

Evidence of the use of dance drugs (ecstasy, amphetamines and LSD) by young members of black and ethnic minority communities is rather limited. It is stated that ecstasy, LSD and amphetamines were regarded as 'white people's drugs' and use by members of black and ethnic minority communities was limited (Gilman 1993; Chaudry *et al.*, 1997). However, stimulant, ecstasy, hallucinogens, LSD and ice (a smokeable form of amphetamines) have been reported to be used by Indians at Bhangra (clubbing) events (Patel *et al.*, 1995; Perera, 1998; Bola & Walpole, 1999). Qat (or kat or khat) was found to be used by the Somali community (Cunningham, 1998; Griffiths, 1998; Fountain *et al.*, 2002); Yemeni communities (Leroy, 2000; Mohammed, 2000); Ethiopians (Fountain *et al.*, 2002); and amongst Arabs from the Middle East (Iran, Iraq, Lebanon and Yemen) (Fountain *et al.*, 2002).

Alcohol misuse

The report on *Health of Minority Ethnic Groups* (National Centre for Social Research, 2001) found that, in England, men and women from all black and ethnic minority groups (except white Irish) were less likely to drink alcohol than the general population and consumed smaller amounts. Overall, the findings show that 7% of men from the general population were non-drinkers, compared with 5% of Irish men, 13% of black Caribbean men,

30% of Chinese men, 33% of Indian men, 91% of Pakistani men and 96% of Bangladeshi men. Higher proportions of women than men were non-drinkers, both in the general population and amongst ethnic minority groups. Of the general population, 12% of women reported being non-drinkers compared with 10% of Irish women, 18% of black Caribbean women, 41% of Chinese women, 64% of Indian women, 97% of Pakistani women and 99% of Bangladeshi women.

On the heaviest drinking day in the previous week (when surveyed) 59% of the general population drank over four units compared with 74% of Irish drinkers, 50% of Indian, 43% of black Caribbean, 21% of Chinese (no figures are available for Pakistani and Bangladeshi men as so few drank in the previous week). For women the proportion of women drinking over three units was 47% for the general population, 56% for Irish women, 36% for Indian women, 35% for black Caribbean women and 30% for Chinese women. In common with the general population, weekly levels of alcohol consumption decrease with age, with the exception of black Caribbean and Indian men. However, these figures also show that a significant proportion of people from the Indian and black Caribbean communities exceed weekly limits and, amongst those who do drink, both men and women report exceeding the daily limits.

A survey (Alcohol Concern, 2001) conducted among 1684 second or subsequent generation men and women in the Midlands from black African, African-Caribbean, black British, Indian Hindu, Indian Sikh, Bengali and Pakistani communities in Birmingham and Leicester found relatively high levels of drinking amongst black communities and male Sikhs. Whilst most Pakistani and Bengali men and women, and Sikh and Hindu women were non-drinkers, amongst African-Caribbean men and women and Sikh men, alcohol was used by most people. Another study of 16–25-year-olds from Pakistani, Indian and Chinese communities in Glasgow shows that higher proportions of the younger members of Asian communities do drink, with 19% of Pakistanis saying they drink, as do 49% of Indians and 73% of Chinese. Interestingly, this study also shows that although young Pakistanis are less likely to drink, those that do drink consume the highest number of alcohol units (on average 13.8 units per week compared with 7.94 for young Indians and 4.76 for young Chinese) (Bakshi *et al.*, 2002). Subhra & Chauhan (1999) point to the fact that although certain of the BME communities place restrictions on the use of alcohol (for religious or cultural reasons) there already exist complex patterns of alcohol use within these communities.

Taken together, the evidence from quantitative surveys strongly indicates that the prevalence of alcohol misuse within the black and ethnic minority groups is increasing, especially amongst the Indian and black Caribbean communities. This has significant implications for service provision. For more comprehensive literature on alcohol in black and ethnic minority groups see Alcohol Concern (2001).

Tobacco

Smoking patterns have been shown to vary between different black and ethnic minority groups according to the data from the 1999 Health Survey for England (Nazroo, 1997; National Centre for Social Research, 2001). Compared with the national prevalence rate of 27% in men, the rates are particularly high in the Bangladeshi (42%), Irish (39%) and black Caribbean (34%) populations. Amongst women, smoking rates are low (at 8% or below) with the exception of black Caribbean (23%) and Irish (31%), compared with the general population. Compared with the general population (in the 8–15 age group), Irish girls were more likely, and Indian, Pakistani, Bangladeshi and Chinese children less likely, to report ever having smoked.

Amongst ethnic minority groups, many types of smokeless tobacco are used, particularly amongst the South Asian population. The survey found that Bangladeshis (both men and women) were more likely than other South Asian groups to report chewing tobacco; 19% of Bangladeshi men and 26% of Bangladeshi women reported chewing tobacco, compared with between 2% and 6% for Indian and Pakistani men and women, respectively. Tobacco is often consumed in combination with other products. Use of paan (a leaf preparation stuffed with betel nut and/or with tobacco or other ingredients), believed to be a risk factor in oral cancer, is high amongst some South Asian ethnic groups. Ready-made mixtures of snuff are known as Gutka or paan masala, which are chewed either on their own or in betel quid. They are prepared by baking and curing a mixture comprising areca nut, lime, spices and tobacco (Pearson & Patel, 1998; Champion *et al.*, 2001).

Special problems and issues

Black and ethnic minority communities are reported to be over represented amongst the lower social classes, with higher unemployment rates, living in poverty, living in poorer housing and with lower employment status, all of which are associated with poor mental health ((Bhugra, 1999; Sashidaran, 2002; Malek & Joughin, 2003). In addition, black and ethnic minority individuals experience high rates of admission to psychiatric in-patient units, are compulsorily detained under the Mental Health Act 1983, have high rates of seclusion and figure disproportionately in the criminal justice arena (Bhat *et al.*, 1996; Davies *et al.*, 1996; Mental Health Act Commission, 2001; Audini & Elliott, 2002).

The report *Inside Outside* (Sashidaran, 2002) acknowledged the problems faced by black and ethnic minority groups in mental health care: that there is an overemphasis on institutional and coercive models of care, professional and organisational requirements are given priority over individual needs and rights, and institutional racism exists within mental health care. This statement is equally applicable to substance misuse service provision and delivery. The marginality and social exclusion experienced by black and ethnic minority groups, compounded by racial discrimination and institutional racism, are likely to be significant in understanding the experiences in these communities and their access to mental health and substance misuse services. The mental health *National Service Framework* (Department of Health, 1999a) states that 'the stigma attached to mental illness can be compounded by racial discrimination, with access to appropriate assessment, treatment and care inhibited'. This statement is equally applicable to substance misuse service provision and delivery. Despite the higher levels of ill health and disability amongst the black and ethnic minority groups they appear to have poorer access to health services (Smaje & LeGrand, 1997). There is a growing notion and increasing national recognition that our nation's health care system is poorly addressing the health care needs of ethnic minority communities and the inequitable access to both substance and mental health services (Department of Health, 1999a, 2005; Sashidaran, 2002; National Treatment Agency, 2003).

In contrast with mental health services, there is evidence to suggest that black and ethnic minority substance misusers, especially those from South Asian communities and women, under present to treatment services (Advisory Council on the Misuse of Drugs, 1998; National Treatment Agency, 2002; Sangster *et al.*, 2002). The low rates of presentation to alcohol and drug services by ethnocultural groups may be due to a multitude of factors that include acculturation, cultural value systems, cultural dissonance, education and literacy, previous experience of persecution, communication difficulties, religio-cultural proscription, discrimination, the lack of understanding of black and ethnic minority cultures, ethnicity of staff, denial of substance misuse by black and ethnic minority communities and lack of understanding of black and ethnic minority culture (Oyefeso & Ghodse, 1993; Rassool, 1995; Khan *et al.*, 1995; Free & McKee, 1998; Perera, 1998; Khan & Ditton, 1999; Alcohol Concern, 2003). In addition, the literature suggests that drug services for black and ethnic minority groups are poorly developed and uncoordinated, and there is a lack of awareness of services and their functions by black and ethnic minority communities (Chantler *et al.*, 1998; Patel, 2000; Sangster *et al.*, 2002). Many agencies are mainstream and ethnocentric in their services to culturally diverse communities, resulting in poor delivery of service in meeting the health needs of these groups (Rassool, 1997).

In summary, research on black and ethnic minority drug users suggests a number of institutional failings in both community and residential settings. The failure to provide equitable and accessible services for black and ethnic minority substance misusers is related to the perceptions of and responses to meeting the needs of these communities. The evidence from the literature has shown that the service provision and delivery are related to 'the image of services and their isolation from the communities, an inability to identify and respond to the distinct patterns of drug use among ethnic minority communities and inability to respond to diverse needs' (Sangster *et al.*, 2002). It has been suggested that patterns of commissioning and service delivery, as well as treatment philosophy, sometimes work against meeting the treatment needs of black and ethnic minority users (National Treatment Agency, 2002). The need to make drug services accessible to black and ethnic minority groups has been recognised by the National Treatment Agency (2002). It stated that 'action to ensure equal access to relevant and appropriate services for the whole population, regardless of age, gender, sexuality, ethnicity, disability or location, will be a theme across all NTA activity' (National Treatment Agency, 2002).

Finally, in relation to dual diagnosis, the Health Advisory Service (2001) recommends that commissioners and providers ensure that all local services are able to meet the diverse needs of the local population and that the services are accessible to black and ethnic minority groups and effective at meeting their needs. Mental health professionals should consider post-traumatic stress amongst clients with co-morbidity and amongst refugees and asylum seekers in particular.

Cultural competence

There is a growing recognition that culture is an important component and determinant of health (Department of Health, 1999a; 1999c). The *National Service Framework for Mental Health* (Department of Health, 1999a) states that mental health services need to develop and demonstrate cultural competence, with staff having the knowledge and skills to work effectively with diverse communities. The provision of culturally competent approaches in working with black and ethnic minority substance misusers has also been advocated by black and ethnic minority drug treatment professionals (Sangster *et al.*, 2002). For nurses, the provision of culturally competent care is both a legal and a moral requirement (Nursing and Midwifery Council, 2004).

The area of cultural competence in general suffers from a lack of agreed definition and is not universally accepted. It is often interrelated, with terms like cultural awareness, cultural sensitivity, cultural appropriateness, cultural specificity and others. Cultural competence is most appropriately viewed as an umbrella term that describes an ability to meet the needs of diverse communities; cultural appropriateness provides the mechanism through which cultural competence is achieved; and cultural sensitivity and cultural specificity form the building blocks for culturally appropriate ways of working (Sangster *et al.*, 2002). Papadopoulos *et al.* (1998) describe cultural competence as the capacity to provide effective health care, taking into consideration people's cultural beliefs, behaviours and needs. A more comprehensive and operational definition is that cultural competence is the integration and transformation of knowledge about individuals and groups of people into specific standards, policies, practices and attitudes used in appropriate cultural settings to increase the quality of services, thereby producing better outcomes (Davis, 1997). In the context of mental health and substance misuse, cultural competence is the willingness and ability of the workforce, services and the system to value the importance of cultural diversity and be culturally responsive in the provision and delivery of quality services to black and ethnic minority groups.

The notion of cultural competence is applied to service provision, service delivery and the system of care. This is a significant development as it provides the basis for moving beyond individually focused anti-racism training and brings into play the culture of organisations, their aims and core competencies, their management structures and their use of monitoring (Chandra, 1996). Services with 'cultural competence', according to Chandra (1996), are those 'perceived by black and ethnic minority users as being in harmony with their cultural and religious beliefs' and offer a range of ways for health purchasers to work towards this with providers. Cross *et al.* (1989) list five essential elements that contribute to an institution or agency's ability to become more culturally competent. These include:

- Valuing diversity
- Having the capacity for cultural self-assessment
- Being conscious of the dynamics inherent when cultures interact
- Having institutionalised cultural knowledge
- Having developed adaptations of service delivery reflecting an understanding of cultural diversity

These five elements should be manifested at every level of an organisation, including policy making, administration and practice. Further, these elements should be reflected in the attitudes, structures, policies and services of the organisation. A summary of the core elements needed in the development and provision of cultural competence drug services for black and ethnic minority communities (Sangster *et al.*, 2002) is provided in Table 9.2.

Nursing approaches: clinical and educational

The Nursing and Midwifery Council in England Code of Professional Conduct: Standards for Conduct, Performance and Ethics (NMC, 2004) points out that nurses and midwives 'are personally accountable for ensuring that you promote and protect the interests and dignity of patients and clients, irrespective of gender, age, race, ability, sexuality, economic status, lifestyle, culture and religious or political beliefs'. Nurses must be aware of their own cultural expectations and not impose these upon communities from different cultures. They need to challenge and confront their own prejudice and negative perceptions of black and ethnic minority groups and to consider the different composition of ethnic and cultural backgrounds of their patients in order to deliver safe and effective care.

Culturally competent nursing approaches are necessary to ensure the best possible access to substance misuse and mental health services and for better health care outcomes. Nurses who are culturally knowledgeable and competent can provide care that ensures that black and ethnic minority groups receive the best and most appropriate health care promotion measures and treatment possible. Due to the significant differences amongst black and ethnic minority communities in lifestyles, health behaviour, disease patterns and mortality levels, appropriate nursing interventions should be tailored to meet the specific health needs of the individual group. Gerrish (2000) has put forward a philosophy of individualised care that incorporates notions of equity and fairness, holism, respect for individuality, establishing partnerships between patients and professionals, and promoting independence. In this framework individualised care entails a holistic assessment of physical, psychological, social and spiritual needs, an assessment approach that can be used across black and ethnic minority groups.

There are major challenges facing addiction and mental health nurses in the provision of culturally competent care to patients from different cultural and ethnic backgrounds. There is a need to recognise the nature and pattern of mental disorders and substance misuse and clinical differences amongst people of different black and ethnic minority groups. These difficulties are accentuated in the recognition and assessment of substance misuse because of cultural variations in presentation symptoms and where a 'dual diagnosis' (substance misuse and psychiatric disorders) is ascribed. Substance misuse and mental health problems should be seen in their social and cultural context. Cultural and religious beliefs should not be applied equally in a stereotypical fashion to members of a particular black and ethnic minority group. There are often differences amongst black and ethnic minority communities and differences between members of the same ethnic group. The focus for nurses is to examine each client's subjective experiences of culture and religious values.

In addition to the client's cultural beliefs, nurses must be aware of their own beliefs, practices and perceptions, as these may have an impact on the care they provide to clients from diverse cultural backgrounds. Burr (2002) identified some stereotypical views of South Asian patients held by qualified and experienced health care professionals and warns against the dangers of imposing one's

Table 9.2 Cultural competence and service delivery in substance misuse services.

- Cultural ownership and leadership (the extent to which race and ethnicity are considered important by a service).
- Symbols of accessibility (something that shows black and ethnic minority people that they are welcomed by a service, for example posters, leaflets, culturally specific newspapers and magazines.
- Familiarity with, and ability to meet, the distinct needs of communities.
- Holistic, therapeutic and social help.
- A range of services.
- Black and ethnic minority workers.
- Community attachment and ownership and capacity building (the process through which the skills and structures needed to provide drug services are developed).

Source: Sangster *et al.*, (2002).

own value systems wittingly or otherwise on others. The imposition of our own values implicitly suggests that underlying these sentiments is the belief that one's own value system is superior to that of others and the expectation that once in England one should think and conduct oneself in keeping with the ways of the majority (Burr, 2002). Respect for the belief systems of others and the effects of those beliefs on health behaviour are critically important to culturally competent care. The main source of problems in caring for patients from diverse cultural backgrounds is the lack of understanding and tolerance and the inability to ask questions sensitively.

Some ethnocentric nursing interventions are clearly biased towards the dominant culture and mainstream counselling may be inappropriate for some black and ethnic minority groups. Studies have shown the predominance of Eurocentric counselling and support by treatment staff and staff ignorance of cultural factors that impact on drug use and drug treatment (Abdulrahim *et al.*, 1994; NTA, 2003). The literature has also shown how ethnocentrism amongst professionals shapes the experience of mental health services by black and ethnic minority users (Littlewood & Lipsedge, 1989). This is also applicable to professionals in the substance misuse services. Many ethnic minorities have very little knowledge or real experience of counselling and counselling process. A client centred approach, as advocated by the literature, may not be the type of approach that the client is looking for. A trans-cultural approach may be more appropriate as part of the therapeutic intervention strategies in the management of dual diagnosis in black and ethnic minority groups. The use of trans-cultural therapy or counselling has been advocated for dealing with mental health and substance use problems. Intercultural therapy and counselling recognises the importance of internal realities of culture (beliefs, values, attitudes, religion and language) for both the therapist and the patient and is sensitive to the external realities of the patient's life (for example poverty, refugee status, racism, sexism).

Recognising and working with the unconscious aspects of culture, the similarities and differences, are considered vital for successful outcome of the therapy (Kareem & Littlewood, 2000). D'Ardenne & Mahtani (1989) stated that 'trans-cultural counselling is not about being an expert on any given culture but a way of thinking about clients where culture is acknowledged and valued'.

However, there is ample evidence to indicate that nurses frequently fall short of providing sensitive and appropriate care to ethnic minority patients. Gerrish *et al.* (1996) demonstrated how, in the early 1990s, nurses in England were inadequately prepared through their education to address the challenge of delivering multi-ethnic nursing care. Whereas the idea of culturally competent nursing has become a recognised theoretical strategy, the elements involved in its application and practices are sometimes only vaguely utilised or understood (Kirkland, 1998). If these policy objectives are to be met, it is essential that nurse education provides students with the opportunity to develop trans-cultural competence. A model to promote the inclusion of cultural competence in nursing and health care sciences education has been developed by Papadopoulos *et al.* (1998). A model of cultural competence is shown in Figure 9.1.

The model consists of four stages. The first stage in the model is cultural awareness and is the basis for a critical examination of our personal values and beliefs. The nature of construction of cultural identity as well as its influence on people's health beliefs and practices is viewed as a learning foundation. Cultural knowledge (the second stage) can be gained in a number of ways. Meaningful contact with people from different black and ethnic minority groups can enhance knowledge around their health beliefs and behaviours as well as raise understanding around the problems they face. An important element in achieving cultural sensitivity (the third stage) is how professionals view people in their care and that clients should be seen as equal partners. This includes trust, acceptance and respect as well as facilitation and negotiation. The achievement of the fourth stage (cultural competence) requires the synthesis and application of previously gained awareness, knowledge and sensitivity. Cultural competence activities include the development of skills in the assessment of need, clinical diagnosis and clinical skills. Practices are responsive to the culture and diversity within the populations served. A most important component of this stage of development is the ability to recognise and challenge racism and other forms of discrimination and oppressive practice. It is argued

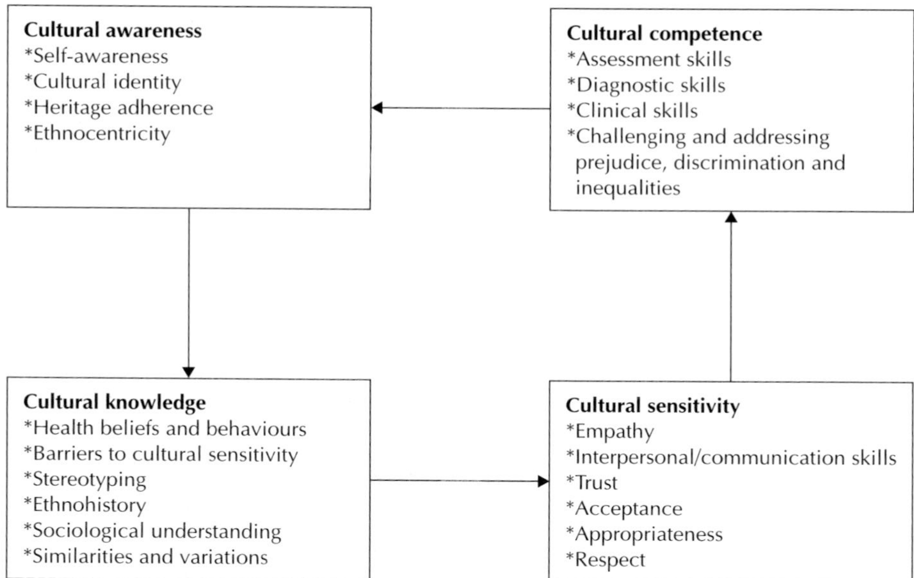

Figure 9.1 The Papadopoulos, Tilki & Taylor model for the development of cultural competence in nursing. Source: Papadopoulos *et al.* (1998).

that this model combines both the multiculturalist and the anti-racist perspectives, and facilitates the development of a broader understanding around inequalities, and human and citizenship rights, whilst promoting the development of skills needed to bring about change at the patient/client level (Papadopoulos *et al.*, 1998).

It is worth pointing out that it is not practical for nurses to have knowledge of all black and ethnic minority groups, but they can learn to appreciate diversity and provide culturally sensitive care to heterogeneous populations. However, nurses should be aware of the culture and traditions of the population they serve, and the goal of the nursing care and interventions is the provision of culturally competent care that diminishes the barriers and improves health outcomes.

Conclusion

The problems and challenges associated with ethnicity, substance misuse and mental health are complex and need a multi-sectorial approach. In mental health, progress and change is dependent on an inclusive process, involving politicians, policy makers and service providers from both statutory and voluntary sectors, service users and carers and, most importantly, black and ethnic minority communities themselves (Sashidaran, 2002). This is equally appropriate in the substance misuse field. In addition, professional and regulatory bodies and educational institutions should establish standards of care and core competencies to promote standards encouraging culturally competent care and to integrate issues of diversity and culture into curricula. Evaluation and monitoring should be an ongoing process.

Substance misuse and mental health, or dual diagnosis, in black and ethnic minority groups in the UK need to be considered in the context of socio-political perspectives and the permeation of racism. The issues related to working with black and ethnic minority groups with mental health problems and substance misuse include language, culture, patriarchy, gender issues, religious beliefs, family pride, health beliefs, stigma, confidentiality, oppression and racism (Rassool, 1997). To work effectively with these client groups does not require one to become an expert in all ethno-cultural groups but to have cultural flexibility, acceptance and understanding; and to perceive the patient or client as an individual (Rassool, 1995). What is considered essential is to develop openness to cultural diversity to the relativity of our own beliefs, values and culture. There is an urgent need to prepare nurses and other health care professionals in mental health and substance misuse fields on cultural competence and race issues to enable them to work in a culturally sensitive manner.

References

Abdulrahim, D., White, D., Phillips, K., Boyd, G., Nicholson, J. & Elliot, J. (1994) *Ethnicity and Drug Use: Towards the Design of Community Interventions*. Vol. 1, AIDS Research Unit, University of East London, London.

Advisory Council on the Misuse of Drugs (ACMD) (1998) *AIDS and Drug Misuse*, Part 1, HMSO, London.

Alcohol Concern (2001) Alcohol Survey: Black and Ethnic Minorities. *Alcohol Concern's Quarterly Information and Research Bulletin*, Alcohol Concern, London.

Alcohol Concern (2003) Alcohol drinking among black and minority ethnic communities (BME) in the United Kingdom. *Alcohol Concern's Quarterly Information and Research Bulletin*, Spring. Alcohol Concern, London.

Audini, B. & Elliott, P.L. (2002) Age, gender and ethnicity of those detained under Part II of the Mental Health Act 1983. *British Journal of Psychiatry*, 180, 222–6.

Bakshi, N., Ross, R. & Heim, D. (2002) *Drug and Alcohol Issues Affecting Pakistani, Indian and Chinese Young People and Their Communities*. Greater Glasgow NHS Board, Glasgow.

Balarajan, R. & Raleigh, V.S. (1992) The ethnic populations of England and Wales: The 1991 census. *Health Trends*, 24, 113–16.

Bhat, A., Carr-Hill, R. & Ohri, S. (1996) *Britain's Black Population: a New Perspective*. Radical Statistics Race Group, Aldershot, Gower.

Bhugra, D. (ed.) (1999) *Mental Health Practice in Multicultural Britain*. Royal College of Psychiatry, London.

Bhugra, D., Baldwin, D.S., Desai, M. & Jacob, K.S. (1999a) Attempted suicide in West London, II. Intergroup comparisons. *Psychological Medicine*, 29 (5), 1131–9.

Bhugra, D., Desai, M. & Baldwin, D. (1999b) Suicide and attempted suicide across cultures. In: *Ethnicity: An Agenda for Mental Health* (Bhugra, D. & Bahl, V., eds) pp. 123–37. Gaskell, London.

Bhugra, D., Desai, M. & Baldwin, D.S. (1999c) Attempted suicide in West London, I. Rates across ethnic communities *Psychological Medicine*, 29 (5), 1125–30.

Bhui, K. (2002) *Racism and Mental Health*. Jessica Kingsley Publishers, London.

Bola, M. & Walpole, T. (1999) *Drugs Information and Communication Needs among South Asians in Crawley*. Executive summary. Youth Action Crawley, Crawley.

Bracken, P.J., Greenslade, L., Griffin, B. & Smyth, M. (1998) Mental health and ethnicity: an Irish dimension. *British Journal of Psychiatry*, 172, 103–5.

Burke, A.W. (1976) Socio-cultural determinants of attempted suicide among West Indians in Birmingham. *British Journal of Psychiatry*, 129, 261–6.

Burr, J. (2002) Cultural stereotypes of women from South Asian communities: mental health care professionals' explanations for patterns of suicide and depression. *Social Science and Medicine*, 55 (200), 835–45.

Champion, J., Bedi, B. & Anees, K. (2001) *Trans-cultural Tobacco Programme*. Educational programme for trading standards and customs and excise officers. National Centre for Transcultural Oral Health, London.

Chandra, J. (1996) *Facing Up to Difference: a Toolkit for Creating Culturally Competent Health Services for Black and Ethnic Minority Communities*. The King's Fund, London.

Chantler, K., Aslam, H., Bashir, C., Darrell, J., Patel, K. & Steele, C. (1998) *An Analysis of Present Drug Service Delivery to Black Communities in Greater Manchester*. Project report, March 1998. Greater Manchester Drug Action Partnership (SRB and Black Drug Workers Forum (BDWF) North West), Manchester.

Chaudry, M.A., Sherlock K. & Patel, K. (1997) *Drugs and Ethnic Health Project: Oldham and Tameside, 1997*. A report to the West Pennine Drug Action Team. Manchester: Lifeline/University of Central Lancashire, Preston.

Cochrane, R. & Bal, S.S. (1989) Mental hospital admission rates of immigrants to England: a comparison of 1971 and 1981. *Social Psychiatry and Psychiatric Epidemiology*, 24, 2–11.

Commission for Racial Equality (2001) *Statutory Code of Practice on the Duty to Promote Race Equality: a Guide for Public Authorities*. Commission for Racial Equality, London.
www.cre.gov.uk

Cross, T., Bazron, B., Dennis, K. & Isaacs, M. (1989) *Toward a Culturally Competent System of Care*, Vol. 1. Georgetown University, Wash.

Cunningham, T. (1998) At home with diversity: race, rehab and drugs. *Drug link*, September/October, 15–17.

Daniel, T. (1993) Ethnic minorities' use of drug services. *Druglink*, 8 (1), 16–17.

D'Ardenne, P. & Mahtani, A. (1989) *Trans-cultural Counselling in Action*. Sage, London.

Davies, S., Thornicroft, G., Leese, M., Higgingbotham, A. & Phelan, M. (1996) Ethnic differences in risk of compulsory psychiatric admission among representative cases of psychosis in London. *British Medical Journal*, 312 (7030), 533–7.

Davis, K. (1997) *Exploring the Intersection Between Cultural*

Competency and Managed Behavioral Health Care Policy: Implications for State and County Mental Health Agencies. National Technical Assistance Center for State Mental Health Planning, Alexandria, Va.

Department of Health (1998a) *Tackling Drugs to Build a Better Britain*. Department of Health, London.

Department of Health (1998b) *Modernising Mental Health Services: Safe, Sound and Supportive*. Department of Health, London.

Department of Health (1999a) *National Service Framework for Mental Health: Modern Standards and Service*. Department of Health, London.

Department of Health (1999b) *Saving Lives: Our Healthier Nation*. Department of Health, London.

Department of Health (1999c) *Reducing Health Inequalities: an Action Report*. Stationery Office, London.

Department of Health (2000) *National Service Framework for Mental Health: Modern Standards and Service Models.* Department of Health, London.

Department of Health (2001) *Safety First: 5-Year Report of the National Inquiry into Suicide and Homicide by People with Mental Illness*. Department of Health, London.

Department of Health (2002) *The Mental Health Policy Implementation Guidance: Dual Diagnosis Good Practice Guide*. Department of Health, London.

Department of Health (2005) *Delivering Race Equality in Mental Health Care: an Action Plan for Reform Inside and Outside Services and the Government's Response to the Independent Inquiry into the Death of David Bennett.* Department of Health, London.
http://www.dh.gov.uk/assetRoot/04/10/07/75/04100775.pdf

Fernando, S. (1989) *Race and Culture in Psychiatry*. Routledge, London.

Fountain, J., Bashford, J., Underwood, S. *et al.* (2002) Update and complete analysis of drug use, consequences and correlates amongst minorities. Cited in: National Treatment Agency (2003) *Black and Minority Ethnic Communities: a Review of the Literature on Drug Use and Related Service Provision*. NTA, London.
www.nta.nhs.uk.

Free, C. & McKee, M. (1998) Meeting the needs of black and minority ethnic groups. *British Medical Journal*, 316, (31 January), 380.

Gerrish, K. (2000) Individualised care: its conceptualisation and practice within a multi-ethnic society. *Journal of Advanced Nursing*, 32, 91–9.

Gerrish, K., Husband, C. & Mackenzie, J. (1996) *Nursing for a Multi-ethnic Society*. Open University Press, Buckingham.

Gerrish, K. & Papadopoulos, I. (1999) Trans-cultural competence: the challenge for nurse education. *British Journal of Nursing*, 8 (21), 1453–7.

Gilman, M. (1993) *An Overview of the Main Findings and Implications of Seven Action Studies into the Nature of Drug use in Bradford*. Home Office Drugs Prevention Team, Bradford.

Griffiths, P. (1998) *Qat Use in London: a Study of Qat Use Among a Sample of Somalis Living in London*. Central Drugs Prevention Unit paper 26. The Stationery Office, London.

Hall, C. (1999) *Drug Use and HIV Infection in South Asian and Middle Eastern Communities in the UK: a Literature Review*. Nat Project, London.

Harrison, L., Sutton, M. & Gardiner, E. (1997) Ethnic differences in substance use and alcohol use related mortality among first generation migrants to England and Wales. *Substance Use and Misuse*, 32 (7/8), 849–76.

Health Advisory Service (2001) *Substance Misuse and Mental Health Co-morbidity (Dual Diagnosis). Standards for Mental Health Services*. Health Advisory Service, London.

Home Office (2000) Race Relations (Amendment) Act 2000. The Stationery Office, London.
www.homeoffice.gov.uk

Iley, K. & Nazroo, J. (2001) Ethnic inequalities in mental health: a critical examination of the evidence. In: *Sociology, Ethnicity and Nursing Practice* (Culley, L. & Dyson, S., eds), pp. 67–89. Palgrave, Basingstoke.

Jones, R. (2002) Black people and mental health services: treading water. *Open Mind*, 114 (March/April), 19.

Kareem, J. & Littlewood, R. (2000) *Intercultural Therapy: Themes, Interpretations and Practice*. Blackwell Publishing, Oxford.

Khan, S., Shabir, G. & Ahmed, I. (1995) *An Investigation into Drugs Issues in the Asian Community in Dudley*. Catalyst Community Services Agency, Blackheath, Birmingham.

Khan, F. & Ditton, J. (1999) *Minority Ethnic Drug Use in Glasgow. Part Two: Special Problems Experienced and Possible Gaps in Service Provision*. Glasgow Drugs Prevention Team, Glasgow.

Khon, M. (1992) *Dope Girls: The Birth of the British Drug Underground*. Lawrence and Wishart, London.

Kirkland, S. (1998) Nurses' descriptions of caring for culturally diverse clients. *Clinical Nursing Research*, 7, 125–46.

Leavey, G. (1999) Suicide and Irish migrants in Britain: identity and integration. *International Review of Psychiatry*, 11, 168–72.

Leitner, M., Shapland, J. & Wiles, P. (1993) *Drug Usage and Drug Prevention: the Views and Habits of the General Public*. HMSO, London.

Leroy, N. (2000) After the goldrush: an unstructured study into visible minority substance misusers not accessing drug services in Granby/Toxteth, Liverpool. *QED Network Journal*.
http://qed.emcdda.org

Littlewood, R. & Lipsedge, M. (1989) *Aliens and Alienists: Ethnic Minorities and Psychiatry*. Unwin Hyman, London.

Lord President of the Council (1998) *Tackling Drugs to Build a Better Britain: the Government's Ten-year Strategy for Tackling Drug Misuse*. Cm 3945. The Stationery Office, London.

Malek, M. & Joughin, C. (2003) *Mental Health Services for Minority Ethnic Children and Adolescents*. Jessica Kingsley Publishers, London.

Mental Health Act Commission (2001) Mental Health Act Commission. *Ninth Biennial Report*. HMSO, London.

Mohammed, S. (2000) *A Gob Full of Khat: a Study of Contemporary Khat Use in Toxteth*. Avaanca Publications, Liverpool/London.

National Centre for Social Research and Dept of Epidemiology and Public Health at the Royal Free and University College Medical School (2001) *The Health of Minority Ethnic Groups '99 (Health Survey for England)*. Office for National Statistics, London.

National Treatment Agency (2001) www.nta.nhs.uk

National Treatment Agency (2002) *Models of Care for Treatment of Adult Drug Misusers*. NTA, London. www.nta.nhs.uk

National Treatment Agency (2003) *Black and Minority Ethnic Communities: a Review of the Literature on Drug Use and Related Service Provision*. NTA, London. www.nta.nhs.uk

Nazroo, J.Y. (1997) *Ethnicity and Mental Health: Findings from a National Community* Survey. Policy Studies Institute, London.

Nazroo, J. & King, M. (2002) Psychosis – symptoms and estimated rates. In: *Ethnic Minority Psychiatric Illness Rates in the Community (Empiric)*, (Sproston, K. & Nazroo, J., eds). National Centre for Social Research, TSO, London.

Neeleman, J. & Farrell, M. (1997) Suicide and substance misuse. *British Journal of Psychiatry*, 175, 303–4.

Nursing and Midwifery Council (2004) *The NMC Code of Professional Conduct: Standards for Conduct, Performance and Ethics*. www.nmc-uk.org

OPCS (2001) *The 2001 Census of Population – Ethnicity and Religion in England and Wales*, Cm. 4253. The Stationery Office, London.

Oyefeso, A. & Ghodse, A.H. (1993) *Addictive Behaviour in Ethnic Minorities*. Paper presented at the National Workshop on Assessing the Health Needs of People from Ethnic Minorities, London.

Oyefeso, A., Ghodse, H., Keating, A. *et al*. (2000) *Drug Treatment Needs of Black and Ethnic Minority Residents of the London Borough of Merton*. Addictions Resource Agency for Commissioners (ARAC) Monograph Series on Ethnic Minority Issues. ARAC, London.

Papadopoulos, I., Tilki, M. & Taylor, G. (1998) *Transcultural Care: a Guide for Health Care Professionals*. Quay Books, Wilts.

Parker, H., Measham, F. & Aldridge, J. (1995) *Drug Futures: Changing Patterns of Drug Use Among English Youth*. Institute for the Study of Drug Dependence (ISDD), Research Monograph 7, London.

Patel, K. (1998) A preliminary enquiry into the nature, extent and responses to drug problems (if any) within the Asian population of Bradford. *Social Work Education*, 8 (1), 39–41.

Patel, K., Pearson, G. & Khan, F. (1995) *Outreach Work Among Asian Drug Injectors in Bradford*. A report to the Mental Health Foundation, Bradford. The Bridge Project, Goldsmith's College, University of London.

Patel, K. Sherlock, K., Chaudry, M. & Buffin, J. (1998) *Drug Use Amongst Asian Communities in Cheetham Hill*. Manchester Lifeline/University of Central Lancashire, Preston.

Patel, K. (2000) Minority ethnic drug use: the missing minorities. In: *Substance Misuse: Its Effects on Families and Child Protection* (Harbin, F. & Murphy-Russell, J., eds). Russell House, Lyme Regis.

Patel, K., Wardle, I., Bashford, J. & Winters, M. (2001) *The Evaluation of Nafas – a Bangladeshi Drug Service*. Ethnicity and Health Unit, Faculty of Health, University of Central Lancashire, Preston.

Pearson, G. & Patel, K. (1998) Drugs, deprivation, and ethnicity: outreach among Asian drug users in a northern English city. *Journal of Drug Issues*, 28 (1), 199–224.

Perera, J. (1996) *Drug Misuse in Bedfordshire: Preliminary Report to Inform Further Assessment Research*. Report to Public Health Specialist and DAT Coordinator. November Action Research Consultancies, London.

Perera, J. (1998) *Assessing the Drugs Information Needs of Asian Parents in North Hertfordshire: a Brief Report to Inform the Planning of a Drugs Education Programme*. Action Research Consultancies, London.

Perera, J., Power R. & Gibson, N. (1993) *Assessing the Needs of Black Drug Users in North Westminster*. Hungerford Drug Project/Centre for Research in Drugs and Health Behaviour, London.

Raleigh, V.S. (1996) Suicide patterns and trends in people of Indian subcontinent and Caribbean origin in England and Wales. *Ethnicity and Health*, 1 (1), 55–63.

Raleigh, V.S., Bulusu, L. & Balarajan, R. (1990) Suicides among immigrants from the Indian Subcontinent. *British Journal of Psychiatry*, 156, 46–50.

Raleigh, V.S. & Balarajan, R. (1992) Suicide levels and trends among immigrants in England and Wales. *Health Trends*, 24 (3), 91–4.

Ram, H. (2000) *Asian Communities Project Report to National Lottery Charities Board*. Dudley Drug Project, The Wavehouse, Dudley.

Ramsey, M. & Spiller, J. (1997) *Drug Misuse Declared: Results of the 1996 British Crime Survey*. Home Office, London.

Ramsey, M., Baker, P., Goulden, C., Sharp, C. & Sondhi, A. (2001) Drug misuse declared in 2000: results from the British Crime Survey. *Home Office Research Study 224*. Home Office Research, Development and Statistics Directorate, Home Office, London.

Rassool, G.H. (1995) The health status and health care of ethno-cultural minorities in the United Kingdom: an agenda for action. *Journal of Advanced Nursing*, 21, 199–201.

Rassool, G.H. (1997) Ethnic minorities and substance misuse. In: *Addiction Nursing: Perspectives on Professional and Clinical Practice*. (Rassool, G.H. & Gafoor, M., eds). Stanley Nelson, Cheltenham.

Sainsbury Centre for Mental Health (2002) *Breaking the Circles of Fear: A Review of the Relationship Between Mental Health Services and the African and Caribbean Communities*. SCMH, London.

Sangster, D., Shiner, M., Sheikh, N. & Patel, K. (2002) *Delivering Drug Services to Black and Ethnic Minority Communities*. DPAS/P16. Home Office Drug Prevention and Advisory Service (DPAS), London. http://www.drugs.gov.uk

Sashidaran, S.P. (2002) *Inside Outside: Improving Mental Health Services for Black and Minority Ethnic Communities in England*. Department of Health, London.

Sheikh, N., Fountain, J., Bashford, J. & Patel, K. (2001) *A Review of Current Drug Service Provision for Black and Ethnic Minority Communities in Bedfordshire*. Final report to Bedfordshire Drug Action Team, August 2001. Centre for Ethnicity and Health, Faculty of Health, University of Central Lancashire, Preston.

Sherlock, K., Patel, K. & Chaudry, M. (1997) Drugs and Ethnic Health Project: Research Report. West Pennine Drug Action Team. Lifeline, Manchester.

Singleton, N., Bumpstead, R., *et al*., (2001) *Psychiatric Morbidity Among Adults Living in Private Households, 2000*. The Stationery Office, London.

Smaje, C. & LeGrand, J. (1997) Ethnicity, equity and the use of health services in the British National Health Service. *Social Science and Medicine*, 45, 485–96.

Sproston, K. & Nazroo, J. (eds) (2000) *Ethnic Minority Psychiatric Illness Rates in the Community (Empiric)*, Quantitative Report. The Stationery Office, London.

Sproston, K. & Nazroo, J. (eds) (2002) *Ethnic Minority Psychiatric Illness Rates in the Community (Empiric)*. National Centre for Social Research, TSO, London. http:officialdocuments.co.uk/document/doh/empiric/empiric.htm
http://www.doh.gov.uk/public/surveys.htm

Subhra, G. & Chauhan, V. (1999) *Developing Black Services: an Evaluation of the African, Caribbean and Asian Services funded by Alcohol Concern's Grants Programme*. Alcohol Concern, London.

Webster, R. (2001) *An Assessment of the Substance Misuse Treatment Needs of Young People in Bedfordshire*. Report to Bedfordshire Health Authority, Bedford.

Whitley, E., Gunnell, D., Doring, D. & Davey Smith, G. (1999) Ecological study of social fragmentation, poverty and suicide. *British Medical Journal*, 319, 1034–7.

Whittington, D. (1999): Nang tien nan: princess opium in Deptford. *Druglink*, September/October, 13–14.

Winstock, A.R., Trivedy, C.R., Warnakulasuriya, K.A.A.S. & Peters, T.J. (2000) A dependency syndrome related to areca nut use: some medical and psychological aspects among areca nut users in the Gujarat community in the UK. *Addiction Biology*, 5, 173–9.

World Health Organization (2003) *International Classification of Diseases – 10*. http://www.who.int/classifications/icd/en/

Wright, S., Bindman, J., Thornicroft, G. & Butcher, M. (2000) *Thematic Review of NHS R & D funded Mental Health Research in Relation to the National Service Framework for Mental Health*. Health Services Research Department, Institute of Psychiatry, London.

10 Vulnerable Young People and Substance Misuse

M. Epling & J. McGregor

Introduction

As young people grow up they may become involved in experimentation and occasional use of alcohol and drugs, usually in specific culturally accepted situations. Experimentation with substances, and with other risk taking behaviours, may be seen as reflecting adolescent normative behaviour. Definitions of use and misuse, or terms such as abuse, depend to some extent on a society's acceptance and tolerance of use (see Chapter 3). Little is actually known about the role of mental health disorders in increasing the risk of children and adolescents for misuse of substances. Stress appears to play a role in both the process and the development of many of the problems young people face. The terms co-morbidity, dual diagnosis and concurrent disorder are often used interchangeably. Young, vulnerable people who use substances, be it drugs and/or alcohol, are a remarkably heterogeneous group. To be exclusive would ignore the diversity.

The drug experience

Setting

Children are in a state of rapid change and growth during their developmental years. Diagnosis and interventions with young people's mental health problems must be viewed with these changes in mind. While some problems are short-lived and may not require intervention, others may be persistent and more serious. Adolescence is the period in life characterised by significant change. Biological, psychological and social learning changes occur at an astonishing rate (Lerner *et al.*, 1980). It is also a time when young people are particularly impressionable and vulnerable to many environmental factors (Fullerton & Ursano, 1994) that positively or negatively influence their future health behaviours. Adults often perceive adolescents as both difficult and disruptive. The developmental tasks during adolescence are to establish a sense of identity, to move from a predominantly family focus to a peer group focus, and to prepare for independence. It is also a period of emerging sexuality.

Services that young people access must reflect their age, ability and maturity. It is no longer the preserve of health care professionals alone to engage and provide care and treatment to young people with substance misuse and mental health problems. All professionals working with young people should be able to respond to substance misuse constructively and according to good practice. Identifying substance misuse and psychosocial needs is crucial to meeting gaps in a young person's knowledge and identifying those children and young people who may be experiencing problems or engaging in risky activity due to their substance use. Progression from childhood through to adolescence is already one of the most confusing and uprooting periods of an individual's life. When a young person approaches a service for help, the network of services should reflect this delicate period of developmental transition.

Drugs

Most young people will enjoy improved health and education, wealth and greater longevity than their parents. A minority of young people 'face a combination of problems' that may increase the psychosocial vulnerability of children and young people (Prosser & McArdle, 1996).

In the UK the risk of drug and alcohol use and misuse is not uniformly distributed through the general youth population. Measham *et al.* (1998) reported on the 'unprecedented rise' in youth drug use in the mid-1990s amongst adolescents from diverse backgrounds, sometimes within the context of the dance culture and against a background of increasing availability and popularity. The drugs predominantly used are cannabis, followed by dance drugs, amphetamines, LSD and ecstasy (methylenedioxymethamphetamine), with a minority using heroin and crack cocaine. This polydrug culture is particularly common among young drug users. However, the *British Crime Survey* (Ramsey & Spiller, 1997) reported that, with the exception of cannabis, levels of use tend to be lower in ethnic minority communities than among whites. British teenagers, along with those in Ireland and Denmark, are among the heaviest teenage drinkers in Europe: they are more likely to drink, to get drunk and to report problems associated with drinking than their counterparts in other European countries. In the UK, more than a third of 15-year-olds report having been drunk at age 13 or earlier. This is true of no more than one in ten French and Italian children (Hibell *et al.*, 2000; Hebbell *et al.*, 2003).

There are a number of 'risk' factors that may make young people vulnerable to drug misuse. 'Curiosity' is often given as the main reason for trying drugs. Of those who experiment with drugs, the majority do not continue to use them on a regular basis. In a small but significant minority, use escalates to intensive levels. Particular groups of young people have much higher levels of drug use than those found in the general national population. These are often young people who have been excluded from school or have truanted, committed a crime, been homeless or run away from home and those whose siblings are drug users (Lloyd, 1998; Swadi, 1999; Goulden & Sondhi, 2001; Hammersley *et al.*, 2003).

Young people who are, or are likely to start, misusing drugs are also very likely to have other health, social or emotional problems as well as problems at home or school (Lerner & Vicary, 1984; Shedler & Block, 1990; Hawkins *et al.*, 1992). There are a range of factors identified as being associated with problematic substance use during adolescence, and/or as playing a role in the later development of drug problems. Chronic substance misuse can seriously affect social competence, impair learning and create a culture of unemployment, alienation and social exclusion. Serious mental health problems in young people often erode a positive self-concept – a situation that is likely to be compounded by substance misuse.

Alcohol and drug use may be associated with increased dropout from school, poor educational attainment, drink and drug driving, antisocial behaviour, early pregnancy and family difficulties. Substance misuse may place a vulnerable young person at greater risk of suicide, depression, conduct disorder, school dropout and poor educational attainment. For these reasons, the use and misuse of licit and illicit drugs amongst young, vulnerable people has become a cause of public and professional concern.

Some authors (Parker *et al.*, 1998) report what has been termed 'normalisation' of substance use – seeing drug and alcohol use as 'normal' exploratory risk taking behaviour. The majority of young people who experiment with drugs cease use in adulthood, with a minority exhibiting continued problems. However, others argue that any sustained use in adolescence predicts later use, and is usually problematic in its own right. Zoccolillo *et al.* (1999) reported that little attention had focused on 'problem' drug use in young people. In fact, he concluded that problem drug use was the 'norm' among the minority that used drugs more than a few times.

Set

If 'vulnerable' young people do use drugs, they start on average at an earlier age than other young people generally do. Young drug users have generally tried an illegal drug by the age of 13 if not before, and are likely to smoke cigarettes and drink alcohol with some degree of regularity. While this does not mean that all of them are experiencing problems related to that drug use, early initiation has itself been shown to be associated with the development of drug problems in later adolescence or adulthood. Early sexual activity also appears to start for many around the same age as their drug use; subsequent pregnancy and parenthood is a cause for concern. This is the period following the transition to secondary school, which studies suggest is a vulnerable time. Several reports speak of young people's progressive disengagement from school during this period, even if not excluded, paralleled with poor levels of supervision in the home.

Vulnerable young people misusing substances display increased service uptake, worsened clinical outcome and increased rates of deliberate self-harm and suicide (Wilens *et al.*, 1997). Longitudinal studies indicate that early severe behaviour problems often characterise the history of those who later misuse substances. Studies of these behaviour problems indicate that the children, usually boys, suffer from a cluster of underlying and often unrecognised developmental vulnerabilities. These include levels of concentration, impulsivity and attention span that are often quite markedly impaired for their age. Some of these young people become so distressed by their failure and by the perceived failure of adults to respond to their distress, that they become angry, antagonistic and mistrustful, rejecting the values of their adult carers.

Many young males will have experienced these patterns of vulnerability and distress. During adolescence, they cannot concentrate, do not see consequences, cannot plan, may be sensation seeking, and through experience they mistrust adults. They often suffer depressive and anxiety symptoms that they do not readily disclose. These young people often value the immediate and illicit rewards afforded by their peer groups. These intrinsic vulnerabilities often stress parents or carers so that the quality of family life deteriorates.

Treatment experience

Early identification, careful assessment and early intervention is crucial to enable appropriate responses. Vulnerable young people are often the most difficult to engage, and require quite intensive, assertive, extended, often inter-agency intervention (Henggeler *et al.*, 1996). A further implication is that treatment will need to address a range of pressing issues in addition to the substance related problem. It is likely that the adversities, such as the experience of being homeless and otherwise socially excluded, further increase risk. Some groups at risk of use and misuse may not be included in school and household surveys. Most of these young people will have mental health problems in addition to high rates of alcohol and drug use/misuse. Among runaways and homeless youths, drug misuse probably contributes to, and exacerbates, their homeless situation and mental health problems.

Setting

Screening, assessment and treatment are not distinct entities, but rather integrated and overlapping parts of the whole process. We take the view that drug treatment should mirror the concept of drug, set, setting (Figure 10.1). The treatment experience should match the drug experience (Figure 10.2). For

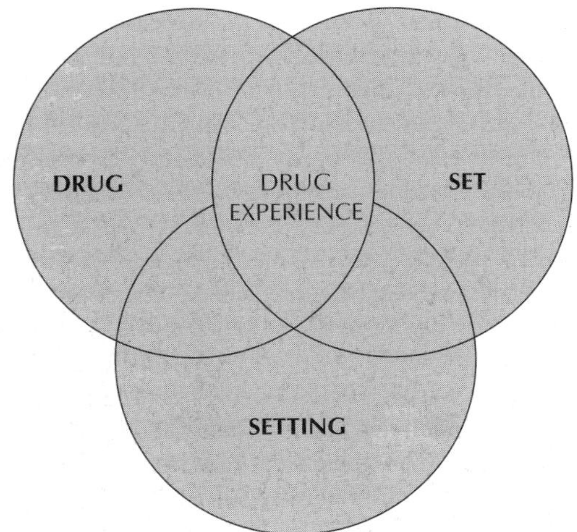

Figure 10.1 Understanding the drug experience. Source: Zinberg (1984).

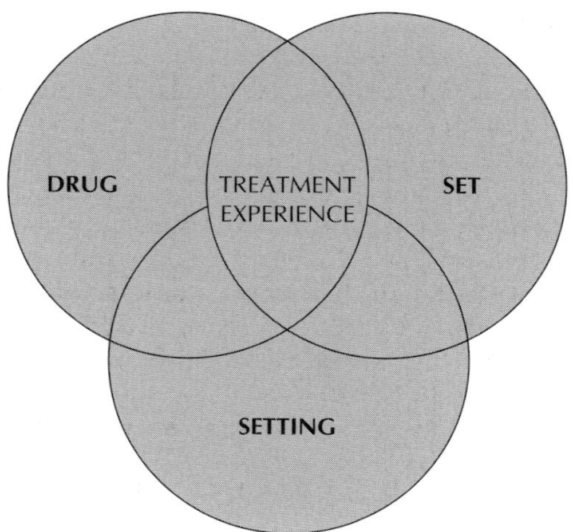

Figure 10.2 Treating the drug experience.

example, if the young person smokes cannabis (**drug**) with their friends (**set**) at a youth club (**setting**) then these should be factored into the treatment experience. Hence, the treatment is preferably experienced as an intervention that may include peers, at the youth club rather than independently attending a sterile, clinical environment that is not youth friendly.

Service providers must carefully adjust the engagement process to fit the young person's needs. This could mean, for example, that treatment could occur in a friend's house. Specific outreach and information strategies go beyond the traditional means of supplying promotional materials and information. It is important to have a spectrum of outreach activities, for example prevention activities, workshops and training. Service philosophy and approach are key elements for effective programmes.

Young people are not a homogeneous group. It is important that service providers enjoy working with young people. Interventions should be based on values of acceptance, non-judgemental approaches, respectful interactions and be sensitive to cultural differences. The location of services and accessibility are critical factors to the success of any treatment. It is important to create an environment that is 'youth friendly' and flexible in terms of hours of operation, for example drop-in, and flexible in terms of location, for example satellites and community based. Few services are adolescent specific. Sometimes, more categorical services are offered, such as sexually transmitted infection or drug and alcohol clinics. Although these clinics may serve a problem specific constituency, they are not usually designed for adolescents and are rarely adolescent friendly. Vulnerable young people require more targeted, locally relevant, comprehensive services.

Set

To properly address the needs of the young people they need to be involved in the planning, implementation and evaluation of services. The promotion of adolescent health care is a collaborative challenge (Bennett & Reed, 1997), requiring health professionals to look beyond the obvious in their dealings with young people, to support families, to create alliances for health and to broaden the horizons of advocacy.

Parents and carers have an important role in supporting young people. Many people are misinformed about substances, are confused by mixed messages in the media or have the knowledge but do not know how to deal with a substance related incident involving someone in their family. Parents and carers may require basic substance information, information on different interventions and how best they can support their child. Services need to consider how parents and carers can be supported so that they can help their child in addressing their substance use. This could be through drug education or parent self-help groups.

Caring, communication, cohesion and supervision aspects of relationships between parents and children have been associated with an effect on a range of substance use and other problematic behaviours amongst young people (Duncan *et al.*, 1995; Mistral & Velleman, 1997). Parental behaviours can be important 'protective factors' against drug use among young people. These include: the development of strong parent–child bonds; effective levels of parent–child communication; and the exercising of parental supervision involving clear rules. Engaging parents is therefore a key area of work for drugs prevention.

UK surveys have shown that up to 90% of parents believe that young people's drug use derives from the need to conform with their peer group (Williams, 1996; Evans *et al.*, 1997; Hiley, 1997). Indeed, family and peer groups may be mutually influential (Parke & Ladd, 1992). Too great an emphasis on peer pressure, however, may lead parents to underestimate their own influence on children, which, though it varies at different ages, has been shown to affect young people's long-term behaviour (Oygard *et al.*, 1995). Family factors impact not only on initiation into substance use but also on problematic use (Health Advisory Service, 1996), and 'a family centred intervention is particularly important in steering young people away from potential drug using careers' (Farrell & Strang, 1991). Involving parents in drug prevention activities may be seen as a way of reinforcing and ensuring consistency, with drug prevention messages delivered via other channels. It can harness parents' concerns about drugs; increase their confidence in talking to their children about drugs; and modify the behaviour of their children.

There has been a developing interest in appropriate and effective responses to adolescent drug and alcohol use and misuse. These should include:

- Attention to the developmental needs of young people
- Any delay in normal cognitive and socio-emotional development should be recognised
- Programmes should involve families
- Not all young people who use drugs will be dependent on them
- The young person in treatment often has multiple needs, including mental health problems, that must be recognised and treated
- Adult programmes should not be a substitute for youth centred approaches

It is crucial to recognise that treatments cannot simply be taken off the shelf. For instance, family therapy might be chosen in a particular case, also with school liaison and agreement about a course of action with a youth worker and a family social worker. Most of the treatment research is US based. Catalano *et al.* (1990) reviewed 29 treatment outcome studies and reported that 'some' treatment was superior to 'no' treatment. Deas & Thomas (2001) reported on ten controlled studies since 1990, with positive effects noted for family therapy. Studies using behavioural and cognitive behavioural therapy were associated with improvements in drug use, school and work attendance.

Influences on outcome include levels of motivation, peer influences, family factors, and pre-treatment severity of legal problems, deviant behaviour, school problems and psychiatric severity. While causal direction is somewhat debated, those adolescents with co-morbid disorders often have poor outcomes and, like adults, demonstrate poor treatment compliance, more chronic psychosocial problems and poor long-term outcome (Westmeyer *et al.*, 1998).

Any substance misuse specific interventions should be embedded in the individual, familial, cultural and developmental background of the young person. Intervention should take into account family attachments, educational needs, physical and psychological health, sexual and physical health, any child protection concerns, peer relationships and psychological distress. Interventions should follow a comprehensive assessment and be part of an overall care and management plan, adapted to the intensity and complexity of the presenting problems. Interventions may range from simple information, advice and support. It may adopt the adolescent's own personal efforts to change without formal treatment. Many young people who use drugs and alcohol, even sometimes problematically and in high-risk situations, gradually cease use. Others, however, continue to use problematically into adulthood. This natural recovery or change may be explained by changes in school, friends, family and other environmental influences that can affect development.

Information and advice

Accurate advice must not only address abstinence, but should also include up-to-date advice and information on responses to intoxication, harm reduction strategies in clubs, overdose and related sexual or physical health. There is considerable evidence from other health and social care fields that this information based approach has useful effects with non-complex presentations (Richmond *et al.*, 1986; Powell *et al.*, 2001). Peer support and advice is a related low-cost intervention that has also proven useful in other health care fields (Shah *et al.*, 2001).

Counselling

Counselling is an intervention that includes a diversity of theoretical models, commonly delivered by community services. The term is often applied to a range of techniques that encompass assessment, engagement and support, the development of therapeutic relationships, self-monitoring, advice and problem-solving techniques, motivational work and relapse prevention. It may apply also to advice on a range of other lifestyle issues such as housing, sexual health and career. It may be attributed to early interventions to reduce use of alcohol and drugs and negative consequences or related problems. According to Wagner *et al.* (1999), components of counselling include information, including substance related education, recognition of problems and self-monitoring, identification of high risk behaviours, family conflict resolution, social supports and alternatives to substance use, a range of coping strategies and advice on relationships.

A great strength of counselling is that potentially it impacts on all relevant aspects of the lifestyle of the young person and not just drug use or misuse. However, whilst it is a commonly applied approach, research on the effectiveness of varieties of counselling techniques for young people's substance use is almost non-existent.

Brief interventions

These interventions may consist of a range of therapies based on the stages of change model: brief advice supported by self-help materials, condensed cognitive behavioural therapy or motivational interviewing. There is good evidence of effectiveness in primary care settings, in A & E and other medical settings, and in educational settings, though evidence in this setting is confined to the USA. Research from the USA has produced some promising results when applied to young people. However, there is an urgent need for research specifically directed to young people in the UK and elsewhere. Ingenuity may be required to identify the settings where young drinkers or drug users may be found.

Individual psychological therapies

Individual psychological therapies such as cognitive and behavioural approaches, motivational interviewing techniques and relapse prevention intervention approaches have received strong empirical support. Moreover, components of these interventions, such as coping skills training, anger management, problem solving, self-monitoring, both alone and together with brief interventions, are in common use but have received little research attention.

Pharmacological therapies

Pharmacotherapy is directed at a number of specific areas: treatment of overdose in emergencies, detoxification, substitution or maintenance therapy, adjuncts to relapse prevention as well as treatment of co-morbid disorders. It should be used in conjunction with a comprehensive plan incorporating a variety of individual interventions (education, psychotherapies) designed to meet the needs of the young person. Prior to prescribing, issues of consent to treatment, involvement of parents, confidentiality and competence of the prescriber must be ascertained. The service must also have appropriate protocols and procedures in place for assessment and titration of drugs, observation and supervised dispensing, and liaison with other agencies.

Little research on the role of pharmacological therapies for addiction has been conducted in adolescents. Both opiates and benzodiazepines have specific pharmacological antagonists; naloxone is useful in emergency settings. General practitioners and paramedics should have naloxone available (Department of Health, 1999). The majority of adolescents are not dependent and so do not generally require detoxification. Some symptomatic treatment, if required, may be useful if there are mild withdrawal symptoms. Correct dosage requires particular care depending on size and age. Furthermore, the possibility of misuse of the medication prescribed must always be considered. The pharmacological management of young drug misusers is very difficult. Many of the medications are not licensed in children.

Despite the fact that controlled research demonstrates the effectiveness of methadone maintenance in adulthood, very few practitioners would see maintenance as a primary goal in adolescents and it is generally not advocated in this population. Nevertheless, there are a small but significant number of young or very young heroin users presenting to services in England. Some may require intervention and have derived benefit from methadone stabilisation and slow reduction (Crome *et al.*, 1999).

Many young people with complex problems co-occurring with substance use have conditions that can be ameliorated by pharmacological means, often as an adjunct to other interventions, or sometimes as the main intervention. The classic example is depressive disorders, which among adolescents, but probably not children, may respond to antidepressant medication. Occasionally, children and young people will present to services with psychotic conditions requiring appropriate pharmacological management. Many young people with complex problems have impaired ability to relate and to communicate, linked with marked attentional problems. There may occasionally be a role for central nervous stimulants in the treatment of these individuals but this is still an area of much discussion.

Family therapies

Functional family therapy, which incorporates current psychological concepts (cognitive, behavioural and systems ideas) in a pragmatic fashion, is a currently recommended form for vulnerable young people (Kazdin, 2001). Family therapies have also been shown to be effective in the management of young people's substance problems and for these reasons should generally be incorporated into any treatment plan if possible (Gilvarry, 2000). Clearly, the extent of involvement will depend on the nature of the problem and the age of the child.

Group therapy

Group therapy has been evaluated, but if groups consist solely of substance using young people, they may be associated with harm. Nevertheless, if groups are selected with care and are heterogeneous, they can be a useful component of interventions. The impact of school based groups in particular have been evaluated in the UK and proved particularly valuable in sustained improvement in general social and behavioural development (Kolvin *et al.*, 1981; McArdle *et al.*, 2001).

Twelve-step approach

This is a philosophy as much as a treatment, often delivered in group settings, and is at the heart of most of the treatment approaches in the USA. However, apart from one research report (Winters, 2000) there is limited evidence for its effectiveness amongst adolescents. The insistence on abstinence as a primary and immediate goal may discourage engagement and retention of some young people. A harm reduction approach may be more acceptable, at least as an interim measure, for many.

Residential settings

A few studies have reported that long-term residential treatments are relatively effective, with length of stay crucial. The most consistent outcome is that of improvement in criminal involvement. Some programmes specifically address substance misuse, though others are more comprehensive, encompassing education and psychological therapies. Consideration could be given to adapting those adolescent units that do exist to deliver substance specific interventions.

Aftercare and follow-up

The purpose of follow-up would be to provide a source of stability, advocacy and a route into additional interventions should the need arise. Contact need not be so frequent so that resources are necessarily very substantial, but tracking mechanisms might be necessary to systematically develop an effective aftercare scheme. A summary of treatment experience is presented in Table 10.1.

Vulnerable populations

Particular groups of vulnerable young people require attention. Some of these, though not all,

Table 10.1 Enhancing the treatment experience.

Treatment modalities
• Information and advice giving • Psychological therapies — Counselling — Brief interventions — Individual psychological therapies • Pharmacological therapies • Family therapy • Group/peer therapy • Twelve-step approach • Residential treatment • Aftercare/follow-up

may include young people in touch with the juvenile justice system, the homeless, young people who are pregnant or who are parents, young asylum seekers, those with multiple (physical and mental health) problems, those who have been and are sexually exploited, the 'hard to engage' and those with learning and other disabilities. Working with vulnerable children and young people can be very complex. Child protection assessments should consider four important parameters:

- The age and maturity of the child
- The degree of seriousness of drug misuse
- Whether harm is continuing or increasing
- The general context in which drug-taking is set

For those in the criminal justice system, treatment for substance use should be delivered alongside other programmes to prevent the possibility of relapse of criminal offences and promote active involvement and social inclusion. Research indicates that those young people who are homeless and often not in touch with services are highly vulnerable and are a difficult population to engage and retain in treatment. They require more assertive outreach services and new methods of service delivery that encourage engagement and retention in services. They may be homeless, have run away from care, be sexually exploited and are often involved in criminal activities. A wide range of techniques need to be in place to facilitate engagement. These might include contact in numerous settings, use of mobile phone contacts, weekend and night hours of contact, mobile physical care units and emergency shelter. Street outreach workers may require time to engage and should focus on immediate needs and care and development of relationships.

Conclusion

Engaging young people

- Identify their concerns, highlight their strengths, lay the foundation for the treatment plan, allow for appropriate referrals, provide feedback and collect data to measure outcomes. Whilst these functions all need to be addressed it is not necessary to do them all during the first interview. Assessment can be accomplished in a variety of ways, for example over the phone, face to face, in groups or in youth recreational facilities.

Needs and barriers to treatment

- Identify the young person's needs and barriers to treatment. It may be useful to involve the people who can contribute to resolving problems in the assessment process, for example family, siblings, community members.
- Drug use history and consequences, physical and mental health, family functioning, peer relations, school and work performance, leisure activities and spiritual life are all important domains that should be considered in the young person's assessment. Often 'staged assessments' are undertaken to provide the time needed for the development of trust. It is important to explain to young people what to expect in the assessment process and what benefits they will be likely to gain.
- Education and awareness groups offer a way to familiarise young people with the process. It will help engage young people in a fun way prior to assessment and will help develop a rapport and a sense of trust with staff.
- Appropriate gender matching between client and service provider may help in the development of a trusting relationship.

Overall, management requires inter-agency working, including housing, addressing family problems, educational needs assessment and delivery of vocational advice, physical and mental health care, as well as substance specific care and interventions. It is no longer the preserve of stand-alone professions to engage and provide care and interventions to young people with substance misuse and mental health problems. Young vulnerable people who use substances, be it drugs and/or alcohol, are a heterogeneous group and it would be excluding to ignore their diversity. Services that young people access must reflect their age, ability and maturity.

References

Bennett, D.L. & Reed, M.S. (1997) Adolescent health care: a collaborative challenge. *Hong Kong Journal of Paediatris*, 2, 108–15.

Catalano, R., Hawkins, J., Wells, E., Miller, J. & Brewer, D. (1990) Evaluation of the effectiveness of adolescent drug abuse treatment, assessment of risks for relapse, and promising approaches for relapse prevention. *International Journal of the Addictions*, 25,1085–140.

Crome, I., Christian, J. & Green, C. (1999) A unique designated community service for adolescents: policy, prevention and education implications. *Drugs: Education, Prevention and Policy*, 7, 87–108.

Deas, D. & Thomas, S. (2001) An overview of controlled studies of adolescent substance abuse treatment. *American Journal of Addiction*, 10, 178–89.

Department of Health (1999) *Drug Misuse and Dependence; Guidelines on Clinical Management*. The Stationery Office, London.

Duncan, T.E., Tildesley, E., Duncan, S.C. & Hops, H. (1995) The consistency of family and peer influences on the development of substance use in adolescence. *Addiction*, 90, 1647–60.

Evans, R., Mallick, J. & Stein, G. (1997) *The Concerns and Needs Expressed by Parents of Children in Kent Schools Regarding Drug Use and Drug Education Strategies.* Report commissioned by Kent County Constabulary on behalf of the Safer Kent Partnership Forum and the East Kent Health Authority. Roehampton Institute, London.

Farrell, M. & Strang, J. (1991) Substance use and misuse in childhood and adolescence. *Journal of Child Psychology & Psychiatry*, 32, 109–28.

Fullerton, C.S. & Ursano, R.J. (1994) Preadolescent peer friendships: a critical contribution to adult social relatedness. *Journal of Youth and Adolescence*, 23 (43), 64.

Gilvarry, E. (2000) Substance abuse in young people. *Journal of Child Psychology and Psychiatry*, 41, 55–80.

Goulden, C. & Sondhi, A. (2001) *At the Margins: Drug Use by Vulnerable Young People in the 1998/99 Youth Lifestyles Survey*. Home Office Research Study 228, Home Office, London.

Hammersley, R., Marsland, L. & Reid, M. (2003) *Substance Use by Young Offenders: the Impact of the Normalisation of Drug Use in the Early Years of the 21st Century*. Home Office Research Study 261, Home Office, London.

Hawkins, J.D., Catalano, R.F. & Miller, J.Y. (1992) Risk and protective factors for alcohol and other drug problems in adolescence and early childhood: implications for substance abuse prevention. *Psychological Bulletin*, 112 (1), 64–5.

Health Advisory Service (1996) *Children and Young People's Substance Misuse Services: The Substance of Young Need*. HMSO, London.

Hebbell, B., Andersson, B., Bjarnasson, T. *et al.* (2003) *IAS Fact Sheet – Young People and Alcohol. ESPAD Report 2003: Alcohol and Other Drug Use Among Students in 35 European Countries*. Produced by Institute of Alcohol Studies, St Ives, Cambs.

Henggeler, S., Pickrel, S., Brondino, M. & Crouch, J. (1996) Eliminating (almost) treatment dropout of substance abusing or dependent delinquents through home-based multi-systemic therapy. *American Journal of Psychiatry*, 153, 427–8.

Hibell, B., Andersson, B., Ahlström, S. *et al.* (2000) *The 1999 ESPAD Report. Alcohol and Other Drug Use Among Students in 30 European Countries*. The Swedish Council for Information on Alcohol and Other Drugs (CAN), Stockholm.

Hiley, J. (1997) *Perceptions of Drug Use*. Report for St Ann's and Sneinton Drug Prevention Project, Nottingham.

Kazdin, A. (2001) Treatment of conduct disorders. In: *Conduct Disorders in Childhood and Adolescence*. (Hill, J. & Maughan, B., eds) Cambridge University Press, Cambridge.

Kolvin, I., Garside, R., Nicol, A., Macmillan, A., Wolstenholme, F. & Leitch, I. (1981) *Help Starts Here: The Maladjusted Child in the Ordinary School*. Tavistock Publications, London.

Lerner, R. (1980) *Adolescent Development*. McGraw-Hill, New York.

Lerner, J.V. & Vicary, J.R. (1984) Difficult temperament and drug use: analyses from the New York longitudinal study. *Journal of Drug Education*, 14, 1–8.

Lloyd, C. (1998) Risk factors for problem drug use: identifying vulnerable groups. *Drugs, Education, Prevention and Policy*, 5 (3).

McArdle, P., Moseley, D., Quibell, T. *et al.* (2001) Randomised trial of school based indicated prevention using group therapy. In: *The Substance of Young Needs*. Health Advisory Service (HAS) review 2001, London.

Measham, F., Parker, H. & Aldridge, J. (1998) The teenage transition: from adolescent recreational drug use to the young adult dance culture in Britain in the mid-1990s. *Journal of Drug Issues*, 28, 9–32.

Mistral, W. & Velleman, R. (1997) *Involving Parents in*

Drug Prevention: a Review of the Literature. Report prepared for the Home Office Drugs Prevention Initiative. Mental Health Research Unit, University of Bath.

Oygard, L., Klepp, K.I., Tell, G.S. & Vellar, O.D. (1995) Parental and peer influences among young adults: ten-year follow-up of the Oslo youth study participants. *Addiction*, 90, 561–9.

Parke, R.D. & Ladd, G.W. (eds) (1992) *Family-peer Relationships: Modes of Linkages*. Lawrence Erlbaum Associates, Hillsdale, NJ.

Parker, H., Aldridge, J. & Measham, F. (1998) *Illegal Leisure: the Normalisation of Adolescent Recreational Drug Use*. Routledge, London.

Powell, T., Yeaton, W., Hill, E.M. & Silk, K. (2001) Predictors of psychosocial outcomes for patients with mood disorders: effects of self-help group participation. *Psychiatric Rehabilitation Journal*, 25 (1), 3–11.

Prosser, J. & McArdle, P. (1996) The changing mental health of children and adolescents: evidence for a deterioration? *Psychological Medicine*, 26, 715–25.

Ramsey, M. & Spiller, J. (1997) *Drug Use Declared: Results of the 1996 British Crime Survey*. Home Office, London.

Richmond, R., Austin, A. & Webster, I.W. (1986) Three-year evaluation of a programme by general practitioners to help patients to stop smoking. *British Medical Journal*, 22, 292 (6823), 803–4.

Shah, S., Peat, J., Mazurski, E., Wang, H., Sindhusake, D. & Bruce, C. (2001) Effect of peer-led programmes for asthma education in adolescence: a randomised controlled trial. *British Medical Journal*, 10, 322 (7286), 583–5.

Shedler, J. & Block, J. (1990) Adolescent drug use and psychological health: longitudinal inquiry. *American Psychologist*, 45, 612–30.

Swadi, H. (1999) Individual risk factors for adolescent substance use. *Drug and Alcohol Dependence*, 55, 209–24.

Wagner, E., Brown, S., Monti, P., Myers, N. & Waldron, H. (1999) Innovations in adolescent substance abuse interventions. *Alcoholism: Clinical and Experimental Research*, 23 (2), 236–49.

Westmeyer, J., Eames, S. & Nugent, S. (1998) Co-morbid dysthymia and substance abuse disorder: treatment history and cost. *American Journal of Psychiatry*, 155, 1556–60.

Wilens, T., Biederman, J., Abrantes, A. & Spencer, T. (1997) Clinical characteristics of psychiatrically referred adolescent outpatients with substance use disorder. *Journal of the American Academy of Child and Adolescent Psychiatry*, 36, 941–7.

Williams, T. (1996) *Integrated Programme: Parents' Surveys. Central Drugs Prevention Unit Internal Memorandum*. November 1996. Home Office, London.

Winters, K.C., Stinchfield, R.D., Opland, E., Weller, C. & Latimer, W.W. (2000) The effectiveness of the Minnesota model approach in the treatment of adolescent drug abusers. *Addiction*, 95 (4), 601–12.

Zinberg, N. (1984) *Drug, Set and Setting; the Basis of Controlled Intoxicant Use*. Yale University Press, New Haven/London.

Zoccolillo, M., Vitaro, F. & Tremblay, R. (1999) Problem drug and alcohol use in a community sample of adolescents. *Journal of American Academy of Child and Adolescent Psychiatry*, 38 (7), 900–7.

11 Meeting Multiple Needs: Pregnancy, Parenting and Dual Diagnosis

F. Macrory

Introduction

The needs of women are central to the Government's programme of reform and investment in public services, and to our commitment to addressing discrimination and inequality. Modernising mental health services is also one of our core national priorities (Department of Health, 2002a). *Women's Mental Health: Into the Mainstream* (Department of Health, 2002a) highlights that women make up over half of the general population, play a significant role in the workforce and assume the major responsibility for home-making, and for the caring of children and other family members. At the same time, many women experience low social status and value. Social isolation and poverty are much more common in women, as is the experience of childhood sexual abuse, domestic violence and sexual violence. Both mental health care and drug treatment services must be responsive to these differences (Department of Health, 2002b).

Problem drug use in the UK is characterised by the use of multiple drugs, often by injection, and is strongly associated with socio-economic deprivation and other factors that may affect parenting capacity (ACMD, 2003). It is typically chaotic and unpredictable, and serious health and social consequences are common. *Models of Care* (National Treatment Agency, 2002) sets out a national framework for the commissioning of adult treatment for drug misuse, expected to be available in every part of England to meet the needs of diverse local populations. It advocates a systems approach to meeting the multiple needs of drug and alcohol users by having explicit links to the other generic health, social care and criminal justice services, including through-care and aftercare.

Hidden Harm: Responding to the Needs of Children of Problem Drug Users (ACMD, 2003) states that parental drug use can, and often does, compromise children's health and development at every stage from conception onwards. The complexity of the situation means it is not possible to determine the precise effects on any individual child. However, a large proportion of the children of problem drug users are clearly being disadvantaged and damaged in many ways, and few will escape entirely unharmed. Risk assessment in itself presents an enormous challenge because of the highly variable course of mental illness, and becomes more problematic when other variables are introduced. Substance misuse is usual rather than exceptional amongst people with severe mental health problems and the relationship between the two is complex (Hull Social Services *et al.*, 2003). Banerjee *et al.* (2001) suggest that when compared with a mental health problem alone, those with a dual diagnosis are more likely to have the following: increased suicide risk, more severe mental health problems, homelessness and unstable housing, and an increased risk of being violent and of victimisation and exploitation. They also state that clients may have more contact with the criminal justice system, family problems and a history of childhood abuse (sexual/emotional/physical). They are also more likely to fall through the net of care, and to be less likely to be compliant with medication and other treatment.

Interventions should, therefore, not just take account of the medical treatment, but the broader social issues that affect their lives and thus potentially their medical condition and mental well-being.

The impact of parental mental illness on family life and children's well-being cannot be overstated. Being labelled with a psychiatric diagnosis profoundly negatively affects the experiences of parents and their family members, adults and children alike (SAMHSA, 1999). Mental illness affects whole families, but there are often powerful tensions between the rights of children to be cared for and protected and the needs of parents who themselves are under stress due to their mental ill health. When pregnancy, motherhood and parenting enter the equation, the situation can become particularly complex. Beck-Sander (1999) reminds us that under UK law, the Children Act 1989 (Department of Health, 1989) leaves us in no doubt that the needs of the child are paramount in all Children Act court proceedings, where a conflict of interest arises between parent and child. Adult and child services must act in accordance with the child centred philosophy behind this Act. However, it is acknowledged that difficulties and conflicts can arise when it is felt that what professional judgement suggests is in the patient's best interests conflicts with the interests or needs of the children for whom they are caring.

Within this chapter these tensions and potential conflicts will be explored in a political and personal context. Whilst dual diagnosis is the focus, the individual complexities associated with both mental illness and substance misuse will necessarily form part of this chapter. The aim is not to provide definitive answers, but to generate discussion about a difficult and sometimes painful part of the responsibilities that professionals must carry when working in this minefield of multiple need.

Dual diagnosis

Daly & Holland (2003) define dual diagnosis as the co-occurrence of mental illness and substance use disorder, where there is a strong correlation between harmful behaviour and substance misuse that is amplified in dual diagnosis. It covers a wide spectrum of substance misuse and mental health problems that may be experienced by an individual at any given time. Harrison (2004) suggests that excessive illicit drug use is common in people with the following mental health problems: antisocial personality disorder, bipolar disorder, schizophrenia and depression.

The importance of the development of quality services for people with co-morbidity cannot therefore be stressed too strongly; research shows that, amongst other things, treatment for substance misuse problems often ameliorates psychiatric and mental health problems. Interventions for people with co-morbidity are also likely to be cost effective: the health care costs of untreated cases are higher than for those left untreated. Substance misuse and mental health treatment providers well recognise that individuals with a dual diagnosis present complicated, chronic, interrelated conditions that often require solutions that are personalised to the specific set of symptoms, level of severity, and other psychosocial and environmental factors (SAMHSA, 2002).

Thus, treatment plans must be individualised to address each person's specific needs, using staged interventions and motivational enhancement to support recovery. However, within this discussion it must also be stated that undiagnosed and untreated mental illness takes its toll on families as well. If one of the co-occurring disorders goes untreated, both usually get worse and additional complications often arise. The combination of disorders can result in poor response to traditional treatments and increases the risk for other serious medical problems, suicide, criminalisation, unemployment, homelessness, and separation from families and communities. As a result, individuals often require high cost services, such as in-patient treatment and accident and emergency care (SAMHSA, 2002). Once within the system, the symptoms of patients suffering from mental disorders may be masked by substance misuse and, conversely, what appear to be mental health problems may be the product of substance misuse. This is well recognised as a complication when evaluation and assessment is being undertaken, particularly if we consider that a dual diagnosis should be the expectation, not the exception, within mental health and drug treatment services.

Pregnancy

Society today still continues to prepare females for the occupation of motherhood, with the media constantly sending out powerful messages that motherhood is the desired state for all women if we want to be 'complete' (Phoenix *et al.*, 1991), but most texts and research on childbirth and motherhood offer paradigms and prescriptions that take little account of women's actual lives. This is especially true when serious mental illness and/or substance misuse is a contributing factor. The experiences of parents with mental illness and substance misuse are similar to those of all parents in many ways. Parents with mental illness routinely describe their relationships with their children and fulfilling the parenting role as extremely important to them (Nicholson, 1998) and may prioritise their children's needs and neglect their own. Their family life may suffer under these circumstances, just as for those living without mental illness or substance misuse problems.

Pregnancy brings a unique set of challenges to adults living with mental illness, and to those involved in their care. Where there is also alcohol and/or drug use present the situation becomes more complex. According to Miller (1990) the percentage of unplanned pregnancies among women with serious mental illness is high, and psychotic denial of pregnancy happens with greater frequency in women who have previously lost custody of their children. Women who are uninformed about issues of psychotropic medication and pregnancy may stop taking their medications unnecessarily, thinking they are protecting the fetus; it is therefore extremely important that there is a holistic approach to treatment that embraces the related issues of substance misuse and mental health. Maternity services must be assertive team players when contributing to multi-agency care plans that are both sensitive and appropriate.

The Confidential Enquiry into Maternal Deaths (CEMD, 2001) is the longest running example of national professional self audit in the world. For the first time, the report *Why Mothers Die 1997–1999* (CEMD, 2001) has been able to fully evaluate other factors that may have played a part in women's deaths. These findings are of great concern, showing that maternal mortality rates among the socially excluded, including women from lower socio-economic classes, very young girls and specific ethnic groups, are higher than among the population as a whole. There has always been a large degree of under ascertainment of deaths from mental illness or substance abuse by this Enquiry. However, a pilot ONS linkage study showed that the CEMD was unaware of over 40 extra deaths from suicide or deaths from violent causes, and another eight where the coroner recorded an open verdict. In addition, 11 unreported women died from an accidental drug overdose. As it is not yet widespread practice for psychiatrists and community mental health or drug support teams to notify such deaths to the Enquiry, this degree of under ascertainment is understandable. But, when all deaths up to one year from delivery are taken into account, the results of the study show that deaths from suicide are not only the leading cause of indirect death, but also the leading cause of maternal deaths overall. Overall, 42 women whose deaths are covered by this report were identified as having psychiatric disorders causing or contributing to their deaths. Key recommendations taken from the Enquiry (CEMD, 2001) are documented in full in Table 11.1.

The case of Dr Daksha Emson dramatically illustrates the above. Dr Emson, a psychiatrist, and her daughter Freya, aged three months, died following an extended suicide in October 2000. The incident took place during a single psychotic episode that was a consequence of her bipolar affective disorder, triggered by her post-natal condition and aggravated by psychosocial stresses (North East London SHA, 2004). Daksha stabbed herself and her baby, covered both of them in accelerant and set it alight. The baby died of smoke inhalation, and Daksha died three weeks later in a burns unit without regaining consciousness.

Eleven deaths in women who were drug or alcohol dependent were also discussed in the Enquiry. In contrast to the other women who died from suicide, these women are characterised by

Table 11.1 Maternal psychiatric deaths: key recommendations (CEMD, 2001).

- Protocols for the management of women who are at risk of relapse or recurrence of a serious mental illness following delivery should be in place in every trust providing services.
- Enquiries about previous psychiatric history, its severity, care received and clinical presentation should be made routinely in a systematic and sensitive way at the antenatal booking clinic.
- The use of the term post-natal depression or PND should not be used as a generic term for all types of psychiatric disorder. Details of previous illness should be sought and recorded in line with the recommendations above.
- Women who have a past history of serious psychiatric disorder, postpartum or non-postpartum, should be assessed by a psychiatrist antenatally, and a plan instituted with regard to the high risk of recurrence following delivery.
- Women who have suffered from serious mental illness, either following childbirth, or at other times, should be counselled about the possible recurrence of that illness following further pregnancies.
- A perinatal mental health team that has the specialist knowledge, skills and experience to provide care for women at risk of, or suffering from, serious postpartum mental illness should be available to every woman.
- Women who require psychiatric admission following childbirth should ideally be admitted to a specialist mother and baby unit, together with their infant. In areas where this service is not available, a transfer should be considered.
- Substance misuse services should be provided, without the need for making an appointment, in antenatal clinics and to improve both the rate of engagement and the compliance with care.
- Future enquiries must require the collection of information from psychiatric services.

Source: CEMD (2001).

their high levels of social adversity, homelessness, poor uptake of services (particularly substance misuse services), poor attendance for either psychiatric or antenatal appointments, and by their youth and single status (CEMD, 2001). Within this context it is additionally important to note that there are a number of health problems and needs that are specific to women in prison, particularly with regard to both substance misuse and mental health. The high levels of drug misuse found among women prisoners, both on remand and sentenced, suggests that points at which women come into contact with the criminal justice system may offer opportunities to provide treatment. However, women do not currently receive equality of experience in the criminal justice system (National Treatment Agency, 2002).

The future provision of health and medical care to prisoners was clearly addressed in the Woolf Report (1991). In particular the working group was tasked to consider the recommendation made by Her Majesty's Chief Inspector of Prisons, in the discussion paper *Patient or Prisoner?* (Ramsbotham, 1996) that the responsibility for providing health care to prisoners should move from the Prison Service to the NHS. Ramsbotham (1996) also pointed out that the health care needs of women, especially those who are pregnant, are not adequately catered for in prison, and concluded that the NHS should assume responsibility for the delivery of all health care, through a purchaser–provider relationship that acknowledges the full and peculiar needs of the Prison Service.

Parenting

Child protection and mental health issues

The interface between child protection and mental health is an arena of professional practice, and legal judgment has had very little formal attention (Weir & Douglas, 1999). Recent concerns about the definition of mental health problems have suggested the need for a revision of this view to incorporate a wider definition of the nature of mental health problems, particularly depression, which has been a feature of major child death enquiries over recent years. The demands of working with parents with mental health problems are some of the most complex in terms of balancing rights, needs and responsibilities. Failure to ensure that the needs of children are addressed at the same time as the care needs of adults are being assessed can result in inappropriate and even dangerous situations arising for children.

As already stated, mental illness affects whole families. There is no doubt that mental illness in parents may represent a risk for their children. The central question today is the extent to which, in the longer term, a parent's mental health problem so reduces their ability to parent that their children's lives become damaged beyond effective repair. When is this point reached? How can this be effectively assessed and managed? These are the issues that all professionals working in the community need to bear in mind, whether they are involved with parents or their children or both (Weir, 1999). Beck-Sander (1999), in discussing ways to reduce conflict between services, suggests that a fundamental caveat of all risk management work is that all risks posed by parents to their children cannot be prevented. At best, risks can only be reduced. It is not even feasible to aim to *identify* all risks, and any service adopting this aim would be doomed to failure. Furthermore, its workers would be over cautious in a vain attempt to avoid any possible harm occurring. She goes on to say that as risk is sometimes unpredictable, harm would eventually occur, and in this event the workers would be vulnerable to scapegoating because the service would view the occurrence of harm necessarily as a service failure. Furthermore, such a service would also be unable to work effectively with other services because of its unrealistic expectations. The task of risk management is therefore to carefully weigh up the harms and benefits in a risk calculation; nevertheless, this can be another source of potential conflict between services. What may appear a 'reasonable risk' (for example, benefits outweigh harms) to one service may appear unreasonable (for example, harms outweigh benefits) to another (Beck-Sander, 1999).

It must be emphasised that people's experiences of mental illness are as different as the people themselves, and that no two individuals have the same experience of mental illness. There are many types of symptoms, from delusions to hallucinations, from apathy to elation, from thought disorder to thought withdrawal (Beck-Sander, 1999). Each symptom may be interpreted in any number of ways, depending on individual factors, such as personality, intellectual ability, social and physical environment, concomitant difficulties and culture. It can therefore be very difficult to anticipate the risks posed by an individual with mental illness unless specific idiosyncratic details are known.

Weir & Douglas (1999) remind us that, at the same time, staff working with children and families need to understand with precision how a particular parent's mental health problem affects his or her parenting ability when they are quantifying the impact of adult mental health problems on individual children. Broadly speaking, they state that the following concerns, as shown in Table 11.2, should be addressed. I suggest that the questions could, and should, be as readily asked of parents with substance misuse problems when making an assessment of parenting capability.

Table 11.2 Concerns: working with children and families.

- When does an adult's mental health pose a conflict of interest within a family?
- When does a parent's mental health pose risks for the safety and well-being of their child?
- How does an adult's parenting capacity become impaired in these circumstances?
- What is a child's capacity to tolerate the changed and often detrimental care that they may receive?
- How can those risks be assessed and how can they be managed?
- Who decides when those risks become acceptable?
- What services need to be available to meet the needs of both adults and children in these circumstances?
- How do professionals working in these circumstances need to be trained and supported?
- What can be done to bridge the gulf between the professionals who are trying to meet the respective needs of children and parents?
- How can the different agencies involved ensure consistent practice and good communication with each other?

Source: Weir & Douglas (1999).

It is very difficult to separate out the effects of specific parental mental disorder, and whilst the severity of the parental illness is an important predictor of difficult behaviour in their children, a high level of psychosocial disadvantage is also of great importance (Sameroff & Seifer, 1990). In understanding risk and protective factors, many disciplines are in agreement about the nature of risk factors that predispose children and adolescents to problem behaviours, and the protective factors that may mitigate against negative outcomes. Children who experience ante/post-natal complications, for example fetal alcohol syndrome, who live in extreme poverty, in constant conflict or who are exposed to multiple traumatic events are at significant risk for developing substance misuse and mental health disorders. As Bernard & Douglas (1999) state, the combination of a parent with severe mental health problems, with or without substance misuse problems, and a child who may be in need of protection demands an almost impossibly high level of skill in risk assessment and decision making.

Child protection and mental health services are arguably the most visible, vulnerable and volatile public services in Britain. The stakes are high, with severe injury or loss of liberty the possible outcomes of professional error. The Zito Trust (1995) is clear that even with regular and good quality supervision, staff may be asked to manage situations for which they do not have sufficient personal or professional training or experience. Where lives are at stake, can we be sure that the present system is good enough?

Whilst risk and protective factors are correlated with the development or absence of mental health and substance abuse problems, Davis (1999) reminds us that correlation does not imply causality. In fact, no one risk factor specifically causes any one disorder and a variety of combinations of risk factors may lead to the same disorder. At the same time, many risk factors are not disorder specific and may relate to a number of negative outcomes, such as mental disorders, post-traumatic stress disorder and substance misuse. Finally, multiple risk factors predict more severe outcomes. Researchers have identified, for example, that children with two or more family risk factors for mental illness are four to ten times more likely to develop a psychiatric disorder than children with no risk factors or only one (Davis, 1999). Biology and heredity are among those risk factors for mental disorders, for example children of parents with depression or schizophrenia are at greater risk of the disease, possibly due to a genetic predisposition. Similarly, 'the greater the number of drug abuse risk factors, the greater the risk for drug abuse' (Glantz & Pickens, 1992; Davis, 1999; SAMHSA, 2002).

The concept of resilience

Over the past 25 years, researchers studying risk factors have identified certain individuals (termed resilient individuals) who are better able to resist destructive behaviours, even in the presence of identified risk factors. Whilst protective factors are typically defined as influences external to a person that contribute to his or her well-being, resilience has been conceptualised as a set of strengths internal to the individual (Wolin & Wolin, 1993). Many protective factors may contribute to a resilient personality. Just as multiple risk factors predict more severe outcomes, multiple protective factors can improve one's chances for positive outcomes (Davis, 1999). It must be noted that risk and protective factors change as a product of an individual's age and developmental stage. Therefore, prevention programmes must be matched to the appropriate developmental stage of the individuals for which they are designed.

However, as Field (1993) reminds us, there is another group of children who seem to cope in the midst of striking adversity. These are the ones who seem to be 'managing' in a situation where the quality and quantity of care they receive is very far from what most children would need. The importance of mental illness in one parent is that it may pose a risk to a child. However, the contribution of the other parent must be considered, and this may be positive or negative. Whilst the factor of resilience is the one quoted most often in relation to children, she finds reliance on children's resilience to be worrying, and liable to lead to false optimism. Emotional abuse may be difficult to identify, but may produce lasting difficulties. Let us now address the real and potential impact of both mental health and substance misuse on the child.

The impact on the child

Over the past 50-plus years there has been a growing awareness of the importance of attachment in infant/carer relationships. Attachment is generally understood to indicate the relationship that develops between an infant and its primary caregiver (usually the mother) during its first few months of life. Our modern understanding began with the pioneering work of John Bowlby (1944, 1951) in which he emphasised that children's experiences of interpersonal relationships were crucial to their psychological development. He argued that the formation of an ongoing relationship between child and primary caregiver was as important to the child's development as other factors, such as the provision of experiences, discipline and child care (Cole & Fearnley, 1998). Bowlby went on to postulate that each infant develops 'an internal working model' about attachment figures, in which the infant's sense of self and others unfolds through interactions with the primary caregiver. Fahlberg (1988) has also suggested that any interruption in the development of a reciprocal relationship between an infant and their primary caregiver, may be experienced as stressful, and may have a detrimental effect on the child's attachment process.

Certain experiences, particularly if met before the age of two, act as risk factors in the development of an attachment disorder (Fearnley & Howe, 1999). These include pre-birth and birth traumas, sudden separations from the primary caregiver, frequent moves between different carers and/or placements, chronic maternal depression/mental illness/substance misuse, and where the primary caregiver has experienced serious childhood trauma that remains unresolved. Severe neglect and physical, emotional and sexual abuse are also significant risk factors. Communication between the parent and the child may also be affected by the disorder, as schizophrenia often causes disturbance in communication. Goodman & Brumley (1990) suggest three possible ways in which having a schizophrenic illness may affect parenting:

(1) Passivity and social withdrawal on the part of the parent
(2) Delusions that may involve the child
(3) Exposure of the child to the incongruent affect often associated with schizophrenia

Lau (1999), in discussing the needs of children and families from different cultures is clear that of particular concern is the finding of parental violence, or potential threats against the children, severe behavioural disturbances (for example drugs/alcohol), self-destructive acts and repeated suicide attempts. She reminds us that it is important to find out what has happened to the exercise of authority, in the traditional extended family, which would normally serve the function of providing a source for mediating family conflict, as well as containing and restraining extreme behavioural disturbance in any one family member. One could argue that in some circumstances, that very exercise of authority denies women the opportunity of the care and support so desperately needed; instead they are hidden from society, ostracised from their family and their rights are denied.

Conclusion

Because outcomes for these families are multiply determined, there are many opportunities and potentially effective strategies for interventions. These must focus on ensuring a safe and stable home environment, reducing parent–child discord and improving communication, developing parenting skills, reducing environmental stressors and supporting children's resilience in order to improve outcomes for parents and children. Efforts to enhance children's understanding of mental illness and parent's understanding of children's needs have also shown promising results (SAMHSA, 2002). Henry & Kumar (1999) remind us that assessing what constitutes 'good enough' parenting is very difficult, and many authors have commented on the fact that parenting remains a very difficult construct to measure because of its complex multidimensional quality (Mrazek *et al.*, 1995).

Adults with mental illness may be caring for adopted children, stepchildren or the children of others in informal arrangements. The issue of who has custody of children is a distinct question of where children live, who is caring for them or the extent and nature of contact or involvement the parents with mental illness have with them. People with co-occurring disorders have lives and families, hopes and dreams, responsibilities and needs. They can be mothers, fathers, grandparents, students, teachers, plumbers or pianists. Too often these individuals pay a high price for having co-occurring disorders: lost dreams, lost families, and in some cases, lost lives (SAMHSA, 2002). Whilst the experiences of adults with mental illness are similar to those of all parents in many ways, the literature has emphasised their unique circumstances, and most commonly, their deficits and failures.

For many women, unresolved issues from their past debilitate presenting behaviours and understanding, especially around relationships. If these needs are not addressed and met, parents with dual diagnosis may never achieve family unity and the goal of good parenting may remain beyond their reach. If it is only within warm, consistent, accepting and reciprocal relationships that children can learn to be empathic and socially competent (Fearnley & Howe, 1999), then the future looks quite bleak for families where drug use and mental illness is present.

Of course it will not always be safe to keep children at home. Maya Angelou, the poet, has put very poignantly the dilemma for those of us who have to intervene in family life: 'How is it possible to convince a child of its own worth after removing him from a family which is said to be unworthy, but with whom he identifies?' (Weir & Douglas, 1999).

Into the Mainstream (Department of Health, 2002a) emphasises the importance of listening to women and taking heed of what they are saying. They want to be listened to, to have their experiences validated, and most of all to be kept safe whilst they recover from mental ill health. They also want importance placed on the underlying causes of their distress in addition to their symptoms, support in their mothering role and their potential for recovery recognised.

Perhaps the most compelling justification for a distinct response to women's health in particular is the fact that it carries a higher individual and social cost than men's. The aim is to promote a coordinated approach so that women with a range of problems and needs can feel assured that the departments and agencies responsible for providing help and support respond to their needs as a whole, rather than in isolation (Department of Health, 2002b). Improvements in services are an investment in the health of future, as well as present, generations. Meaningful and effective interventions have the great potential to positively impact on physical and mental health, parenting in the long term, reduce the need for children to be placed in care, and help to break the present cyclical nature of drug use, mental illness, poverty and despair.

References

ACMD (Advisory Council on the Misuse of Drugs) (2003) *Hidden Harm: Responding to the Needs of Children of Problem Drug Users*. The report of an inquiry by the Advisory Council on the Misuse of Drugs. www.drugs.gov.uk

Banerjee, S., Clancy, C. & Crome, I. (2001) *Co-existing Problems of Mental Disorder and Substance Misuse (Dual Diagnosis): an Information Manual. Final Report to the Department of Health*. Royal College of Psychiatrists, Research Unit, London.

Beck-Sander, A. (1999) Working with parents with mental health problems: management of the many risks. Chapter 8. In: *Child Protection and Adult Mental Health: Conflict of Interest?* (Douglas, A. & Weir, A., eds) Butterworth-Heinemann Press, Edinburgh.

Bernard, J. & Douglas, A. (1999) The size of the task facing professional agencies. Chapter 11. In: *Child Protection and Adult Mental Health: Conflict of Interest?* (Douglas, A. & Weir, A., eds). Butterworth-Heinemann Press, Edinburgh.

Bowlby, J. (1944) Forty-four juvenile thieves: their characters and home life. *International Journal of Psycho-Analysis*, 25, 19–52.

Bowlby, J. (1951) *Maternal Care and Mental Health*. WHO Monograph Series, no.2. World Health Organization, Geneva.

CEMD (2001) *The Confidential Enquiry into Maternal Deaths: 'Why Mothers Die' 1997–1999*. National Institute for Clinical Excellence, London.

Cole, J. & Fearnley, S. (1998) *Attachment Therapy: a Preliminary Report of an Attachment Therapy Model Being Pioneered at the Keys Attachment Centre as a Treatment for Children Assessed as Having an Attachment Disorder*. Available from Keys Attachment Centre, Rawtenstall, Lancashire.

Daly, C. & Holland, M. (2003) Dual diagnosis. Co-morbid mental illness and substance misuse: a managed practice network of service provision in Manchester. Draft 6. Unpublished.

Davis, K.L. (1999) Risk and protective factors for alcohol abuse and dependence. *Journal of Neuropsychopharmacology: 5th Generation of Progress*. (In SAMHSA Report to Congress, 1999).

Department of Health (1989) *The Children Act 1989*. HMSO, London.

Department of Health (2002a) *Women's Mental Health: Into the Mainstream. Strategic Development of Mental Health Care for Women*. Department of Health, London.

Department of Health (2002b) *Mental Health Policy Implementation Guide: Dual Diagnosis Good Practice Guide*. www.Department of Health.gov.uk/mentalhealth/dualdiagnosis.htm

Fahlberg, V. (1988) Fitting the pieces together. British Association for Adoption and Fostering. In: *Attachment Therapy: a Preliminary Report of an Attachment Therapy Model Being Pioneered at the Keys Attachment Centre as a Treatment for Children Assessed as Having an Attachment Disorder* (Cole, J. & Fearnley, S., eds). Available from Keys Attachment Centre, Rawtenstall, Lancashire.

Fearnley, S. & Howe, D. (1999) Disorders of attachment and attachment therapy. *Adoption and Fostering*, 23 (2), 19–30.

Field, I.M. (1993) Enhancing parent sensitivity. In: *At Risk Infants: Interventions, Families and Research* (Anastonion,

N.J. & Harel, S., eds) pp. 81–9. Paul Brooks Publishing, Baltimore, Md.

Glantz, M. & Pickens, R. (1992) *Vulnerability to Drug Abuse. Proceedings of Annual Meeting of American Psychological Association*, xvi, p. 533 (Books: Call no. RC 563.2 V 85 1992). American Psychological Association, Washington, DC.

Goodman, S.H. & Brumley, H.E. (1990) Schizophrenia and depressed mothers: relational deficits and parenting. *Journal of Developmental Psychology*, 12, 31–9.

Harrison, A. (2004) *Proposal: Development of a Consultant Nurse Post in Dual Diagnosis*. Avon and Wiltshire Mental Health Partnership NHS Trust. University of the West of England, Bristol.

Henry, L.A. & Kumar, R.C. (1999) Risk assessments of infants born to parents with a mental health problem or a learning disability. Chapter 6. In: *Child Protection and Adult Mental Health: Conflict of Interest?* (Douglas, A. & Weir, A., eds). Butterworth-Heinemann Press, Edinburgh.

Hull Social Services, East Riding of Yorkshire Council, Hull and East Riding Community Health NHS Trust (2003) Dual Diagnosis Strategy (A Secondary Response to the Department of Health Guidelines on Dual Diagnosis). Unpublished.

Lau, A.Y.-H. (1999) Understanding the needs of children and families from different cultures. Chapter 9. In: *Child Protection and Adult Mental Health: Conflict of Interest?* (Douglas, A. & Weir, A., eds). Butterworth-Heinemann Press, Edinburgh.

Miller, L.J. (1990) Psychotic denial of pregnancy: phenomenology and clinical management. *Hospital and Community Psychiatry*, 41 (11), 1233–7.

Mrazek, D.A., Mrazek, P. & Kimnert, M. (1995) Clinical assessment of parenting. *Journal of the American Academy of Child and Adolescent Psychiatry*, 34, 272–82.

National Treatment Agency (2002) Models of Care for the Treatment of Drug Misusers. NTA, London.

Nicholson, P. (1998) *Post-natal Depression, Psychological Science and the Transition to Motherhood*. Routledge Press, London.

North East London Strategic Health Authority (2004) Report of an Independent Inquiry into the Care and Treatment of Daksha Emson MBBS and her daughter Freya.
www. nelondon.nhs.uk

Phoenix, A., Woollett, A. & Lloyd, E. (eds) (1991) *Motherhood: Meanings, Practices and Ideologies*. Sage Publications, London.

Ramsbotham, D. (1996) *Patient or Prisoner? A New Strategy for Health Care in Prisons: a Discussion Paper*. Home Office, London.

Sameroff, A.J. & Seifer, R. (1990) Early contributions to developmental risk. In: *Risk and Protective Factors in Development of Psychopathology* (Rolf, J., Mastern, A.S., Cichetti, D., Nueehterlein, K.H. & Weintraub, S., eds). Cambridge University Press, Cambridge.

SAMHSA. US Department of Health and Human Services (1999) *Report to Congress on the Prevention and Treatment of Co-occurring Substance Abuse Disorders and Mental Disorders*. Substance Abuse and Mental Health Services Administration (SAMHSA), National Institute of Mental Health, Rockville, Md.

SAMHSA. US Department of Health and Human Services (2002) Substance Abuse and Mental Health Services Administration (SAMHSA), National Institute of Mental Health, Rockville, Md.

Weir, A. (1999) An introduction to the issues: a new holistic approach outlined. Chapter 1. In: *Child Protection and Adult Mental Health: Conflict of Interest?* (Douglas, A. & Weir, A., eds). Butterworth-Heinemann Press, Edinburgh.

Weir, A. & Douglas, A. (eds) (1999) *Child Protection and Adult Mental Health: Conflict of Interest?* Butterworth-Heinemann Press, Edinburgh.

Wolin, S.J. & Wolin, S. (1993) *The Resilient Self: How Survivors of Troubled Families Rise Above Adversity*. Villard Books, New York.

Woolf, Justice & Tumim, Judge, S. (1991) *Prison Disturbances April 1990: Report of an Enquiry by The Rt. Hon. Lord Justice Woolf and His Hon. Judge Stephen Tumim (The Woolf Report)*. Cm. 1456. HMSO, London.

Zito Trust (1995) *Learning the Lessons*. Mental Health Inquiry Reports published in England and Wales between 1969 and 1994 and their recommendations for Improving Practice. The Zito Trust, London.

Part 3

Context and Approaches

Chapter 12 Addiction and Mental Health Nursing: a Synthesis of Role and Care in the Community

Chapter 13 Shared Care and Inter-professional Practice

Chapter 14 Primary Care and Dual Diagnosis

Chapter 15 Dual Diagnosis In Acute In-patient Settings

Chapter 16 Dual Diagnosis in a Forensic Setting

Chapter 17 Models of Care and Dual Diagnosis

12 Addiction and Mental Health Nursing: a Synthesis of Role and Care in the Community

K. Moore & G.H. Rassool

Introduction

Dual diagnosis developments have been formalised in the contents of the White Paper *Tackling Drugs to Build a Better Britain* (Cabinet Office, 1998). The *National Service Framework for Mental Health* (NSF) (Department of Health, 1999) clearly identifies 'dual diagnosis patients' as a population with higher rates of illness and a greater risk of stigmatisation and exclusion from existing service provision. In the past few years, most health authorities have included dual diagnosis personnel within their commissioned mental health or substance misuse provisions. Assertive outreach became an identified focus for treatment strategies, and funding for dual diagnosis services was made available through specific grant projects. The development of community based practices targeting vulnerable groups such as dual diagnosis have been outlined in standard one of the NSF; such practices are beginning to evolve in selected locations in the UK.

However, overall services for this complex group remain marginalised. Within the *National Service Framework for Mental Health* (NSF) (Department of Health, 1999) and the *Models of Care for Substance Misuse* (National Treatment Agency, 2002), development of community based practices has been outlined. New drug subcultures have been described when discussing the coexistence of substance misuse and mental health problems, and the development of services within the UK. There has been an increasing exposure of mental health patients to a wide range of licit and illicit substances following the emphasis and movement of treatment services from hospital based into community settings (Moore & Rassool, 2002). In many cases the failure of services to recognise dual diagnosis as a problem led to the development of significant treatment gaps whereby dual diagnosis patients were unable to access either service due to philosophical treatment differences (Gafoor & Rassool, 1998).

While it has been said that both addiction and mental health nurses are in ideal positions to offer positive interventions to dual diagnosis patients, there remain several key factors that have hindered progression in this area. The effect of stigmatisation in relation to the independent problems of alcohol, illicit drugs and mental health continue to be significant for individuals with dual diagnosis. There is an even greater risk of stigmatisation and exclusion from services for those individuals (Byrne, 2000; Department of Health, 2002; National Treatment Agency, 2002). Besides, there remains both a lack of knowledge about substance misuse and dual diagnosis within nursing professions and a negative attitude towards substance misusers (Royal College of Psychiatrists, 2001; Rassool, 2002).

The concept that dual diagnosis patients are

difficult to work with could be considered a reflection of the inability of general mental health nursing practices to adapt and grow. Factors that affect our ability as practitioners to challenge and implement new practices are related not just to personal beliefs, but are significantly influenced by difficulty in understanding the language of change desired, the imposition of change, a lack of desire for change decreasing the likelihood of staff to initiate new practices or not seeing the model as useful (Pediani, 2000). Community nursing staff need to be supported in viewing working with dual diagnosis patients as simple, understandable, potentially successful and enjoyable. Nurses, in the many different aspects of care within all health settings, can and do make both subtle and profound changes in the lives of dual diagnosis patients.

Where are we now? Developing community oriented services

In recent times, dual diagnosis developments centred on studies from the USA that outlined the development and testing of community interventions (Zweeban, 1993). Since then, there has been a growing impetus from the British Government, coupled with changing health needs of the population, to address dual diagnosis. Community services oriented towards services for substance misusers and mental health problems emerged from this socio-cultural and political shift. This resulted in the increased number of statutory and non-statutory agencies working with dual diagnosis and gave rise to many different modalities of approach and service provision. Further guidance in *Dual Diagnosis: Good Practice Guide* (Department of Health, 2002) highlighted four models of community practice in the field. These models included: liaison (Kingston CDAT dual diagnosis service), joint collaborative work (Haringey dual diagnosis team), training and liaison (COMPASS, Birmingham) and outreach, training and consultancy (Mid-Cheshire dual diagnosis team). The good practice guide highlighted the need for services being developed to be based on local needs, emphasising the need to deliver integrated treatment, utilising skilled training, liaison and support. However, how does this work in practice?

High levels of vulnerability, social isolation and homelessness are found in dual diagnosis, and when concerns are raised regarding mental health, many supervised hostels, mental health or substance misuse agencies state that they are not able to offer the needed services. This is perhaps one of the most frustrating aspects of community dual diagnosis work. Concerns about mental health issues, psychopharmacology of mental health, drug dealing, and drug and alcohol use on premises, combined with a general housing shortage, have often placed the service users outside any criteria established for different levels of housing or supported accommodation. Mental health practice in the community is driven by the community programme approach (CPA) (Department of Health, 2000). This predominantly means that interventions are based on the level of risk to the individual and the general public, whereas addiction services are driven by public health and criminal justice agendas. Assessment of presenting problem or need is one of the critical elements of any treatment intervention and, at the most basic level, asking questions that relate to either substance misuse or mental health will assist the clinician in determining the treatment pathway that the service user could access. Abou Saleh (2004) promotes the routine screening of all patients presenting to substance misuse and mental health services, whilst others argue that there is an inherent difficulty in distinguishing between symptoms presenting in dual diagnosis (Rassool, 2002).

Nurses provide comprehensive and ongoing assessments in all aspects of their work. In clinical activities, broad nursing skills are used, in combination with the art of incorporating the level and nature of risks in the presentation, and the history and current nature of the type and frequency of psychoactive substance(s) used. There are a number of screening tests that can be useful but the selection can in itself be confusing. In initial detection and assessment of substance use and misuse, the use of self-report, informant/familial report and laboratory tests are the most frequent combinations used. Assessments of this nature are dependent on the ability of the individuals to understand and describe their perceptions of the events they are experiencing. At all levels of nursing practice, and in all fields from general practitioners, practice nurses to community mental health and specialist community practitioners there are opportunities to assess and intervene with emerging and established dual diagnosis problems. Every presentation is an opportunity to provide basic assessment and interventions.

Primary care presentations that include stress, anxiety, panic, distress or loss as psychological factors, with physical complications such as poor sleep, appetite and concentration, are key triggers for nurses to probe for problematic substance use. Minimal interventions using skilled communication, building trust, taking a non-judgemental stance and active listening are the key nursing interventions. The provision of basic drug, alcohol or mental health information appropriate to the presenting need, and tailoring approaches to the individual are also recommended. For some dual diagnosis patients at the less chaotic end of the spectrum, gentle understanding and information can sometimes be enough to provoke positive lifestyle changes. Evidence based practice requires that all formulations for nursing care are based on fact. In dual diagnosis, a combination of current behaviours, mood and psychological changes for both mental health and substance misuse enables comprehensive treatment programmes to be developed. An additional requirement for nurses is the development of a working care plan; as providers of care, skills such as basic drug and alcohol education, and a broad understanding of how different categories of drugs affect mental health states is essential. Individual care programmes need to meet the criteria for CPA, and require that nurses develop techniques that operate within different settings and at many different levels of patient sophistication. The level of severity of the mental health problems in combination with the substance use and the numbers of professionals involved indicate which level of CPA is needed.

Addiction nursing as a specialty

Historically, occupational labels such as alcohol nurse, drug dependency nurse, chemical substance nurse, specialist nurse in addiction and community psychiatric nurse (addiction) have been ascribed to those working with substance misusers (Rassool, 1997). It was not until the mid-1980s that addiction nursing as a clinical specialty, within the broader framework of mental health nursing, began to put down its clinical and academic roots. The concept of addiction nursing was introduced in the literature in the UK by Rassool (1996, 1999, 2000). It is defined as a specialist branch of mental health nursing concerned with the care and treatment interventions aimed at those individuals whose health problems are directly related to the use and misuse of psychoactive substances and to other addictive behaviours such as eating disorders and gambling (Rassool, 1997). It is argued that, although the concept of addiction nursing may be criticised on the grounds that it is too medically oriented and substance focused, other ascribed labels are too generic and lack the distinctive professional representation of the nature and roles of addiction nurses (Rassool, 1997). Thus, the scope of professional practice in addiction nursing and mental health nursing incorporates the activities of clinical practice (nursing, a range of psychosocial intervention strategies including complementary therapies), education, policy-making, research and all other pursuits through which nurse practitioners contribute to the care and interests of clients.

Addiction nurses practice in both residential and community settings and have an excellent track record in developing innovative health care initiatives and community oriented programmes for substance misusers, and many of the key developments in recent years have been nurse led. These include smoking cessation clinics, mobile methadone clinics, outreach work with drug-using commercial sex workers, satellite clinics for homeless drinkers and development of multi-professional, postgraduate educational programmes in addictive behaviour (Gafoor & Rassool, 1998; Rassool, 2000). The massive expansion of community services for substance misusers, such as the development of community drug/alcohol teams, drug alcohol liaison teams, day care programmes, street agencies, outreach work and needle exchange schemes has heralded the potential development of addiction nursing as a community specialty (Rassool, 1999).

Working in community settings

Community mental health and addiction nurses are currently undergoing significant changes in order to meet the modernisation agendas of mental health act reforms and national service frameworks for mental health and substance misuse. However, if dual diagnosis is to be successfully mainstreamed into the daily business of mental health there are several factors (Kennedy & Griffiths, 2003) that must be addressed by all staff involved:

- Management
- Support
- Leadership style of the teams involved
- The ability of the organisation to adapt
- The level of empowerment staff feel within the process
- Attitudes to risk and innovation

In order to achieve the mainstream agenda, there needs to be an investment in bringing staff together to find an agreed commonality and shared responsibility, with an emphasis given to sharing core skills (Barnes *et al.*, 2002). Care in the community means that as nurses we are involved in complex roles that enable health care resources of individuals, families and communities, often in circumstances that are unstructured, chaotic and where delivery is a necessity (Clarke, 1999). The management of dual diagnosis in community settings poses significant demands on services and staff; however, there are several key principles that cross boundaries. Dual diagnosis is the norm, rather than the exception; many patients do not often acknowledge that they have combined mental health and substance misuse problems; and finally, abstinence as the first treatment priority is often off-putting, creating barriers to engaging in meaningful treatment.

Clinical practice in risk management is one of the key issues within community working, and this remains a thorny issue for dual diagnosis. Community nursing of this client group requires that safety is one of the most important issues, regardless of which model of treatment is being provided. It is understandable that many practitioners have concerns in working with dual diagnosis. However, the obstacles must balance information on violence, fear and prejudice from systems that exclude dual diagnosis patients from engaging in treatment. For nurses in these teams some differences in presentation can be expected. Understanding the therapeutic roles that nurses play in dual diagnosis work must also be considered in the light of their responsibilities to the individual, in relation to risk. Initiating the use of the Mental Health Act and the potential for readmission to hospital under section can present nurses with professional and personal conundrums when they are building a therapeutic alliance at the same time. Staff in the community must work within this delicate balancing act, to achieve non-judgemental and therapeutic relationships, whilst at the same time being potentially 'punitive' by making professional judgements that affect liberty.

Pathways mapping dual diagnosis patients

Entry into treatment usually starts, in most cases, with the general practitioner, accident and emergency department or self-help agencies. Many primary care teams will provide situational assessment and treatment, and any assessment or intervention in relation to dual diagnosis is opportunistic. In many cases only situation treatment is offered at the time of the event, and there may not be a professional view as to further interventions, or a referral to another, more specialist, team or agency. When nurses in primary care settings offer brief interventions, many patients do not attend for follow-up; dual diagnosis patients are no different. However, they have been described in literature as characteristically poor at treatment compliance (Department of Health, 2002).

Many staff feel frustrated when patients do not seem interested in changing their behaviour (Hunt, 1995). One of the key challenges faced by addiction or mental health nurses is to facilitate change in others, and this means that we must understand the problems from the patient's perspective. This is not an easy task, as in order to become health promoters, we must acknowledge and accept the judgements we make based on our own norms and values, ensuring, where possible, limited transference of such values (Crogan, 2005). An understanding of Prochaska & DiClemente's cycle of change (1986) is useful in increasing knowledge of change and motivation processes over time. This helps focus nursing interventions away from using direct persuasion and coercion into support and facilitation of change. Nurses in community settings may need to take a more proactive and persistent view to engage patients in treatment, by enhancing motivation and contemplation of change.

One key aspect of dual diagnosis intervention is the development and enhancement of motivation. Addiction nurses have many of the key skills central to the model, including the ability to express empathy, roll with resistance, support self-efficacy and use discretion (Hunt & Pearson, 2001). Using the Osher & Kofoed (1989) multi-staged framework of therapeutic interventions, the first task is to engage the patient in treatment. It is not simply a case of offering an appointment; often there can be significant amounts of work and planning to achieve contact with the patient. Indeed multiple attempts at contact can sometimes be the case. Consideration of different times, days and venues, negotiated with the patient where possible, can make the first meeting more successful and provide a positive start to engaging in treatment.

When the initial engagement and assessment has been completed, consideration will need to be given to individual needs. Treatment approaches need to be varied, as dual diagnosis patients have a broad spectrum of mental health and substance misuse presentations that are often complicated by additional social and physical factors. Some dual diagnosis patients may have a sophisticated understanding of the interactions between their mental health, whilst others may have significant difficulties with describing their experiences and lack insight into their mental health. There is therefore no one approach that can be promoted as the model of choice; rather, using a patient centred approach, and flexible use of nursing skills and strategies, individual plans can be developed with the patient to meet their needs (Kavanagh *et al.*, 2003).

Community nursing of dual diagnosis patients within different team philosophies continues to utilise the broad skills of medico-nursing practice, education and psychotherapeutic interventions. Whilst some nursing interventions are predetermined by access to tools like rapid illicit drug testing kits and breathalysers, psycho-educational strategies such as harm reduction embody nursing practice regardless of setting. Psychotherapeutic interventions by nursing staff can be found in the recognition of characteristics and consequences of substance misuse and mental health sequelae, with the implementation of nursing actions that address these consequences. Addiction nurses have the ability to link this to the potential for the reduction of harm. Additionally, interventions such as support programmes, psychodynamic/person centred approaches, motivational inteviewing, group work, family work, cognitive and behavioural programmes, are key features of nursing approaches and practices for individuals with dual diagnosis.

Active treatment in dual diagnosis encapsulates interventions that are already being successfully provided by mental health teams, and that target different levels of severity. Integrated strategies that address both the mental health and substance misuse issues are led by the dual diagnosis patient and reflect their needs. At this point in treatment, it is important to agree short-term and intermediate goals, aimed at reducing harm. Motivation and relapse prevention are ongoing elements that need to be supported throughout the treatment event by staff. Techniques that can be used in different combinations include education, use of objective testing (blood and urine testing, diary work), life and decision balance sheets, exploring barriers to change, reframing events and supporting, where appropriate, the use of medication regimes (Department of Health, 2002). Active treatment can also include discussion of preventative primary health care issues, one-to-one counselling interventions, including assertive interventions and social support interventions. Working on life skills management, liaison services, social activities, peer support, support groups and relapse prevention work is all in a day's work for nurses. Regardless of the combination of interventions agreed, there are no quick solutions, and different people respond in different ways to the same treatment.

New teams and new roles in the community

Despite the development of new teams for crisis, outreach and early intervention, there continue to be more commonalities than differences in the nursing roles. The primary role of addiction nursing and mental health nursing exemplifies the contribution they can make to comprehensive patient care in many different settings. However, with the nature of the work undertaken, and the composition of the teams, the blurring of roles is highly apparent. Many of the everyday tasks nurses undertake involve certain core skills, including assessment, counselling, relapse prevention and coordination of whole team responses to patient care. In the past, such coordination of care was dependent on the profession of the individual in charge of the allocation process, and which staff member was able to see the patient.

Guidance by the Department of Health (2002) explicitly outlines the development and roles that underpin each team, and includes the management of co-morbidity (dual diagnosis), but does little to provide any focus for interventions that are useful and effective. For nurses working within crisis teams, the presentation of dual diagnosis patients can be somewhat different from patients managed in more traditional community mental health teams (CMHTs). The essence of nursing care in this team will be in relation to acute distress or crisis, levels of intoxication, or those with high expressed emotional needs who are at high risk of self-harm or suicide. The delivery of dual diagnosis care needs to reflect the ability of staff to work rapidly, using flexible, but secure, approaches in home environments. Treatment in crisis can begin at any time of the day, and nursing staff need to be able to understand the role and impact that substance misuse can have on mental health and, conversely, the effect mental health can have on drug and alcohol use within a crisis presentation.

Nursing staff in crisis teams need to have a sound understanding of basic drug and alcohol awareness, assessment skills for substance misuse, knowledge of dual diagnosis and management principles for substance misuse problems. Interventions made by staff in these circumstances are short, and staff may only have planned interventions for up to two weeks that are predominantly based on the level of risk presenting, and whilst they may be able to find treatment success for the crisis, in complex cases, full resolution of the dual diagnosis may not be possible. Nurses in crisis teams face similar conundrums to their CMHT counterparts; in many cases the crisis team is the gatekeeper to psychiatric beds, and working in home environments means that staff must have the ability to work not only with individuals, but potentially with family systems.

Assertive outreach nurses, by comparison to staff from crisis teams, have significantly more treatment time with the dual diagnosis patient. Work in this area is seen as long-term engagement and treatment. Although a team approach is taken with a shared workload, nurses will need to have knowledge of dual diagnosis, and will need to expand their use of engagement skills to include substance misuse and motivational work. In addition, the task of identifying early warning signs of relapse and relapse prevention for both mental health and substance misuse are key elements of care and care coordination. As treatment progresses and patients begin to achieve their goals, staff will need to begin to incorporate specific management strategies for mental health and substance misuse problems. Underlying this work is the ongoing assessment and management of risk within community settings and the utilisation of community re-socialisation and support systems.

Early intervention teams are another area of mental health care where dual diagnosis is a prominent feature. Although these teams are specifically aimed at first episode psychosis, statistically the patient population is younger, and in relation to substance misuse may be more likely to have recreational or regular substance use. In this type of work, nurses need to have a sound understanding of recreational drug use, and how these drugs may influence or impact on the initial presentation. In tandem with this, staff will need to have the ability to complete an assessment in relation to drug use, and be able to understand the events as they relate to and influence each other. Critical in this team is the ability to take non-judgemental approaches, assess risk and enhance engagement with the team. Like their counterparts in assertive outreach, crisis and CMHT, the work is completed in home environments and not just with the individual, but often with the family as a whole.

Nursing roles: commonalities and differences

There are more commonalities than differences in the nursing roles of addiction nurses and mental health nurses. The primary role of addiction nurses or mental health nurses exemplifies the contribution that they can make to comprehensive patient care by performing clinical interventions from triage to counselling, psychotherapy to case management (Greenman, 1994). Due to the nature of the work and the composition of many community drug and alcohol teams, decisions regarding whether a client is seen by a nurse, medical practitioner or psychologist have, in the past, often depended upon which discipline was in charge of the allocation process and which staff member had a vacant slot (Gafoor, 1997). This phenomenon is no different in community mental health teams.

A comparison of the primary roles within addiction nurses, mental health nurses and the team in dual diagnosis is outlined in Table 12.1. This highlights many similarities for each discipline, and the considerable number of transferable roles and skills that are shared. It also illustrates that within the new nursing roles within mental health settings, work on dual diagnosis is a central feature. What is important to note are the subtle differences in the focus of dual diagnosis work that is being undertaken in the different teams and how nurses have both individual and team responsibilities.

Table 12.1 Comparison of nursing roles.

	Psychiatric nursing	Addiction nursing	Dual diagnosis nursing
Assessment	Concerned primarily with mental health presentation: • Presenting factors, history of presenting factors • Treatment compliance • Section of Mental Health Act, including specialist assessments such as forensic and eating disorders • Risk to self and others • Level of insight into mental health • Current mood • Current behaviour • Use of psychotropic medications • Use of drugs and alcohol • Brief intervention • Motivational interviewing	Concerned primarily with illicit drug use: • Drug/s of choice • Amount and frequency • Risks around substance misuse • Risk related to behaviours to support substance misuse • Level of insight into substance use and effects of use • Motivations to change • Relapse prevention	Concerned with substance misuse in the presenting mental health: • Drug/s of choice currently used, including psychotropic medications • Amount and frequency of substance misuse • History of substance misuse in relation to occurrence of psychiatric symptoms • Risks related to the use of drugs and alcohol, including the implication for harm to self or others and risk behaviours related to obtaining drugs or alcohol • Level of insight into both mental health and substance misuse • Current mood • Current behaviour • Motivation for change
Medication	Concerned with psychotropic medications: • Effects • Side effects • Overdose • Actions and interactions • Supervised consumption • Administration of depot medications • Medication compliance	Concerned with illicit and licit substances, including prescription medications: • Effects of drugs and alcohol • Side effects of drugs and alcohol • Withdrawal effects of drugs and alcohol • Overdose and accidental overdose • Supervised consumption of methadone • Administration of detoxification medications • Additional substance misuse during substitute prescribing	Concerned with psychotropic and prescribed medications: • Effects of illicit substances and prescribed medications • Actions and interactions of prescribed and non-prescribed medications • Side effects of both substances of abuse and prescribed medications • Overdose and accidental overdose • Administration of medication for detoxification • Supervised consumption of methadone • Medication compliance, including additional substance use during substitute prescribing

Table 12.1 (*cont'd*)

	Psychiatric nursing	Addiction nursing	Dual diagnosis nursing
Health checks	• Weight • Height • Urine testing for basic analysis • Sleep patterns • Dietary intake • Hygiene patterns	• Substance misuse either by urine testing or via breathalyser • Injecting sites for damage • Hepatitis and HIV testing can be offered • Requests for full blood counts/liver function tests and confirmation of substance misuse	• Weight • Height • Urine testing for basic analysis and substance misuse • Breath testing for alcohol use • Hygiene at initial presentation • Injection sites for damage • Dietary intake • Requests for full blood counts/liver function tests and confirmation of substance misuse
Nursing care offered	• Risk assessments for harm to self and others • Ongoing mental health assessments • Active role in the community programme approach • Key worker responsibility for outpatients • Administration of medications including depot medications • Individual counselling/individual support/group work • Work on insight into mental health and development of strategies related to activities of daily living • Support of relatives/partners and other family members • Development of structured programmes and care plans enhancing mental health • Simple wound dressings	• Supervision of methadone consumption and where applicable on site injecting clinics • Harm minimisation of substance use • Counselling specific to the use and reduction of drugs and alcohol • Supervision of home detoxification programmes • Administration of methadone prescriptions • Community care funding assessments for in-patient treatment • Simple wound dressings • Individual/group counselling	• Risk assessments for harm to self and others • Supervision of medications including methadone and psychotropic prescriptions • Individual supported counselling • Outreach work to enhance engagement within local services • Harm minimisation for substance misuse and harm to self or others • Counselling specific to mental health and substance misuse • Supervision of outpatient detoxification for substance misuse • Administration of methadone prescriptions • Adjunctive role in community programme approach/community care funding assessments • Development of care plans to optimise patient care • Simple wound dressings

These are comparisons of roles and not exhaustive lists.
Source: adapted from Moore & Rassool (2002).

Dual diagnosis nursing can thus be seen as a synthesis of principles of care management from both addiction and mental health nursing (Moore & Rassool, 2002). In community settings, there is now a pathway of care from entry in mental health, treatment in crisis, to ongoing or highly specialist substance misuse/dual diagnosis care. A central feature of dual diagnosis nursing in the community is the implementation of programmes with multidisciplinary teams, working with practitioners from general practice, addiction teams and acute mental health teams to provide specialist care. Working with each other will ensure that there is support and expertise for helping this complex client group and demonstrates how nurses take important roles in the provision and coordination of care without working in isolation.

Problems and issues

Patients with coexisting mental health and substance misuse problems present great challenges for nurses and other health care professionals. There are several problems and issues regarding the engagement of and interventions for patients with dual diagnosis. Many individuals may have had difficulty engaging with psychiatric services due to the substance use, or failed at addiction treatment by defaulting on the prescribed programme. This group of patients are often thought of as 'difficult to treat', non-compliant or non-attenders. Patients often face the prejudice of having not just a mental health problem or substance misuse problem and, as such, can be doubly rejected (Department of Health, 1999). There are additional prejudices that can add to this picture: ethnicity, culture, gender, education and social status are factors that influence diagnosis and the perceived levels of risk made by professional groups. In working with the dual diagnosis population our own fears and prejudices about the complexity of the physical, emotional, moral and ethical problems must be examined.

In bridging the gap between mental health and substance misuse it is common to encounter the difficult area of 'responsibility' and 'confidentiality'. Dual diagnosis teams run the risk of being seen to be ultimately responsible for all dual diagnosis clients, whether they are appropriate for addiction or mental health services, or not. Abdication of responsibility for this client group can be due to concerns of risk, and an inability to deal with the duality of the presenting problems, or lack of expertise with this complex client group. Risk has been highlighted as a growing concern within community nursing management of dual diagnosis. Recent literature has suggested that dual diagnosis patients are regarded as high-risk patients for violence and criminal behaviour, and even in homicides (Scott *et al.*, 1998; Ward & Applin, 1998). It is understandable that many practitioners have concerns about working with this client group. However, the obstacles must balance information on violence, fear and sometimes prejudice from systems that exclude them from engaging. Whilst it can be argued that the nature of dual diagnosis may compound the level of risk, the full extent of violent behaviour and dual diagnosis continue to be assessed. Clinical practice of risk management at service level remains a thorny issue, a combination of mental health and substance misuse risk assessments would be important components of any comprehensive dual diagnosis work. Community nursing of this client group requires that in a similar vein to community mental health, safety is one of the most important components of day-to-day working, regardless of which model the dual diagnosis service is based on.

Confidentiality as a core principal service provision continues to remain a difficult issue for health care professionals and substance misuse services, who have a long history of strict guidelines on both confidentiality and breach of confidentiality. Conversely, many mental health services have joint agreements with statutory agencies regarding information sharing. This one issue has the potential to cause working agreements to collapse if it is not explored and addressed in the early stages of any planned development for working within hospital and community settings.

There are inherent difficulties in working with dual diagnosis in homeless populations. Community substance misuse services provide community care assessments for detoxification and rehabilitation; however, there is no provision that has enabled funding for dual diagnosis patients to attend specialist centres for treatment. Additionally, there is a distinct lack of in-patient detoxification and residential rehabilitation services for this client group. Whereas substance misuse patients can enter into rehabilitation that addresses their ability not only to remain drug free but also offers rehabilitation into the wider community, this is not so with dual diagnosis patients and may result in inappropriate admissions to acute psychiatric services.

One of the most important considerations in community services for dual diagnosis is how all teams and services work together; collaboration and joint working practices can provide a comprehensive care package for dual diagnosis patients (Teague *et al.*, 1995; Shwartz *et al.*, 1997; Mueser *et al.*, 1998). Many services developed in the USA, and more recently in the UK, are based on case management, with the belief that this would reduce the number of crisis episodes and admissions (Shwartz *et al.*, 1997). Breslow *et al.* (1996) studied an evaluation of the impact by managed care systems and found that whilst managed care patients continued to require emergency services, patients who were not case managed required more interventions and showed more psychotic symptoms and substance use.

Conclusion

Both addiction and mental health have well developed and established services; however, these services have developed different focuses for treatment. Substance misuse services make attempts at engaging the service user to seek help, and see the individual as responsible for the actions and choices they make: psychiatry does not (Moore & Rassool, 2002). Severe and enduring mental illness is often seen as the individual not being able to make safe choices, and at times not being responsible for their actions. These philosophies form the basis of treatment services, and in the case of psychiatry the ability to detain an individual under the Mental Health Act (1983) to ensure treatment. Whilst both substance misuse and mental health services have dual diagnosis patients in treatment programmes, there are a significant number who fall between the service provisions due to the severity of their problems. This gives rise to the 'revolving door syndrome' for dual diagnosis patients who are seen as inappropriate to either service. Dual diagnosis services attempt to bridge this gap in the current service arrangements by addressing both the substance misuse and the mental health problems.

So whose patient is it anyway? Who is responsible for providing dual diagnosis services? All services have a role to play; whilst some may argue that specific services need to be established, it is unlikely that separate funding of specific services will become available. Regardless of which agency takes a lead, nurses play a central role in the development of dual diagnosis practice, including designing and implementing a combined approach to working in dual diagnosis. Individual case management works in parallel with nominated key worker care programme approach (CPA) systems, allowing for flexible working practices in all settings, including assertive outreach programmes, which can be extended to joint working agreements with other agencies. The community responses to the health and social care needs of patients with mental health problems and substance misuse have, in the past, failed to provide adequate and accessible services. To some extent, this group has been marginalised by professionals and by society at large.

References

Abou Saleh, M.T. (2004) Dual diagnosis: management within a psychosocial context. *Advances in Psychiatric Treatment*, (10), 352–60.

Barnes, A., Murray, M., Ritchie, F. & Jones, M. (2002) Dual diagnosis: developing the skill base. *Mental Health Practice*, 5 (7), 16–19.

Breslow, R., Klinger, B. & Erickson, B. (1996) Characteristics of managed care patients in a psychiatric emergency service. *Psychiatric Services*, 47 (11), 1259–61.

Byrne, P. (2000) Stigma of mental illness and ways of diminishing it. *Advances in Psychiatric Treatment*, 6, 65–72.

Cabinet Office (1998) *Tackling Drugs To Build a Better Britain. The Government's 10-Year Strategy for Tackling Drug Misuse*. Cm. 39459. The Stationery Office, London.

Clarke, C. (1999) Revisiting the concepts of community care and community health nursing. *Nursing Standard*, 14 (10), 34–6.

Crogan, E. (2005) An introduction to behaviour change among clients. *Nursing Standard*, 19 (30), 60–2.

Department of Health (1999) *National Service Framework for Mental Health: Modern Standards and Service Models*. Department of Health, London.

Department of Health (2000) *The Mental Health Implementation Policy Implementation Guide*. Department of Health, London.

Department of Health (2002) *Mental Health Policy Implementation Guide. Dual Diagnosis: Good Practice Guide*. Department of Health, London.

Gafoor, M. (1997) Substance misuse and mental health. In: *Addiction Nursing: Perspectives on Professional and Clinical Practice* (Rassool, G.H. & Gafoor, M., eds), pp. 152–8. Stanley Thornes, Cheltenham.

Gafoor, M. & Rassool, G.H. (1998) The coexistance of psychiatric disorders and substance misuse: working with dual diagnosis patients. *Journal of Advanced Nursing*, 27, 497–502.

Greenman, D. (1994) The role of the addictions nurse specialist in adult psychiatry. *Perspectives on Addictions Nursing*, 5 (3), 3–4.

Hunt, P. (1995) Dietary counselling: theory into practice. *Journal of the Institute of Health Excellence*, 33 (1), 4–8.

Hunt, P. & Pearson, D. (2001) Motivating change. *Nursing Standard*, 16 (2), 45–52.

Kavanagh, D., Mueser, K. & Baker, A. (2003) Management of co-morbidity. In: *Co-morbid Mental Disorders and Substance Use Disorders: Epidemiology, Prevention and Treatment* (Teesson, M. & Proudfoot, H., eds). National Drug and Alcohol Research Centre, New South Wales, Sydney, Australia.

Kennedy, P. & Griffiths, H. (2003) 'Mental health': collaborative challenges care culture. *Psychiatric Bulletin*, 27, 164–6.

Moore, K. & Rassool, G.H. (2002) A synthesis of addiction and mental health nursing: an approach to community interventions. In: *Dual Diagnosis: Substance Misuse and Psychiatric Disorders* (Rassool, G.H., ed.). Blackwell Publishing, Oxford.

Mueser, K.T., Drake, R.E. & Wallach, M.E. (1998) Dual diagnosis: a review of aetiological theories. *Addictive Behaviours*, 23 (6), 717–34.

National Treatment Agency (2002) *Models of Care for Substance Misuse*. National Treatment Agency, London.

Osher, F. & Kofoed, L. (1989) Treatment of patients with psychiatric and psychoactive substance abuse disorders. *Hospital Community Psychiatry*, 40 (10), 1025–30.

Pediani, R. (2000) Changing practice: are memes the answer? *Nursing Standard*, 1 (14), 36–40.

Prochaska, J.O. & DiClemente, C.C. (1986) Towards a comprehensive model of change. In: *Treating Addictive Behaviours: Processes of Change* (Miller, W.R. & Heather, N., eds). Plenum, New York.

Rassool, G.H. (1996) Addiction Nursing and Substance Misuse: A Slow Response to Partial Accommodation. Editorial in *Journal of Advanced Nursing*, 24 (2), 425–7.

Rassool, G.H. (1997) Addiction nursing – towards a new paradigm: the UK experience. In: *Addiction Nursing – Perspectives on Professional and Clinical Practice* (Rassool, G.H. & Gafoor, M., eds), p. 11. Stanley Thornes, Cheltenham.

Rassool, G.H. (1999) Addiction nursing: a community oriented approach. In: *Current Issues in Community Nursing* (Littlewood, J., ed.), pp. 91–118. Churchill Livingstone, Edinburgh.

Rassool, G.H. (2000) Addiction: global problem and global response: complacency or commitment? Editorial in *Journal of Advanced Nursing*, 32 (3), 505–8.

Rassool, G.H. (2002) Substance misuse and mental health: an overview. *Nursing Standard*, 16 (50), 46–52.

Royal College of Psychiatrists (2001) *Changing Minds Campaing*. RCP, London.

Scott, H., Johnson, S., Menzies, P. *et al.* (1998) Substance misuse and risk of aggression and offending among the severely mentally ill. *British Journal of Psychiatry*, 172, 345–50.

Shwartz, M., Baker, G., Mulvey, K. & Plough, A. (1997) Improving publicly funded substance abuse treatment: the value of case management. *American Journal of Public Health*, 87 (10), 1659–64.

Teague, G., Drake, R. & Ackerson, T. (1995) Evaluating the use of continuous treatment teams for persons with mental illness and substance abuse. *Psychiatric Services*, 7, 689–95.

Ward, M. & Applin, C. (1998) *The Unlearned Lesson. The Role of Alcohol and Drug Misuse in Homicides Perpetrated by People with Mental Health Problems*. Wynne Howard Books, London.

Weaver, T., Charles, V., Madden, P. & Renton, A. (2002) *Co-morbidity of Substance Misuse and Mental Illness Collaborative Study*. National Treatment Agency, London.

Zweeban, J. (1993) Dual diagnosis: key issues for the 1990s. *Psychology of Addictive Behaviours*, 7 (3), 168–72.

13 Shared Care and Inter-professional Practice

A. Simpson

Introduction

The majority of mental health professionals that have experience of working with people with a dual diagnosis will have witnessed endless games of professional 'ping-pong'. Services for mentally ill people bat the referral across to drug or alcohol agencies, only to see the dazed and confused client knocked swiftly back across the invisible service line by a drug worker keen to keep substance misuse services free of people with mental illness. Often, after numerous discussions behind closed doors as to the suitability of this particular 'referral', the unseen, and often much maligned, individual has long since disappeared, having 'fallen through the net' of professional provision, thus unwittingly confirming their supposed unreliability and lack of motivation. Months or years later, the same rejected individual reappears at the doors of less discriminating voluntary services or, all too frequently, is delivered through the swing doors of the local casualty department.

Fortunately, as dual diagnosis has become increasingly commonplace and recognised it has been acknowledged that a range of different agencies and workers need to work together in order to provide skilled and effective care for people with a combination of substance misuse problems and mental illness. Government policy in England now requires high quality, patient focused, integrated care for people with dual diagnoses to be delivered within 'mainstream' services. Drug and alcohol services will continue to treat people with substance misuse problems, but are also required to advise and work closely with colleagues in primary care and mental health services, often providing collaborative approaches to treatment, care and support (Department of Health, 2003a).

But cross-agency and inter-professional working does not necessarily come easily and there is evidence to suggest that misunderstandings and tensions frequently diminish the undoubted benefits that effective joint working can bring to both service users and staff. These difficulties are even more likely to exist where managers and workers operate within organisations that adhere to different, even contradictory philosophical beliefs and clinical approaches. This is often the case between psychiatric and substance misuse services or where staff in statutory services work alongside those from the voluntary sector. Organisations may exhibit different attitudes and adopt contrary stances towards treatment regimes, harm minimisation, communication, management of aggression, risk and safety, and issues of confidentiality.

This chapter will outline some of the benefits of shared care, inter-professional collaboration and teamwork. It will also explore some of the tensions and difficulties frequently reported and suggest some of the measures that can and should be taken to minimise conflict and maximise cooperation, coordination and the provision of effective, integrated teamwork. For the purposes of this chapter, the term teamwork will be be used interchangeably with inter-professional or collaborative practice. It is defined to include any situation where professional or non-professional workers from different disciplines or agencies are required to work closely with the service user and each other in order to ensure that health and social care needs are met. The issues discussed will be applicable whether staff work in primary care, in hospitals, in community services, or across any or all of these. First, I will outline the policy framework that underpins inter-professional practice for people with a dual diagnosis.

Case management, the care programme approach and dual diagnosis

Case management aims to target resources at those most in need, reduce duplication and disorganisation in service provision, and ensure the coordinated delivery of a range of services to vulnerable and needy people. The exact shape and nature of case management is determined by the design and philosophy of the system created to deliver it and the context in which it operates (Intagliata, 1982). Since the early 1990s, services for people with mental illness in England have operated within the framework of the care programme approach (CPA), a loosely defined form of case management (Simpson *et al.*, 2003a).

The essential motivation underpinning the CPA is commendable. It is intended to provide a seamless service for mentally ill people, addressing both health and social care needs through an integrated and coordinated approach. When implemented well it enables multidisciplinary staff to provide an agreed plan of care, whilst minimising inter-professional conflict and maximising opportunities for joint working. But the CPA was not well implemented or resourced and was unaccompanied by appropriate training. It was associated with political and media attacks on community care, copious paperwork and bureaucratic procedures, and was seen as part of an emerging 'blame culture'. This led to patchy service provision, little enthusiasm amongst staff and minimal impact on service users and carers (Simpson *et al.*, 2003b).

In response to the uneven implementation of the CPA and concerns that there was too much focus on the administrative aspects, the policy was reformed (Department of Health, 1999). People with a dual diagnosis were explicitly identified to be included under the CPA for the first time, whether they were located in mental health or substance misuse services. This entitles them to an assessment of their health and social care needs and the allocation of a named care coordinator who develops a plan of care in consultation with the service user, their family or informal carers and various care providers. This written care plan, which should consider and reflect the service user's culture, ethnicity, gender and sexuality, is given to the user. Copies are sent to the GPs, family carers and all health and social care staff involved. This might include workers in voluntary agencies, staff in hostels or supported accommodation, as well as workers in mental health and substance misuse services.

The care coordinator ensures that contact is maintained with the user and that the agreed services and interventions are delivered. The care plan should be regularly reviewed and modified as and when needs and circumstances change. Risk assessment and management is an essential and ongoing part of the CPA process and should include consideration of risk of neglect, exploitation and harm from others, self-harm, suicide and anything that threatens the safety of others. Alongside an increased propensity to suicide (Appleby *et al.*, 1999) and aggression (Taylor & Gunn, 1999; Walsh & Fahy, 2002), substance misuse also raises potential child protection concerns that may require specialist assessment and support (Department of Health, 2003b).

People with more complex needs, such as dual diagnosis, receive the 'enhanced' version of the CPA (see Table 13.1). Enhanced care plans should include instructions on what to do in a crisis and details of how to contact someone during non-office hours. They should also incorporate contingency plans so that continuous care and support is provided even when key personnel are not available, whether through sickness, holidays or any unforeseen situations (Department of Health, 1999).

Although there is variable evidence concerning the effectiveness of the CPA, the evidence for case

Table 13.1 Characteristics of those people more likely to be on the 'enhanced' level of the care programme approach (CPA).

- Multiple care needs, including housing, employment, finances, etc., requiring inter-agency coordination
- Contact with a number of agencies (including the criminal justice system)
- More frequent and intensive interventions, perhaps with medication management
- Mental health problems coexisting with other problems such as substance misuse
- More likely to be at risk of harming themselves or others
- More likely to disengage from services

management approaches generally is more positive, if not without controversy and disagreement (Simpson *et al.*, 2003a). The key factors identified in the provision of effective case management are identified in Table 13.2. Without doubt, an assertive approach to engagement and intervention, involving a high level of persistent outreach, is likely to be a key component of the work with people with a dual diagnosis. This is especially so for those who are frequently readmitted to hospital, who are chaotic, homeless, or resistant to psychiatric and substance misuse services. Other aspects of case management, such as providing advice and support to obtain appropriate accommodation, finances and employment are also likely to be crucial aspects of the work. The use of specific evidence based psychosocial interventions (Baguley & Baguley, 1999), including those specifically addressing substance misuse, should also be an important component of the care coordinator's role. However, there can be tensions in this regard unless organisational factors, such as excessive workload and lack of clinical supervision, are addressed (Grant & Mills, 2000; Simpson, 2005).

Importantly, the successful discharge of individual responsibilities under case management can only be achieved when clinicians are working as part of a good team. Effective teamwork is absolutely imperative when the nature of work with users requires a high level of communication and cooperation or interdependence between workers in order to 'get the job done' (Onyett, 2002). This lies at the heart of successful work with people with a dual diagnosis of mental illness and substance misuse.

Benefits of shared care and effective teamwork

Summarising research in private and public sector organisations, West (1999) argued that teams are seen as the most effective way of delivering services, with positive effects on performance, quality, efficiency, profits, staff turnover and redundancy. In mental health services, community mental health teams (CMHTs) are generally perceived to be the

Table 13.2 Factors identified in effective case management approaches.

Reasonable caseloads for case manager and team	Persistent, assertive approach for challenging and resistant service users
Clinical role for case manager and use of psychosocial interventions	Team planning, input and support with good team leadership
Development of therapeutic relationship with users	Medication management (essential with dual diagnosis)
Long-term relationship with users, responsive to changing needs	Encourage engagement with 'mainstream' community services
Help with accommodation, finances, employment, legal system, etc.	Psycho-education and support with families and other carers
Aim to maximise self-determination of users	Focus on individuals' strengths, interests and resources
Majority of contact in community settings, not office or hospital	Extended out-of-hours service and 24-hour emergency access
Support with and development of daily living skills	Ongoing training, development and supervision of workers

Source: adapted from Simpson *et al.* (2003a).

most appropriate delivery system for effective community care (Department of Health, 2002). Advantages include multidisciplinary assessment of needs, access to a wide range of skills and disciplines, continuity of care, shared responsibility for clients and decisions, professional support and improved management of workload. CMHT care for people with severe mental illness helps services maintain contact with users, reduces the risk of suicide, cuts the time spent in hospital and is popular with patients (Tyrer *et al.*, 2002).

Features that appeared to be key to effective interdisciplinary teamwork were identified by Proctor-Childs *et al.* (1998) and include:

- A commitment to a shared philosophy of teamwork that has been consciously worked through
- Leadership with a vision, supported by senior professionals who cascade those beliefs to their own discipline
- A focus on user led work that encourages reflection on practice
- A high level of role understanding facilitated by joint working practices, which enhance role visibility
- Joint care planning and goal setting that allows exploration of professional values and beliefs
- The sharing of knowledge, skills and information, which develops 'team knowledge'

Effective interdisciplinary working requires each profession to understand what other staff are doing and why. It incorporates an appreciation of how other disciplines understand knowledge and the methods by which it is gained and used. Conflict resolution, including an appreciation of the difference between responsibility and accountability, is also central. A study of seven health and social care teams in various settings found clear benefits for service users where teams worked in this more integrated, collaborative fashion (Miller *et al.*, 2001). Benefits include:

- Continuity of care, where professionals 'carry over' interventions initiated by colleagues
- Consistency of approach and reduction of ambiguity with a high level of shared, agreed knowledge provided to users
- Appropriate referrals to team colleagues based on an understanding of each other's roles
- A holistic approach derived from joint planning and working
- High levels of constructive problem solving

However, they found that 'fragmented' working, in which individual professionals often worked well but not as part of a team focus, was much more commonplace. Where this occurred, many aspects of patient management, such as problem solving, decision making and responsibility for actions were related to single professional groups. Partly as a result, communication between team members was relatively brief and tended to involve giving of information rather than sharing of professional perspectives. In such teams, role understanding was superficial, with staff unable or unwilling to develop an in-depth understanding of each other's roles. Professionals reinforced the 'mono-professional' nature of clinical practice by actively protecting role boundaries. Team leadership was often problematic and tended to create an unsafe environment in which communication and learning was stifled and multi-professional collaboration unsupported. As a result, skills and knowledge remained within individual professional groups and the benefits of teamworking were rarely discussed, realised or demonstrated (Miller *et al.*, 2001).

Effective teamworking is strongly related to the quality of teamwork. A major three-year study of over 400 health care teams in England and Scotland, including 113 CMHTs, found that effective teams were those that had clear team objectives, enabled higher levels of participation, had a greater emphasis on quality and high support for innovation (Borrill *et al.*, 2000). The better the level of communication in meetings and the more integration between different staff, the better and more innovative were the approaches to patient care. More reflective CMHTs were also found to be more innovative. Reflective teams are those that 'reflect upon their objectives, strategies, processes and their organisational and wider environments, plan to adapt to their tasks, and make changes accordingly' (West, 1999).

Team leadership was again found to be important. Where there was lack of clear leadership, team members reported low levels of effectiveness and this was associated with poor quality team working, less participation by members and lack of clarity about objectives. In all types of health care teams studied, Borrill *et al.* (2000) also found that better team functioning was associated with better mental health amongst staff. In contrast, staff in teams with poor leadership and low levels of communication reported higher levels of stress and psychological ailments.

The findings from these studies suggest that any attempt to establish shared care arrangements for people with dual diagnoses will need to ensure a number of key factors are in place. These include:

- Safe environments and meetings in which effective sharing of information and professional knowledge takes place
- Structures and support that enable high levels of constructive participation, joint planning of care and decision making
- Multi-professional support for strong, consensual leadership that considers, includes, values and unites the different professions
- Clear aims and objectives for the team with an underpinning philosophy of high quality user focused care, team reflexivity and responsiveness

These will be absolutely crucial for the success of shared care projects and the provision of effective, innovative care for people with dual diagnoses. However, there is plentiful evidence that numerous barriers and difficulties are likely to threaten integrated working unless these are recognised, considered and addressed. I shall consider these now.

Problems with inter-agency and inter-professional practice

Attempts to establish multidisciplinary teamworking in health and social care have faced numerous difficulties, with the potential benefits often not realised (Leathard, 1994; West & Poulton, 1997). Barriers, often predicated on issues of hierarchy, social class and gender, include communication difficulties, power imbalances, interpersonal and inter-professional conflict, differing leadership styles, inequalities in status and pay and various organisational factors (Leathard, 1994; Firth-Cozens, 1998). The tendency for professional workers to protect their individual positions rather than work cooperatively is always likely to be a key obstacle to the successful working of multidisciplinary teams (Beeforth *et al.*, 1990).

Doctors in particular, being the dominant profession, have a lot to lose through inter-professional collaboration and may understandably resist any loss of their power or authority (Mackay *et al.*, 1995). Inter-group stereotypes also hamper effective team working (Carpenter, 1995), and tend to underpin some of the 'games', tactics and negotiations that have characterised communication and interactions between doctors and nurses over the years (Stein, 1978; Allen, 1997; Wicks, 1998). Relations between nurses and social workers can also be difficult (Edwards & Garrety, 1998) with each bringing their own historical allegiances, suppositions and strong ideological differences (Brown, 1989; Bywaters, 1989; Dalley, 1989). It has even been suggested that community mental health teams were, at least partly, created to contain and resolve the tensions between professional groups without explicitly addressing the fundamental differences in culture and practice that exist between the different agencies and professions (Peck, 1995; Onyett *et al.*, 1997). The addition of substance misuse workers with another set of approaches, ideas and philosophies can only add to the inter-professional fun and games.

Professional groups tend to hold different views about the role and importance of teams, with psychiatrists and psychologists, in particular, often experiencing high levels of conflict over issues of leadership, responsibility and philosophical approaches (Mistral & Velleman, 1997). A range of views are essential to a multidisciplinary approach, but where destructive differences are not addressed those in inferior hierarchical positions tend to feel alienated, with the potential loss of their knowledge and input to the team (Cott, 1998). The *Confidential Inquiry into Homicides and Suicides* found that inter-professional disagreements were often detrimental to the care of the user, with the potential for tragic consequences (Royal College of Psychiatrists, 1996).

Research into community psychiatric nurses (CPNs) working in CMHTs found that CPNs in teams marked by more problematic inter-professional dynamics did not participate or communicate as readily in team meetings (Simpson, 2004). They and other team members, including social workers and occupational therapists, became inhibited, and their ability to discuss and coordinate the care of their clients was severely hampered. Where there was a perceived lack of safety in the team meetings, CPNs and others failed to disclose and discuss important information about service users that included issues of serious risk. When psychiatrists acted disrespectfully, or when they undermined the contribution of other professionals, staff tended to reduce their participation, withdraw from meetings and assume defensive or even obstructive positions within the team. There is enormous potential for such interdisciplinary tensions to erupt in teams drawn from different agencies and professions to meet the needs of people with dual diagnoses.

Other research has found that staff working within multidisciplinary teams are often reluctant to comply with operational directives aimed at facilitating inter-agency working. They adhere to their own professional cultures and there is an absence of a strong philosophy of care shared by all groups. Factors originating in training and maintained by professional socialisation can undermine attempts to establish and sustain inter-professional collaboration (Norman & Peck, 1999). Staff, particularly psychiatrists and psychologists, often express concerns over the loss of autonomy and revert to their own professional groups for 'protection'. Norman & Peck (1999) suggested that CPNs were less concerned over loss of autonomy as they had always worked within hierarchies. However, this is contradicted by other research in which CPNs greatly resented the loss of clinical autonomy that came with CMHT working. CPNs closely managed by a combination of psychiatrists, team managers and senior managers expressed concerns about the dilution of their role and the impact on professional boundaries (Kashi & Littlewood, 2000). CPNs felt that they were being 'redirected towards traditional activities [and] controlled by psychiatrists', and experienced 'increasing professional rivalry and suspicions within the practice arena' (Kashi & Littlewood, 2000). In my own study, CPNs often reported concerns that their traditional psychotherapeutic role was being subsumed by the need to address social care needs previously associated with the social worker role (Simpson, 2005); a finding reported elsewhere (Miller & Freeman, 2003).

Role substitution, or generic working, leads to concerns that 'role boundaries are muddled, resulting in unclear lines of accountability and responsibility and deskilling' (Norman & Peck, 1999). There are also concerns that such moves reduce the range of skills available within a team to meet users' needs. This can create increased adherence to professional culture, defensive manoeuvres and inflexible demarcation as roles are stoutly defended.

In a study of three CMHTs, Brown *et al.* (2000), reported that different team members saw role boundaries differently. Some wanted to work towards removing role boundaries in order to develop interdisciplinary teamwork, whilst others expressed concern that the erosion of boundaries would result in role confusion and the development of 'generic' mental health workers. In such a model, all team members would be doing the same or 'meddling' in each other's areas of expertise, when they saw it as a strength and an advantage that the CMHTs could offer service users a variety of skills and approaches from different professional backgrounds. So, there was a dichotomy between those who thought it important that different professions maintained their separateness, whilst others within the same teams believed that it was beneficial for professional roles to 'blur' or develop to incorporate skills and knowledge from team colleagues. A third point of view wanted team members to concentrate on what they were each good at and to recognise and communicate the limits of their own knowledge and expertise.

Clearly, in the light of these findings, any attempt to introduce new roles such as substance misuse worker, or to redefine existing roles or responsibilities, need to be considered and implemented skilfully. This is particularly so at a time of enormous change, in which many professionals feel under threat and are uncertain of their professional status and futures (Kennedy & Griffiths, 2000).

Structure and procedures

Team structures and procedures are also important. In the study by Brown *et al.* (2000), decisions had been made to introduce a level of 'democracy' in the running of the teams, so, for example, a 'rolling chair' for team meetings was introduced with a different person chairing or taking minutes each week. However, this lack of clear structure left most people unhappy, feeling ill-equipped and unprepared for such tasks. As a result, the meetings and the team itself were experienced as insufficiently stable or secure, creating a 'sense of inadequacy' rather than empowerment (Brown *et al.*, 2000). Several staff members were required to work across different teams, which also undermined the coherence of the teams studied. The authors suggested that contrary to the aims of the management, attempts to remove boundaries were having the effect of reinforcing them. Similarly, difficulties were also identified in my study of seven CMHTs, when teams lacked clear objectives or there was a lack of structure or agreed procedures (Simpson, 2004). Inadequate arrangements for accepting referrals, allocating work within teams and running the team meetings led to repetition of work and time wasting as the same issues were continually rehashed. It also created resentment and suspicion when workers perceived that others were 'not pulling their weight' or were not subject to the same organisational demands and strictures. Other studies in both hospital and community health and social care settings have stressed the importance of boundaries and structures in the maintenance of workers' psychological safety and security (Menzies, 1960; Bowers, 1992; Bray, 1999). Such personal security, it has been argued, is essential in allowing staff to feel secure in their work with service users and will be particularly so with the challenges faced in working with people with dual diagnoses.

Onyett *et al.* (1997) stressed the need for organisational managers to ensure that multidisciplinary teams have clear aims and objectives and good internal structures for operational management. Ovretveit (1993; Ovretveit *et al.*, 1997) made similar recommendations for the design and planning of teams, and suggested that whilst personalities are important, lack of operational structure makes it difficult for even the 'most willing and cooperative of people to collaborate with others' (Ovretveit, 1993). He explained how there are usually organisational or structural explanations for difficulties within teams that are frequently blamed on 'personality clashes'. For example, issues like a team leader not being able to get the information needed from a team member, or a team never confronting or making difficult decisions, are often explained in terms of the personalities involved. Or a legitimate concern about the quality of another team member's work is reduced to a 'conflict of personalities', when there were not agreed arrangements in place for monitoring and support, or for properly addressing and raising such issues without 'personalising' them (Ovretveit, 1993).

As well as conflict within teams, there is also enormous potential for conflict between the team and the parent organisation, even more so when teams are answerable to a variety of statutory and voluntary organisations. Conflicting boundaries within therapeutic organisations tend to be problematic, especially where governmental or managerial policies are at odds with the therapeutic priorities held by the clinicians and service users. In certain circumstances teams can become united in their conflict with organisations, but in such situations it is rare that the needs of either the team or the service users will prevail (Pietroni, 1995). Tension between clinical teams and organisations was identified in focus groups of 'experts' in mental health that included practitioners, educators, academics, service users and carers. Staff saw the risk aversive organisational culture of NHS trusts as obstacles to delivering effective care (Warner *et al.*, 2001).

The potential for disagreements about issues of risk is likely to be magnified when working with people with dual diagnosis. The potential for risky scenarios is greater and the chance that staff from different agencies will share perspectives on how best to assess, predict and manage risky behaviours is likely to be remote. It is important that staff are aware of these potential inter-professional 'hot-spots' and are able to discuss and agree a pragmatic, shared approach. One issue that often complicates such discussions is that of patient confidentiality, which is discussed next.

Confidentiality

Issues around confidentiality and disclosure are often difficult for mental health staff. The number of people and agencies involved in the care of people using mental health services can be surprising. Alongside immediate staff that may include GPs, psychiatrists, various nurses and health care assistants, occupational therapists, psychologists, social workers and advocates there can be a range of other people and agencies involved, each acquiring and passing on sensitive client information. Other staff that might frequently be involved could include benefits and financial advisers, social security staff, housing officers and housing support workers. Szmukler & Holloway (2001) have outlined just how difficult, if not impossible, it is to maintain client confidentiality in mental health services given the vast range of agencies involved. The addition of substance misuse services simply magnifies the problem. Alongside the addition of drug and alcohol workers, needle exchange staff and counsellors, it is not unusual for people with substance misuse problems to have contact with the police, probation officers, solicitors and court officials.

Staff working in these agencies might have quite different expectations regarding what constitutes confidential information. There might be difficult situations where information considered personal and confidential by one person is considered absolutely crucial information that needs to be passed on and documented by others before key decisions can be made. For example, discussions over the allocation of accommodation would involve consideration of previous criminal and other risky behaviour in order to consider the safety of other residents in shared accommodation or neighbourhoods. It would not be untypical for such issues to be factors in the lives of people with drug and alcohol histories.

Issues of confidentiality can be particularly complex and challenging for staff working with people who misuse illicit substances. The position concerning knowledge of possible illegal behaviour by clients and the responsibilities of service providers and their staff to act on that knowledge has become more sensitive and grievous following the case of the 'Cambridge Two' in the late 1990s (Simpson, 2000). The director and manager of a day centre for homeless people in Cambridge, England, were jailed for five and four years respectively when the courts found that they had not taken sufficient steps to prevent the selling of illicit drugs on or in the vicinity of their premises. The severe sentences passed on two experienced and respected workers have serious implications for staff in a range of health and social care settings. People who have a drug addiction often sell small amounts to their friends as a way of financing their drug use. The judge's ruling in this case says that if staff are aware of the trading of drugs and do not take action to prevent it they are guilty of 'knowingly permitting' the supply of the drug and could face prosecution and a hefty jail sentence.

In such a complex environment and when dealing with such potentially devastating situations, it is imperative that staff working jointly with people with a dual diagnosis ensure that they have an unambiguous and agreed understanding of where their responsibilities lie. There should be a clear policy and guidelines on the sharing and disclosure of client information with particular attention paid to potential risk factors and criminal activity.

Conclusion

It is now recognised that a range of different agencies and workers are required to work together in order to provide skilled and effective care for people with a combination of substance misuse problems and mental illness. The evidence suggests that service users and staff stand to benefit from well planned, integrated teamwork. It is also clear that there are numerous tensions and difficulties that, if not considered and addressed, hold the potential to derail any attempt at establishing shared care and teamwork. Consider the following essential points:

- Encourage open discussion of roles and responsibilities between mental health staff and substance misuse workers and establish an agreed, written operating policy, which should include a review date.
- Encourage role shadowing and sharing in order to develop knowledge and understanding of each other's roles, skills and underpinning philosophies.
- Establish regular team teaching sessions or 'master classes', in which one or more members lead an exploration of their professional contribution to the care of service users.
- Establish a mechanism for discussing and resolving disputes and differences of opinion. If you have a procedure you will be less likely to use it. If you do not have one, disagreements often become intractable arguments.

- Identify and discuss areas of potential conflict and seek compromise and agreement, for example referral criteria, admission and discharge criteria, abstinence versus harm minimisation, risk assessment and management, confidentiality.
- Establish clear leadership and organise regular reviews of working practices, procedures and policies. Use the arrival of new staff or the introduction of new national or local policies to reflect on the aims and purpose of the team.

References

Allen, D. (1997) The nursing–medical boundary: a negotiated order? *Sociology of Health and Illness*, 19 (4), 498–520.

Appleby, L., Shaw, J., Amos, T. & McDonnel, R. (1999) *Safer Services: National Confidential Inquiry into Suicide and Homicide by People with Mental Illness*. Department of Health, London.

Baguley, I. & Baguley, C. (1999) Psychosocial interventions in the treatment of psychosis. *Mental Health Care*, 2 (9), 314–17.

Beeforth, M., Conlan, E., Field, V., Hoser, B. & Sayce, L. (1990) *Whose Service is it Anyway? Users' Views on Coordinating Community Care*. Research and Development in Psychiatry, London.

Borrill, C., West, M., Shapiro, D. & Rees, A. (2000) Teamworking and effectiveness in health care. *British Journal of Health Care Management*, 6 (8), 354–71.

Bowers, L. (1992) Ethnomethodology 11: a study of the community psychiatric nurse in the patient's home. *International Journal of Nursing Studies*, 29 (1), 69–79.

Bray, J. (1999) An ethnographic study of psychiatric nursing. *Journal of Psychiatric and Mental Health Nursing*, 6, 297–305.

Brown, B., Crawford, P. & Darongkamas, J. (2000) Blurred roles and permeable boundaries: the experience of multidisciplinary working in community mental health. *Health and Social Care in the Community*, 8 (6), 425–35.

Brown, R. (1989) Social work in mental health teams: the local authority field social worker. In: *Social Work and Health Care: Research Highlights in Social Work 19* (Taylor, R. & Ford, J., eds), pp. 47–57. Jessica Kingsley Publishers, London.

Bywaters, P. (1989) Social work and nursing: sisters or rivals? In: *Social Work and Health Care: Research Highlights in Social Work 19* (Taylor, R. & Ford, J., eds), pp. 33–46. Jessica Kingsley Publishers, London.

Carpenter, J. (1995) Doctors and nurses: stereotypes and stereotype change in inter-professional education. *Journal of Inter-professional Care*, 9 (2), 151–61.

Cott, C. (1998) Structure and meaning in multidisciplinary teamwork. *Sociology of Health and Illness*, 20 (6), 848–73.

Dalley, G. (1989) Professional ideology or organisational tribalism? In: *Social Work and Health Care: Research Highlights in Social Work 19* (Taylor, R. & Ford, J., eds), pp. 102–17. Jessica Kingsley Publishers, London.

Department of Health (1999) *Effective Care Coordination in Mental Health Services: Modernising the Care Programme Approach*. A Policy Booklet. HMSO, London.

Department of Health (2002) *Mental Health Policy Implementation Guide: Community Mental Health Teams*. Department of Health, London.

Department of Health (2003a) *Mental Health Policy Implementation Guide: Dual Diagnosis Good Practice Guide*. Department of Health, London.

Department of Health (2003b) *What To Do If You're Worried a Child is Being Abused (Summary)*. Department of Health, London.

Edwards, K. & Garrety, C. (1998) Learning to work with social workers. *Nursing Times Learning Curve*, 2 (7), 4–5.

Firth-Cozens, J. (1998) Celebrating teamwork. *Quality in Health Care*, 7 (Suppl), S3–S7.

Grant, A. & Mills, J. (2000) The great going nowhere show: structural power and mental health nurses. *Mental Health Practice*, 4 (3), 14–16.

Intagliata, J. (1982) Improving the quality of community care for the chronically mentally disabled: the role of case management. *Schizophrenia Bulletin*, 8 (4), 655–74.

Kashi, R. & Littlewood, J. (2000) Politics and practice. *Mental Health Nursing*, 20 (4), 10–16.

Kennedy, P. & Griffiths, H. (2000) *Discussion Paper: an Analysis of the Concerns of Consultant General Psychiatrists about their Jobs, and of the Changing Practices that May Point Towards Solutions*. Northern Centre for Mental Health, Durham.

Leathard, A.E. (1994) *Going Inter-professional: Working Together for Health and Welfare*. Routledge, London.

Mackay, L., Soothill, K. & Webb, C. (1995) Troubled times: the context for inter-professional collaboration? In: *Inter-professional Relations in Health Care* (Soothill, K., Mackay, L. & Webb, C., eds), pp. 5–10. Edward Arnold, London.

Menzies, I.E.P. (1960) A case-study in the functioning of social systems as a defence against anxiety. *Human Relations*, 13, 95–121.

Miller, C., Freeman, M. & Ross, N. (2001) *Inter-professional Practice in Health and Social Care: Challenging the Shared Learning Agenda*. Arnold, London.

Miller, C. & Freeman, M. (2003) Clinical Teamwork: the impact of policy on collaborative practice. In:

Inter-professional Collaboration: From Policy to Practice in Health and Social Care (Leathard, A., ed.), pp. 121–32. Routledge, London.

Mistral, W. & Velleman, R. (1997) CMHTs: the professionals' choice? *Journal of Mental Health*, 6 (2), 125–40.

Norman, I.J. & Peck, E. (1999) Working together in adult community mental health services: an inter-professional dialogue. *Journal of Mental Health*, 8 (3), 217–30.

Onyett, S. (2002) *Teamworking in Mental Health*. Palgrave, London.

Onyett, S., Standen, R. & Peck, E. (1997) The challenge of managing community mental health teams. *Health and Social Care in the Community*, 5 (1), 40–7.

Ovretveit, J. (1993) Coordinating Community Care: Multidisciplinary Teams and Care Management. Open University Press, Buckingham.

Ovretveit, J., Mathias, P. & Thompson, T.E. (1997) *Inter-professional Working for Health and Social Care*. Macmillan, Basingstoke.

Peck, E. (1995) On the team. *Health Service Journal*, (6 April), 28–9.

Pietroni, M. (1995) The nature and aims of professional education for social workers: a post-modern perspective. In: *Learning and Teaching Social Work: Towards Reflective Practice* (Yellowy, M. & Henkel, M., eds), pp. 34–50. Jessica Kingsley Publishers, London.

Proctor-Childs, T., Freeman, M. & Miller, C. (1998) Visions of teamwork: the realities of an interdisciplinary approach. *British Journal of Therapy and Rehabilitation*, 5 (12), 616–35.

Royal College of Psychiatrists (1996) *Report of the Confidential Inquiry into Homicides and Suicides by Mentally Ill People*. Royal College of Psychiatrists, London.

Simpson, A. (2000) What price confidentiality? *Nursing Times*, 96 (9), 35.

Simpson, A. (2004) Coordinating care for people with severe mental illness (Unpublished PhD thesis). University of Brighton, Brighton.

Simpson, A. (2005) Community psychiatric nurses and the care coordinator role: squeezed to provide 'limited nursing'. *Journal of Advanced Nursing*, 52 (6), 689–99.

Simpson, A., Miller, C. & Bowers, L. (2003a) The history of the care programme approach in England: where did it go wrong? *Journal of Mental Health*, 12 (5), 489–504.

Simpson, A., Miller, C. & Bowers, L. (2003b) Models of case management and the care programme approach: how to make the CPA effective and credible. *Journal of Psychiatric and Mental Health Nursing*, 10, 472–83.

Stein, L. (1978) The doctor-nurse game. In: *Readings in the Sociology of Nursing* (Dingwall, R. & McIntosh, J., eds), pp. 107–17. Churchill Livingstone, London.

Szmukler, G. & Holloway, F. (2001) Confidentiality in community psychiatry. In: *Confidentiality and Mental Health* (Cordess, C., ed.), pp. 53–70. Jessica Kingsley Publishers, London.

Taylor, P.J. & Gunn, J. (1999) Homicides by people with mental illness: myth and reality. *British Journal of Psychiatry*, 174, 9–14.

Tyrer, P., Coid, J., Simmonds, S., Joseph, P. & Marriott, S. (2002) Community mental health teams (CMHTs) for people with severe mental illnesses and disordered personality (Cochrane Review). In *The Cochrane Library* (Issue 1). Update Software, Oxford.

Walsh, E., Buchanan, A. & Fahy, T. (2002) Violence and schizophrenia: examining the evidence. *British Journal of Psychiatry*, 180, 490–5.

Warner, L., Hoadley, A. & Ford, R. (2001) Obstacle course. *Health Service Journal*, 111 (5775), 28–9.

West, M. (1999) Communication and teamworking in healthcare. *NTresearch*, 4 (1), 8–17.

West, M.A. & Poulton, B.C. (1997) A failure of function: teamwork in primary health care. *Journal of Interprofessional Care*, 11 (2), 205–16.

Wicks, D. (1998) *Nurses and Doctors at Work: Rethinking Professional Boundaries*. Open University Press, Buckingham.

14 Primary Care and Dual Diagnosis

R. Lawrence

Introduction

Substance misuse has a high prevalence amongst patients with mental health problems and vice versa. Primary care services have been identified as being particularly important in provision of care in terms of contributing to identification, assessment, engaging in treatment, referral to specialist services and the offering of a continuity that clients with complex issues associated with dual diagnosis require (Chilton, 2005; Gerada, 2005). This chapter will consider the prevalence of dual diagnosed clients presenting to primary care, clinical presentations and implications for assessment, service developments, the provision of general and specific services and treatment within primary care, liaison with specialist services, and training needs within the primary care team, to ensure a high quality of care and practitioner development.

Dual diagnosis in primary care

Estimates for dual diagnosis in substance misusing and mental disorder populations are high. One third of heavy drinkers have associated mental health problems and half of dependent drug takers have mental health problems of varying severity (Department of Health, 1999a). In a study of community mental health teams and substance misuse treatment centres in four inner-city areas, 44% of CMHT clients reported previous year problematic drug use and/or harmful alcohol use, and 75% of drug service clients had a previous year psychiatric disorder (Weaver *et al.*, 2003). High rates of dual diagnosis have also been identified in homeless and prison populations (Farrell *et al.*, 1998).

Primary care teams are therefore becoming increasingly involved in the provision of care for substance misusers and by implication those with dual diagnosis. A Department of Health review concluded that all drug misusers need to have access to primary care services, and that GPs are well placed to identify and offer advice to drug misusers who may not be in touch with specialist services (Department of Health, 1996). The review identified a dual role for GPs providing treatment: the provision of general medical services and specific treatment for substance misuse, including identification, referral, harm minimisation and undertaking of shared care with a specialist service. Although it is not always appropriate for many dual diagnosed patients to be managed within a shared care model, all patients require general medical care from a GP (Department of Health, 1999a). In a survey by Strang *et al.* (2005) half of responding GPs in England and Wales had seen a drug user in the preceeding month, with half of these prescribing substitute medications. Across the country, it is estimated that 32% of GPs are involved in care of drug users. Increased involvement in care provision for substance misusers, together with the fact that a significant proportion of GP consultations (one in four) are with people suffering with mental health problems (Department of Health, 2000) means that primary care teams are seeing more patients with dual diagnosis. Frisher *et al.* (2004) estimate that the average GP practice in 1993 had a statistical figure of 3.5 dual diagnosed patients, increasing to 6.8 by 1998, with (by extrapolation) increases to 11.3 for 2003 and 14 by 2006. Where primary care teams are working with particularly vulnerable populations or in inner-city areas the prevalence of dual diagnosis may further be increased.

Dual diagnosis is defined as a concurrent existence of substance misuse and one or more psychiatric disorders (Gafoor & Rassool, 1998; Department of Health, 2002). However, the relationship between the disorders can be complex and dynamic, and there may be diagnostic uncertainty on presentation. In addition, the implications of these concurrent disorders means that the individual is at increased risk of physical health problems, homelessness, isolation, unemployment and debt. The individual can therefore present in primary care with what can be termed multiple morbidity (Gerada, 2005), experiencing a range of problems that need addressing, as well as mental health and substance misuse issues.

Treatment provision for dual diagnosed patients in the UK has been influenced in recent years by three developments: enhancing of service provision specifically for the dual diagnosed and publishing of good practice guidelines (Department of Health, 2002), increasing provision of shared care for drug misusers in general, and the development of a commissioning framework for adult substance misuse treatment, *Models of Care* (National Treatment Agency, 2002). Development of a commissioning framework for treating alcohol misuse will further shape service provision.

Three types of treatment service models for treating dual diagnosis have been identified (Department of Health, 2002): serial treatment, where one disorder is treated before another; parallel treatment, where there is concurrent treatment but from separate service providers; and integrated treatment, where the psychiatric and substance misuse problems are treated by the same staff team. Serial treatment can be disadvantaged through problems identifying the primary and secondary diagnosis, and poor outcomes can occur for treating the primary diagnosis due to delays in treating the secondary diagnosis (Crawford *et al.*, 2003). Shaner *et al.* (1998) reviewed cases of diagnostic uncertainty for chronically psychotic cocaine abusers and concluded that it was frequently difficult to distinguish schizophrenic symptoms from chronic substance induced psychosis. Therefore clinicians should consider initiating treatment for both disorders with clarification of diagnosis developing once the patient is stabilised. Minkoff (1989) proposed a model in which both diagnoses are seen as primary, to allow for the integration of concurrent treatment. It is suggested that an integrated treatment approach by one team appears to deliver better outcomes than serial or parallel care (Department of Health, 2002). There have been methodological problems in comparing treatments, for example differences in definitions and diagnosis, treatment delivery and changes in patterns of substance use (Crawford *et al.*, 2003; Jeffery *et al.*, 2004). There is an opinion that further evidence based research with well designed controlled clinical trials is required to support the assertion, as clinical studies so far have not demonstrated a clear advantage over standard care (Jeffery *et al.*, 2004). Integrated treatment services, where available, are focused on treatment for those who are severely mentally ill.

Finch (2004) notes that guidance on the management of dual diagnosis has focused mainly on the severely mentally ill group. Dual diagnosis clients present within primary care with substance misuse and mental health problems ranging from mild to severe. Whether they are referred to specialist services (mental health or substance misuse services), or are managed within primary care will depend on the severity of the problems.

Shared care and care plan approach

The mental health service should take the lead in the treatment of the severely dual diagnosed with patients being on the care plan approach (Department of Health, 2002). Finch (2004) notes that a significant proportion of dual diagnosed patients presenting to primary care services, particularly those that are mainly opiate users, suffer mild to moderate mental health disorders (anxiety or panic disorder, depressed mood, personality difficulties). These are not severe enough to be managed by a community mental health team under the care plan approach. In these instances responsibility for management will mainly lie within the primary care team, normally sharing care with a substance misuse specialist service (whether that is within the primary care team with GP prescribing and linked drug/alcohol workers, or in liaison with a specialist prescribing and/or counselling service). It is important that primary care practitioners know the level of co-morbidity their service can deal with, when to ask for additional support and the referral procedures for the appropriate specialist services. In addition, if the patient is not under the care plan approach there should still be a form of care plan and coordination (National Treatment Agency, 2002). In joint working, clarification and agreement for all key aspects of the treatment process must be achieved for effective care delivery (Checinski, 2002). The treatment approach needs to be flexible and tailored to the patient (Flanagan, 2002) and close collaboration and communication between teams is required. When there are potentially several services involved in treatment delivery the primary care practitioner can play a role in ensuring clients do not fall between services by facilitating coordination between different care providers (Gerada, 2005).

Shared care is a model that can be applied to any close cooperative work between agencies/services in the provision of treatment. With regards to substance misuse the Department of Health (1996) defined it as:

> 'The joint participation of specialists and GPs (and other agencies as appropriate) in the planned delivery of care for patients with a drug misuse problem, informed by an enhanced information exchange beyond routine discharge and referral letters. It may involve the day-to-day management by the GP of the patients' medical needs in relation to his or her drug misuse. Such arrangements would make explicit which dimension was responsible for different aspects of the patients' treatment and care. These may include prescribing of substitute drugs in appropriate circumstances.'

The shared care model has developed in different ways according to local conditions and includes GPs providing normal medical services in close liaison with a specialist drug/alcohol service, GPs prescribing substitute medication in liaison with specialist services and GPs providing care supported by primary care based drug/alcohol workers.

Research indicates 'good' outcomes are equally likely for primary care and specialist services in terms of reduction in drug use, reducing injecting related risks, reduced crime, retention in treatment and improvements in physical and psychological health (Lewis & Bellis, 2001; Gossop *et al.*, 2003). Some evidence also suggests that those treated in primary care are more likely to be immunised against hepatitis B (Lewis & Bellis, 2001). A key to the success of shared care is the level of specialist support available to the GP and primary health care team, ease of access to support and close collaboration between parties. There should be development of local shared care guidelines incorporating standardised assessment, treatment, referral protocols, roles, responsibilities, support mechanisms, monitoring and evaluation, arrangements, identification of knowledge and training needs, and strategies to develop this. For psychiatric co-morbidity the primary care team should have access to medical/clinical leadership and/or advice from mental health specialists even if the patients' mental health will be primarily managed within the primary care team (Department of Health, 2002).

Models of care and primary care settings

Models of Care (National Treatment Agency, 2002) sets out a national framework for commissioning of adult treatment for drug misuse. It describes services for drug users as being grouped into four tiers (see Chapter 17):

- Tier 1: non-substance specific services requiring an interface with drug and alcohol treatment services, for example primary care, general medical services, community pharmacists
- Tier 2: open access drug and alcohol treatment services with aims of engagement in treatment and reducing drug-related harm
- Tier 3: structured community based drug

treatment services (incorporating substitute prescribing and counselling)
- Tier 4: in-patient or specialist services, for example rehabilitation centres, day programmes, in-patient detoxification, liver specialists

Primary care services that are non-substance specific can mainly be located in tier 1 and can act as access points for referral and treatment. Primary care based drug/alcohol drop-in services can be placed in tier 2, and shared care schemes can be placed in tier 3. When substance misuse is identified the tier 1 care provision plays an important part in liaising and interfacing with treatment offered at other tiers and, as such, spans across the tier framework.

Models of Care suggests the treatment principle should be harm minimisation, with there being a reduction in various forms of drug-related harm until the user is ready and able to come off drugs. A range or hierarchy of goals have been identified for treatment:

- Reduction of health, social and other problems directly related to drug misuse
- Reduction of harmful or risky behaviours associated with drug misuse
- Reduction of health, social or other problems not directly attributable to drug misuse
- Attainment of controlled, non-dependent, or non-problematic drug use
- Abstinence from main problem drugs
- Abstinence from all drugs

The harm minimisation approach and treatment goal range/hierarchy can inform the delivery of treatment undertaken by the primary care team.

Assessment and treatment

Primary care teams can offer general services and also interventions specifically for substance misusers and the dual diagnosed as detailed below:

- Assessment and treatment of physical illness and referral on to other medical services
- Assessment and treatment of mental health problems and referral to psychiatric services
- Identification of drug/alcohol problems, assessment and referral to appropriate services

Practitioners should be alert to opportunities for identification and screening for substance misuse. If a patient is presenting with needle marks, skin infections secondary to scratching, cellulitis, skin ulcers and abscesses then possible substance misuse should be explored. If a patient is presenting for analgesia or sedatives then substance misuse history may be explored if the patients' history is not known. If a patient is presenting with anxiety or affective disorder substance use can be checked for. Alcohol use should be routinely discussed, whether or not physical or mental problems associated with alcohol misuse or dependency are evident. Early detection of problem drinking and subsequent brief interventions can lead to positive behaviour changes (Sims & Iphofen, 2003). When screening for substance use it is important to undertake it in a non-threatening, empathic, non-judgemental manner and environment (Chilton, 2005).

- General health promotion and advice together with substance specific advice when misuse is identified. Practitioners should familiarise themselves with the physical and mental health consequences of particular substances to advise users. Advice on the harm that can occur for different methods of drug administration, for example injecting and snorting should be provided. Overdose awareness should be discussed.
- Screening for blood borne viruses (hepatitis B and C and HIV) or referral to specialist clinics for this. One third of patients with dual diagnosis may be sero-positive for HIV, hepatitis B or C (Department of Health, 2002). It is recommended that drug users should be offered immunisation against hepatitis B, whether or not they are injecting drugs, as non-injectors can move on to injecting (Coffey & Young, 2005). It is also recommended that there is no need to carry out pre-vaccination testing for hepatitis B, as the patient may disengage before being immunised. The Royal College of General Practitioners (RCGP) guidelines recommend vaccinating all injecting drug users against hepatitis A, and that hepatitis B vaccination should be offered to partners and children. For hepatitis C diagnosed patients there should be liaison with specialist services regarding treatment (Department of Health, 2001). There should also be care and advice to help patients move

away from behaviour that may result in acquiring or spreading HIV, and there should be facilities to provide condoms (ACMD, 1988).
- Family planning advice.
- Advice and screening (or referral on) for sexually transmitted diseases.
- Abscess dressing and wound care by the practice nurse.
- Midwifes and health visitors are important in providing support to dually diagnosed mothers, in advising them on effects of substances on pregnancy and impact on childcare, monitoring mental health and general stability, liaison with mental health teams, substance misuse services, social services, as well as antenatal and paediatric services.
- The primary care team can act as a resource to support family members (Copello *et al.*, 2000).
- Pharmacists can be a point of contact for general health information. They can provide a needle exchange service and in shared care schemes can provide supervised dispensing of opiate substitute medication if necessary. Drug interactions and adverse reactions can be monitored. They may also be able to identify the misuse of over-the-counter medications.
- Dental services can provide support to substance misusers whose lifestyles have caused neglect of teeth or whose substance misuse has directly caused teeth problems, for example ecstasy use causing grinding down of teeth.

When assessing patients, practitioners should be aware of groups warranting specific attention (Department of Health, 2002):

- Young people: substance misuse is a major contributing factor in the development of mental health difficulties for this group.
- Homeless people: there are high levels of concurrent disorders (Farrell *et al.*, 1998), and homelessness almost trebles a young person's chance of developing mental health problems (Department of Health, 2002).
- Offenders also have higher rates of dual diagnosis (Farrell *et al.*, 1998) and can be particularly vulnerable to fatalities: drug-related mortality among newly released offenders is high in the immediate post-release period, with risk of mortality much higher than the general population (Farrell & Marsden, 2005).
- Women: it is suggested that substance misusing women are more likely to present with psychological difficulties than associated substance misuse, tend to access drug/alcohol services later than men, are more likely than other women or men to have experienced sexual, physical and/or emotional abuse, and can be deterred from accessing services for help due to fears of having their children removed (Crawford *et al.*, 2003).
- People from ethnic minorities: the Department of Health (2002) notes that severe mental illness and substance misuse can present differently across cultures and ethnic groups. Services should therefore seek to be suitable and sensitive to the needs of each ethnic group (see Chapter 9).

In the assessment practitioners should clarify the following:

- The reason for presentation.
- Substances of misuse and the pattern, methods, context and severity of use. Full details of use in the previous four weeks, together with a substance misuse history starting from first use of substances should be gathered. Whether or not patients are sharing needles, pipes and other using equipment should be explored. Urine screening and alcohol breath tests will also provide further clarification.
- A physical examination should be undertaken and a medical and psychiatric history taken.
- A mental state examination should be provided which will cover appearance, behaviour, speech, mood, thoughts, cognitive state and insight (Gelder *et al.*, 2003).
- Family history of physical/mental illness/ substance misuse should also be noted.
- Personal history (including details of relationships and children).
- Sexual behaviour.
- Forensic history.

There may be diagnostic uncertainty as restlessness, paranoia, anxiety and irritability might indicate intoxication with stimulants, hallucinogens or opiate withdrawal. Depression can be caused by withdrawal from stimulants, or by alcohol or sedative drugs. Delusions and hallucinations can be caused by stimulant or hallucinogen use. Such presentations will affect the eliciting of information from the client. There should be ongoing risk assessment covering risk of suicide/self-harm, risk of self-neglect, risk to others, risk from others and other risks identified. Phillips (2000) notes significantly higher rates of violence for dual diagnosis when compared to single diagnostic groups. The assessment should identify factors contributing to a high risk and how substance use features in this, and this should be discussed and reviewed with the patient (Martino *et al.*, 2002). The risk assessment should also identify those professionals that need to be informed of the assessment. The style of intervention can also change towards crisis intervention and management as risk levels increase (Martino *et al.*, 2002).

In provision of treatment GPs should be aware of particular influences substances may have on mental health presentation. Opiates may mask symptoms (Maremmani *et al.*, 2003), cannabis use may worsen the prognosis for schizophrenic disorders (Hall, 1998) and exacerbate symptoms of psychosis (Iversen, 2003), cocaine may cause depressive symptoms and paranoid delusions (Gafoor & Rassool, 1998) and in the absence of stimulants delusional symptoms may subside. There may be diagnostic uncertainty when symptoms present, for example for some cannabis users acute psychotic reactions occur in clear consciousness and are indistinguishable from schizophrenic like psychosis (Harrison & Abou Saleh, 2002). Primary care treatment providers need to decide how to manage this uncertainty as part of the care plan. Substance misuse can also create adverse complications for mental health treatment compliance and Poole & Brabbins (1996) note that it is associated with increased rates of relapse in the chronically mentally ill.

If prescribing methadone, there may be a need to provide a higher stabilisation dose than for non-co-morbid clients. The reasons for this are not established. Features of some co-morbid opiate users include polydrug use, more chaotic lifestyle and persistent psychiatric symptoms, which may raise the stabilisation level required (Maremmani *et al.*, 2000). Methadone may also mask the presentation of psychotic symptoms due to its anti-dopaminergic qualities suppressing the hyperactive dopaminergic system in schizophrenic disorders. As methadone is reduced there may be a re-emergence of symptoms (Levinson *et al.*, 1995; Schifano, 2002; Maremmani *et al.*, 2003). There is also a risk of major depressive episodes during or shortly after methadone tapering; therefore, it should be undertaken more slowly than for non-co-morbid clients, and caution must be exercised with dosages of antipsychotics and antidepressants if required, given the possible interactions with methadone (Maremmani *et al.*, 2003). Practitioners should be aware of the possible lethal interaction of methadone with other drugs, for example tricyclic antidepressants (Agath, 2004). Where there is moderate depression or anxiety prior to starting methadone or buprenorphine treatment, the effects of stabilisation on the medication should usually be awaited before specific psychiatric treatment is undertaken (Seivewright, 2000). For cocaine users, SSRI antidepressants should be used only if underlying depression is confirmed and stimulant use is stopped (Shapiro, 2004). If cocaine use continues SSRIs should be used with caution due to the risk of the rare occurrence of serotonergic syndrome.

Evidence based treatment

Spencer *et al.* (2002) notes reviews by Drake *et al.* (1998) and Siegfried (1998) that indicate that more successful treatments for dual diagnosis clients involve cognitive behavioural approaches such as relapse prevention (Marlatt & Gordon, 1985) and motivational interviewing (Miller & Rollnick, 1991). Martino *et al.* (2002) and Graham (2004) describe tailored models of cognitive behavioural integrated approaches that combine treatment for both disorders and explore the connection between them. It is important to establish the motives and expectations for substance use and gain an understanding of the clients' drug using knowledge and practice (Phillips & Labrow, 2000; Spencer *et al.*, 2002). Although there may be some self-medication for relief of mental disorder symptoms or negative side effects of medication, other reasons such as enhancement of mood, social interaction and coping strategies will inform a tailored treatment plan. Motivational interviewing can help the client identify harms associated with use, and stages of change theory and a harm reduction approach can help match viable treatment interventions for each substance the client is using. The degree to which specialist cognitive behavioural therapy is available for the primary care team is limited. Therefore, brief psychological interventions such as motivational interviewing and solution focused brief interventions, together with the development of a therapeutic relationship are important to keep the patient engaged in treatment.

Training and development

To ensure a high standard of service delivery it is necessary to identify staff training needs and implement an organisational strategy to meet training requirements. The training should cover shared care for treatment of general substance misuse, with additional specific training focusing on dual diagnosis.

The Department of Health (1999a) recommends that local shared care guidelines should incorporate identification of skills, knowledge, training needs and strategy. The proposed training curriculum should cover background issues, the role of shared care schemes and primary care in treating dual diagnosis, treatment issues, prescribing in primary care, roles of different agencies and inter-agency protocols, and other health issues relevant to substance misuse, for example blood borne viruses. Where possible, formal recognition of competence should be made. The training should be compatible with national training standards such as those detailed in *Drug and Alcohol National Occupational Standards* (Skills for Health, 2005). The training should incorporate three main strands: inter-agency collaboration and information exchange through inter-agency training, theoretical and skills based training, together with supervision and practice development (Department of Health, 2002).

Training programmes should take into account the different levels of involvement within primary care teams to ensure that all team members (clinical and non-clinical) have the opportunity of development (Department of Health, 1999a). Heuston *et al.* (2001) highlighted that managers and receptionists wish to receive and should have training and support for their contribution to managing substance misusing clients. This would include training concerning mental health issues and would have the additional benefit of contributing to general staff training for patients with mental health problems. Training delivery to specific staff groups should be flexible and creative to facilitate as high attendance as possible.

Ford & Ryrie (2000) showed that GP training for substance misuse increased the level of treatment activity, together with GP confidence and willingness to treat. The Royal College of General Practitioners has developed training for general and enhanced GP involvement in the treatment of substance misusers (RCGP, 2005) and issued treatment guidelines for opiate substitute prescribing and crack and cocaine use (Ford *et al.*, 2004; Shapiro, 2004; Ford *et al.*, 2005). This peer training and support can significantly enhance treatment delivery. Local areas can incorporate additional training requirements for dual diagnosis into the training programmes, forums and peer support meetings that have the RCGP training scheme as their base.

Conclusion

Presentations to primary care services of patients with dual diagnosis are increasing. Management of such patients can be challenging due to the complex and problematic relationship between mental health and substance use, associated physical and social problems that can develop, and instability that can adversely affect treatment compliance. Episodes of co-occurring disorders can be acute or chronic in nature. There can be diagnostic uncertainty, with establishment of a primary and secondary diagnosis sometimes only being clarified once stability is achieved. Both disorders are associated with chronic relapses, which can then trigger the occurrence of the other disorder.

To effectively manage cases there should be clear protocols, lines of communication and care pathways developed between primary care and specialist services. Specialist services should take the lead in the management of the severely mentally ill. Whether or not management of mildly to moderately mentally ill patients remains within primary care, the support of specialist services should be readily available. Treatment of substance misuse should be within a local shared care framework, with either primary care or specialist services being the lead treatment coordinator, depending on the severity of misuse and local shared care guidelines. Co-occurring disorders cannot be treated in isolation from one another. There should be concurrent treatment, with care planning and coordination also addressing other needs of the patient. Primary care should liaise with other agencies and can play an integral part in screening, identification, referral, treatment provision, monitoring and liaison.

Treatment can range from brief cognitive behavioural interventions delivered in the context of general medical care, to specific targeted interventions involving prescribing and counselling. The development of a therapeutic relationship is important and facilitates engagement with treatment. An understanding of the potential dynamic between substance use, mental health and medication will inform treatment. To ensure a high quality of service delivery, identification of skills and knowledge requirements should be undertaken across the different levels of primary care staff involved with dual diagnosis patients. Programmes should be developed to promote training. This should include inter-agency collaboration, local care pathways, treatment philosophy and method, and be compatible and interlinked with national and professional training programmes and standards. This approach can enable the primary care team to meet the challenges involved in providing care for the dual diagnosed patient.

References

ACMD (Advisory Council on the Misuse of Drugs) (1988) *AIDS and drug misuse, Part 1*. HMSO, London.

Agath, K. (2004) Management of dual diagnosis patients in primary care. *Substance Misuse Management in General Practice Newsletter*, 8, 6–7.

Checinski, K. (2002) Treatment strategies and interventions. In: *Dual Diagnosis: Substance Misuse and Psychiatric Disorders* (Rassool, G.H., ed.), pp. 134–47. Blackwell Science, Oxford.

Chilton, J. (2005) The complex world of dual diagnosis, nursing and primary care. In: *Substance Misuse in Primary Care* (Winyard, R., ed.), pp. 149–77. Radcliffe Publishing, Oxford.

Coffey, E. & Young, D. (2005) *Guidance for Hepatitis A and B Vaccination of Drug Users in Primary Care and Criteria for Audit*. Royal College of General Practitioners, London.

Copello, A., Templeton, L., Krishman, M., Orford, J. & Vellman, R. (2000) Methods for reducing alcohol and drug-related family harm in non-specialist settings. *Addiction Research*, 18, 471–84.

Crawford, V. (1996) Co-morbidity of substance misuse and psychiatric disorders. *Current Opinion in Psychiatry*, 9 (3), 231–4.

Crawford, V., Crome, L.B. & Clancy, C. (2003) Coexisting problems of mental health and substance misuse (dual diagnosis): a literature review. *Drugs: Education, Prevention and Policy*, 10 (Supplement), S1–S74.

Deehan, A., McCambridge, J., Ball, D.M. & Strang, J. (2002) Increasing practice nurse access to alcohol training. *Drug and Alcohol Review*, 21 (3), 281–6.

Department of Health (1996) *Task Force to Review Services for Drug Misusers: Report of an Independent Review of Drug Treatment Services in England*. Department of Health, London.

Department of Health (1999a) *Drug Misuse and Dependence – Guidelines on Clinical Management*. The Stationery Office, London.

Department of Health (1999b) *National Service Framework for Mental Health*. The Stationery Office, London.

Department of Health (2000) *The NHS Plan. A Plan for Investment. A Plan for Reform*. Department of Health, London.

Department of Health (2001) *Hepatitis C – Guidance for Those Working With Drug Users*. Department of Health, London.

Department of Health (2002) *Mental Health Policy Implementation Guide: Dual Diagnosis Good Practice Guide*. Department of Health, London.

Drake, R.E., Mercer-McFadden, C., Mueser, K.T., McHugo, G.J. & Bond, G.R. (1998) Review of integrated mental health and substance abuse treatment for patients with dual disorders. *Schizophrenia Bulletin*, 24 (4), 589–609.

Farrell, M., Howes, S., Taylor, C. *et al.* (1998) Substance misuse and psychiatric co-morbidity: an overview of the OPCS National Psychiatric Morbidity Survey. *Addictive Behaviours*, 23 (6), 909–18.

Farrell, M. & Marsden, J. (2005) *Drug-related Mortality Among Newly Released Offenders 1998–2000. Home Office Research, Development and Statistics Online Report 40/05* (online) available from: http://www.homeoffice.gov.uk/rds/onlinepubs1.html (8 December 2005)

Finch, E. (2004) Dual diagnosis in the context of mild to moderate mental health problems. *Substance Misuse Management in General Practice Newsletter*, 8, 7.

Flanagan, M. (2002) The challenge of shared care. In: *Dual Diagnosis: Substance Misuse and Psychiatric Disorders* (Rassool, G.H., ed.), pp. 97–107. Blackwell Science, Oxford.

Ford, C. & Ryrie, I. (2000) A comprehensive package of support to facilitate the treatment of problem drug users in primary care: an evaluation of the training component. *International Journal of Drug Policy*, 11 (6), 387–92.

Ford, C., Morton, S., Lintzeris, N., Bury, J. & Gerada, C. (2004) *Guidance for the Use of Buprenorphine for the Treatment of Opioid Dependence in Primary Care*, 2nd edn. Royal College of General Practitioners, London.

Ford, C., Barnard, J., Bury, J. *et al.* (2005) *Guidance for the Use of Methadone for the Treatment of Opioid Dependence in Primary Care*. Royal College of General Practitioners, London.

Frisher, M., Collins, J., Millson, D. & Crome, I. (2004) Prevalence of co-morbid psychiatric illness and substance misuse in primary care in England and Wales. *Journal of Epidemiology and Community Health*, 58 (12), 1036–41.

Gafoor, M. & Rassool, G.H. (1998) The coexistence of psychiatric disorders and substance misuse: working with dual diagnosis patients. *Journal of Advanced Nursing*, 27 (3), 497–502.

Gelder, M., Mayou, R. & Geddes, J. (2003) *Psychiatry*. 2nd edn. Oxford University Press, Oxford.

Gerada, C. (2005) Drug misuse and co-morbid illness: 'dual diagnosis'. In: *RCGP Guide. The Management of Substance Misuse in Primary Care* (Gerada, C., ed.), pp. 317–28. Royal College of General Practitioners, London.

Gossop, M., Stewart, D., Browne, N. & Marsden, J. (2003) Methadone treatment of opiate dependent patients in general practice and specialist clinic settings: outcomes at 2-year follow-up. *Journal of Substance Abuse Treatment*, 24 (4), 313–21.

Graham, H.L. (ed) (2004) *Cognitive-Behavioural Integrated Treatment (c-BIT)*. John Wiley and Sons Ltd, Chichester, UK.

Hall, W. (1998) Cannabis use and psychosis. *Drug and Alcohol Review*, 17, 433–4.

Harrison, C.A. & Abou Saleh, M.T. (2002) Psychiatric disorders and substance misuse: psychopathology. In: *Dual Diagnosis: Substance Misuse and Psychiatric Disorders* (Rassool, G.H., ed.), pp. 43–5. Blackwell Science, Oxford.

Heuston, J., Groves, P., Al Nawad, J., Albery, I., Gossop, M. & Strang, J. (2001) Caught in the middle: receptionists and their dealings with substance misusing patients. *Journal of Substance Use*, 6 (3), 151–7.

Iversen, L. (2003) Cannabis and the brain. *Brain*, 126 (6), 1252–70.

Jacka, D., Clode, D., Patterson, S. & Wyman, K. (1999) Attitudes and practices of general practitioners training to work with drug-using patients. *Drug and Alcohol Review*, 18 (3), 287–91.

Jeffery, D.P., Ley, A., McLaren, S. & Siegfried, N. (2004) Psychosocial treatment programmes for people with both severe mental illness and substance misuse (Cochrane Review). In: *The Cochrane Library, Issue 1, 2004*. John Wiley and Sons Ltd, Chichester, UK.

Krausz, M., Degkwitz, P., Kuhne, A. & Verthein, U. (1998) Co-morbidity of opiate dependence and mental disorders. *Addictive Behaviours*, 23 (6), 767–83.

Levinson, I., Galynker, I. & Rosenthal, R.W. (1995) Methadone withdrawal psychosis. *Journal of Clinical Psychiatry*, 56 (2), 73–76.

Lewis, D. & Bellis, M. (2001) General practice or drug clinic for methadone maintenance? A controlled comparison of treatment outcomes. *International Journal of Drug Policy*, 12 (1), 81–9.

Maremmani, I., Zolesi, O., Aglietti, M. *et al.* (2000) Methadone dose and retention during treatment of heroin addicts with axis I psychiatric co-morbidity. *Journal of Addictive Diseases*, 19 (2), 29–41.

Maremmani, I., Pacini, M., Lubrano, S., Lovrecic, M. & Perugi, G. (2003) Dual diagnosis heroin addicts. The clinical and therapeutic aspects. *Heroin Addiction and Related Clinical Problems*, 5 (2), 7–98.

Marsden, J., Gossop, M., Stewart, D., Rolfe, A. & Farrell, M. (2000) Psychiatric symptoms among clients seeking treatment for drug dependence. Intake data from the National Treatment Outcome Research Study. *British Journal of Psychiatry*, 176, 285–9.

Marlatt, G.A. & Gordon, J.R. (eds) (1985) *Relapse Prevention: Maintenance Strategies in the Treatment of Addictive Behaviours*. Guilford Press, New York.

Martino, S., Carroll, K., Kostas, D., Perkins, J. & Rounsaville, B. (2002) Dual diagnosis motivational interviewing: a modification of motivational interviewing for substance abusing patients with psychotic disorders. *Journal of Substance Abuse Treatment*, 23, 297–308.

Matheson, C., Pitcairn, J., Bond, C.M., van Teijlingen, E. & Ryan, M. (2003) General practice management of illicit drug users in Scotland: a national survey. *Addiction*, 98 (1), 119–26.

Miller, W.R. & Rollnick, S. (eds) (1991) *Motivational Interviewing: Preparing People to Change Addictive Behaviour*. Guilford Press, New York.

Minkoff, K. (1989) Integrated treatment models of dual diagnosis of psychosis and addiction. *Hospital Community Psychiatry*, 40, 1031–6.

Minkoff, K. (2005) *Comprehensive Continuous Integrated System of Care (CCISC) – Psychopharmacology Practice Guidelines for Individuals with Co-occurring Psychiatric and Substance Use Disorders (COD)* (online) available from: http://www.kenminkoff.com/article1.html (20 November 2005).

National Treatment Agency (2002) *Models of Care for the Treatment of Drug Misusers. Part 2: Full Reference Report*. Department of Health, London.

Phillips, P. (2000) Substance misuse, offending and mental illness: a review. *Journal of Psychiatric and Mental Health Nursing*, 7, 483–9.

Phillips, P. & Labrow, J. (2000) Dual diagnosis – does harm reduction have a role? *International Journal of Drug Policy*, 11, 279–83.

Poole, R. & Brabbins, C. (1996) Drug induced psychosis. *British Journal of Psychiatry*, 168, 135–8.

Royal College of General Practitioners (2005) *RCGP Certificate Level Training for the Management of Drug Misuse in the Primary Care Setting* (online) available from: http://www.rcgp.org.uk/drug/certificate.asp (22 November 2005)

Royal College of Psychiatrists and Royal College of General Practitioners (2005) *Roles and Responsibilities of Doctors in the Provision of Treatment for Drug and Alcohol Misusers*. Royal College of Psychiatrists and Royal College of General Practitioners, London.

Schifano, F. (2002) European dimension of dual diagnosis. In: *Dual Diagnosis: Substance Misuse and Psychiatric Disorders* (Rassool, G.H., ed.), pp. 58–65. Blackwell Science, Oxford.

Seivewright, N. (2000) *Community treatment of drug misuse: more than methadone*. Cambridge University Press, Cambridge.

Seivewright, N. & Ford, C. (2003) Co-morbidity of substance misuse and mental illness in community mental health and substance misuse services. *British Journal of Psychiatry*, 183, 304–13.

Shaner, A., Roberts, L.J., Eckman, T.A. *et al.* (1998) Sources of diagnostic uncertainty for chronically psychotic cocaine abusers. *Psychiatric Services*, 49 (5), 684–90.

Shapiro, H. (ed.) (2004) *Guidance for Working with Cocaine and Crack Users in Primary Care*. Royal College of General Practitioners, London.

Siegfried, N. (1998) A review of co-morbidity: major mental illness and problematic substance use. *Australian and New Zealand Journal of Psychiatry*, 32 (5), 707–17.

Sims, J. & Iphofen, R. (2003) Primary care assessment of hazardous and harmful drinkers: a literature review. *Journal of Substance Use*, 8 (3), 176–81.

Skills for Health (2005) *Danos Standards – What are DANOS?* (online) available from: http://www.skillsforhealth.org.uk/danos/standards.php?page=2 (1 December 2005)

Spencer, C., Castle, D. & Michie, P.T. (2002) Motivations that maintain substance use among individuals with psychotic disorders. *Schizophrenia Bulletin*, 28 (2), 233–47.

Strang, J., Sheridan, J., Hunt, C., Bethanne, K., Gerada, C. & Pringle, M. (2005) The prescribing of methadone and other opioids to addicts: national survey of GPs in England and Wales. *British Journal of General Practice*, 55, 444–51.

Weaver, T., Madden, P., Charles, V. *et al.* (2003) Co-morbidity of substance misuse and mental illness in community mental health and substance misuse services. *British Journal of Psychiatry*, 183, 304–13.

15 Dual Diagnosis In Acute In-patient Settings

J. Gallagher & S.J. Scott

Introduction

Substance misuse in society has reached epidemic proportions and this increase is inevitably reflected in patients with mental health problems who are admitted to psychiatric wards (Williams & Cohen, 2000). As pointed out by Gafoor & Rassool (1998) the number of individuals who have coexisting substance misuse and psychiatric disorders within the UK is increasing. Krausz (1996) emphasises this point by stating that:

> 'the coincidence of severe mental illness and addiction is and will be one of the most important clinical challenges in psychiatry in the coming years which will also point to structural weaknesses in the treatment system between psychiatric and addiction treatment'.

Progress towards community based mental health provision has led to an increase in pressures and demands on acute in-patient settings (Baker, 2000) due to raised bed occupancy (up to 104%) and the changing nature of the patients served. Patients with serious mental illness and those with complex behavioural and social problems, including substance misuse, are now the norm within acute in-patient settings (Sainsbury Centre for Mental Health, 1998a). The aims of this chapter are to examine the prevalence of dual diagnosis in in-patient settings and describe the identification and assessment of substance misuse in acute care settings. Barriers to engagement and treatment are also discussed.

In-patient settings

Within acute in-patient settings schizophrenia is common, accounting for 60% or more of the population (Baker, 2000). Co-presenting substance misuse within this group is up to three times that in the average population at roughly 37% (Cantwell *et al.*, 1999) and is more prevalent in younger clients (Hambrecht & Hafner, 2000). Cantor-Graae *et al.* (2001) reported higher lifetime prevalence rates of 40–60%. Due to this high level of co-morbidity between substance misuse and schizophrenia, dual diagnosis is now often considered the norm rather than the exception in acute in-patient settings (Smith & Hucker, 1993). In most studies the prevalence of cannabis use is equivalent to alcohol use at about 30–40% (Hambrecht & Hafner, 2000) and misuse continues before and after hospital discharge (Sevy *et al.*, 2001). The prototypical dual diagnosis patient in an acute in-patient setting is therefore a young schizophrenic male with co-morbid substance misuse, probably cannabis or alcohol.

Despite this prototypical group, a heterogeneous group of patients with dual diagnosis emerges from the major national epidemiological studies in Australia (Teesson *et al.*, 2000) and in the USA (Regier *et al.*, 1990). Dual diagnosis patients have varied mental health problems (depression, social phobia, schizophrenia, manic depression and severe anxiety disorders) and misuse a number of substances (including cannabis, alcohol, amphetamines, cocaine and opiates) (Watkins *et al.*, 2001). Poly-substance misuse is common in this group of clients (Teesson *et al.*, 2000). Although Australian epidemiological patterns may not be directly replicated in the UK it is likely that there is considerable overlap. This heterogeneous presentation makes it necessary to conclude that even with seemingly prototypical patients we must consider each unique patient's pattern of mental health and substance misuse issues.

The patterns of interaction between substance misuse, mental health and social exclusion demonstrate a need for complex theoretical formulations of the individual's problems. As with any other complex client an integrated approach to understanding is necessary (Barker, 1997; Watkins *et al.*, 2001). From this position it is the whole picture that is developed rather than the assessment tools adopted that will allow treatment to be mutually planned and implemented. Only by applying appropriate theory to each individual illness narrative (Barker, 2001) can a clear picture of the interaction of the biological, the personal (psychological) and the social begin to occur and the voyage to recovery commence (Stevenson & Fletcher, 2002). The assessment conducted when working with patients with complex conditions must therefore focus on these issues as well as the tools used. A summary of the relationship between substance misuse and mental health is presented in Table 15.1.

Table 15.1 Summary of the relationships between substance misuse and mental health.

Stressors + physiological vulnerability + poor coping (including substance misuse) = relapse into mental illness + symptom management (drug use) = vulnerability + chaotic behaviour = exclusion and labelling = hospitalisation + boredom = further substance misuse to relieve boredom and reduce medication side effects = further labelling and increasing exclusion.

The problems for acute care

Patients with psychosis and substance misuse problems tend to have longer stays in hospital, have more re-admissions and are less likely to be compliant with medication and other treatments. They have increased rates of suicide, HIV and other physical illnesses and have poorer overall social functioning. These findings highlight the need to provide more effective interventions to enable high quality care that addresses both the substance misuse and mental health problem simultaneously, using an integrated approach (Drake *et al.*, 2001).

Despite the clear needs, this client group are not treated effectively within any setting. In-patient care focuses on 'diagnosis and control' and in terms of mental illness alone this reduces opportunities to meaningfully engage patients in their own recovery (Sainsbury Centre for Mental Health, 1998a; Kovisto *et al.*, 2003). Rassool (2002) suggests that services, both substance misuse and mental health, at best address the co-morbid issues separately (not integrating) and at worst ignore one aspect of the problem totally. The consequence of this is that substance misuse is often left untreated in acute settings and mental illness is left untreated in substance misuse services. Exclusion of certain clients from services appears to militate against a holistic client focused approach.

Whilst substance misuse workers traditionally use a long-term recovery perspective, accepting a relapse–recovery pattern over an extended period of time (Watkins *et al.*, 2001) acute in-patient services have been increasingly franchised to treat illness and promote rapid discharge policies to ease pressure on beds (Baker, 2000). Early intervention material talks about prevention of a relapse profile which can worsen outcome (Birchwood *et al.*, 2000). This means that patients who display 'revolving door' pathology and need a longer journey to recovery challenge existing service models and evidence based treatments for schizophrenia. Patients with co-morbid substance misuse are both revolving door and longer stay (Watkins *et al.*, 2001). Further, a relapse–recovery pattern is a central part of their journey to health (Miller & Rollnick, 2002). Conflict therefore exists between a pressure to stabilise an illness and discharge a patient on the one hand and a focus on longer term recovery including relapse on the other.

Qualitative research into training needs in acute in-patient settings suggests that staff are motivated and keen to work with this client group but often feel unprepared when dealing with the challenges they face (Ryrie & McGowan, 1998). Richmond & Foster (2003), utilising the Substance Abuse Attitude Survey (Chappel *et al.*, 1985), identified beliefs that impact negatively on treatment, including low optimism and low permissiveness in mental health staff. These attitudes mean that staff will feel treatment is unlikely to succeed if substance misuse is present. This can lead to an attitude of low permissiveness and a punitive confrontational approach to drug use. Patients in this situation may feel excluded and stigmatised within mental health services, leading to a cycle of stigmatisation, alienation and social exclusion (Sayce, 1999; Sainsbury Centre for Mental Health, 1998b).

Overall, the present system of care, the in-patient ethos and skills mix in acute in-patient provision can mitigate against an effective service for this patient group and highlights conflicts that exist between best practice and service delivery models.

Considering the government agenda

The Government's *Dual Diagnosis Good Practice Guide* (Department of Health, 2002) states that in-patient services and others such as assertive outreach must develop the skills necessary to work with both substance abuse issues as well as mental illness (Department of Health, 2002). The document also recognises a clear need to develop integrated treatment approaches. Despite this clear distribution of responsibility (Department of Health, 2002) no clear guidance is given about underlying service level, and service ethos issues, although some guidance is given in terms of treatment and training. The treatment model suggested by the guidance focuses on the New Hampshire Team community treatment approach to dual diagnosis (Drake *et al.*, 2001).

The model of engagement, motivation action stage and relapse prevention demands a long-term approach, years rather than months, delivered by staff who have a good knowledge of both mental health problems and substance misuse problems. The aim is to maintain patients in their own community. The relapsing–recovery pattern in dual diagnosis patient profiles means that at various stages individuals may require in-patient treatment. The present whole system approach to patient management (Department of Health, 1999) places in-patient admission as one step on the whole journey to recovery, rather than the whole journey itself. Acute in-patient settings will be primarily involved in engaging clients and working to help them understand the present episode of relapse in the broader picture. Relapsed clients can be at any stage of change (Prochaska & DiClemente, 1984; Prochaska *et al.*, 2002) and continuity of treatment, including relapse learning and prevention is also sometimes the focus of acute in-patient work within a whole system of services, all helping the client on their journey to social and psychological recovery (Maslin *et al.*, 2001).

The bridge between these recovery based community models and an existing in-patient focus on diagnosis and stabilisation is, however, still problematic and we need to consider the means by which we can engage with clients across the service boundaries we have created to implement this whole system relapse–recovery approach. This clearly has implications for acute care in terms of the service delivery process and its integration with community teams.

Detecting substance misuse in acute mental health patients

Substance misuse problems within mental health settings are frequently undetected and underdiagnosed (Annath *et al.*, 1989; Shaner *et al.*, 1993). Barnaby *et al.* (2003) found that more than 50% of 200 patients admitted to six acute psychiatric wards, over three months, had their substance misuse history ignored. Lack of identification is one cause of poor outcome. Such findings are in contradiction to the *Dual Diagnosis Good Practice Guide* (Department of Health, 2002), which states: 'Individuals with dual problems deserve high quality patient focused care. This should be delivered within mental health services'. Poor assessment mitigates against this. An important consideration in the failure to detect dual problems within psychiatric ward settings is related to lack of knowledge and competence in the nursing and medical staff in detecting substance misuse. This is a point raised by Carey & Correia (1998) who highlight that this lack of knowledge, along with the lack of substance specific assessment in mental health treatment settings are possibly the most significant obstacles.

Patients who have a sensitivity to substances that interact with their mental health status rarely present a full substance misuse history that indicates dependency. Signs of intoxication or withdrawal may not be apparent; however, the substance misuse is still significant in the person. Understandably, these patients are overlooked by a less knowledgeable assessor. Even biomedical methods of detecting substance misuse, such as the analysis of blood, breath and urine for the metabolites of misused substances may be 'insensitive' with this patient group, as metabolites may remain in a person's system for only a limited time, often up to just three days (Hawks & Chiang, 1986) and this does not therefore detect intermittent usage. Indirect methods of detecting prolonged substance misuse, such as raised liver enzymes or enlarged liver, may also be absent due to the relatively low doses of substances that negatively compromise the patient's mental state but do not overtly impact upon their physiological status. It follows that if nurses are to make accurate assessments of patient's substance misuse diagnosis they must recognise that the DSM-IV criteria for substance dependence and DSM-IV for substance misuse (APA, 1994) may exclude many people who have a dual diagnosis issue. This is because even small doses of alcohol and other psychoactive drugs, which would not cause the average person any significant problems may be problematic for individuals who have a severe mental illness.

A study by Moore *et al.* (1989) suggested that clinicians are more likely to diagnose substance use disorder amongst clients who comply with their concept of a typical alcohol and drug misuse patient. This may explain why certain groups of substance misuse patients who do not meet this stereotype are diagnosed less frequently than others. Even if symptoms of a substance misuse support a diagnosis they are often ignored and a diagnosis is withheld (Hansen *et al.*, 2000). Milling *et al.* (1994) found that one third of the patients in a mental hospital with a clear indication of substance misuse disorder did not have this recorded in official documents. This was supported by Barnaby *et al.* (2003) who also identified that 53% of people recognised as having a substance misuse problem did not have this formally recorded. A lack of knowledge of effective interventions for substance misuse, compounded by a pessimistic view of outcomes for the client group may be the main reason that diagnosis is not recorded. Schwartz & Taylor (1989) and Appleby *et al.* (1997) suggest that substance misuse disorders tend to be ignored if previous attempts to treat the patient have been unsuccessful.

Assessing the client's needs in an acute care environment

The assessment process itself may not be rigorous enough to identify substance misuse behaviour as it is geared to a relatively high level of substance misuse. A single interview can misattribute symptoms and fail to identify either substance misuse or a psychiatric problem. Williams & Cohen (2000) state that:

> 'the needs of the co-morbid clients are clinically complex and multi-focal, and the failure of many treatment programmes to provide clinicians time and opportunity for multi-level assessment may contribute to the failure to identify these clients'.

Single early interviews may be compounded by the acute stage of the patient's problem. Assessment should therefore be seen as a process rather than a one-off event.

One tool that may be useful in screening for substance misuse problems with patients with mental health problems is the Addiction Severity Index (ASI) (McLellan *et al.*, 1980). This assesses the patient's substance use against a psychiatric dimension. Appleby *et al.* (1997) state that the ASI is the most widely used instrument to assess substance misuse, and that findings from studies to evaluate its effectiveness in dual diagnosis support its use in this. The Dartmouth Assessment of Lifestyle Instrument (DALI) (Rosenberg *et al.*, 1998) was developed to identify substance misuse in dual diagnosis in-patients (Carey & Correia, 1998). Preliminary reports suggest it is reliable over time and across interviewers, and is more sensitive (has the ability to detect a substance misuse disorder if it is there), and specific (able to accurately identify people who do not have substance disorder).

Table 15.2 Summary of the models of treatment suggested that may facilitate dual diagnosis working.

Dual diagnosis guidelines (D of H, 2002)	Motivational interviewing (Miller & Rollnick, 2002)	COMPASS/STOP (Kavenagh *et al.*, 1998; Maslin *et al.*, 2001)	Psychosocial intervention (Sainsbury Centre, 2002)	Interpersonal nursing narrative approaches (Barker, 2001)
• Engagement	• Engagement	• Engagement	• Engagement	• Engagement
• Assessment	• Building motivation	• Developing a shared formulation	• Assessment	• Hearing the client's story
• Persuasion • Motivation	• Responding to change • Responding to resistance	• Information sharing • Substance intake goals • Reduction of high risk behaviour	• Shared understanding • Psycho-education	• Empowering education
• Treatment	• Enhancing confidence	• Reducing symptoms • Alternative activities • Assertive substance refusal • Impulse control	• Medication managed • Cognitive behavioural therapy for psychosis • Family interventions	• Planning • Recovery
• Relapse prevention	• Strengthening commitment • Relapse learning	• Relapse prevention	• Early warning signs and relapse prevention	• Relapse • Recovery

Assessment at this stage of our knowledge and development needs to use a continuing process that is exploratory, non-confrontational but that aims to clarify what, when and how the person is using substances and the interaction between their substance misuse, mental health and social situation. At present we are some way off from developing a tool capable of gathering this kind of information; therefore, tools should be considered part of an ongoing process of information gathering only.

Several approaches to substance misuse issues have been developed for community based delivery (Prochaska & DiClemente, 1984; Miller & Rollnick, 1991) and applied to people with dual diagnosis (Drake *et al.*, 2001; Maslin *et al.*, 2001; Rassool, 2002; Dumaine, 2003). These models are complemented by community based collaborative psychosocial approaches developed for the treatment of psychosis (Chadwick *et al.*, 1996; Barraclough & Tarrier, 1997; Sainsbury Centre for Mental Health, 2002), particularly those models related to early interventions (Birchwood *et al.*, 2000) and applied to patients with dual diagnosis (Kavanagh *et al.*, 1998; Maslin *et al.*, 2001; Sainsbury Centre for Mental Health, 1998b). Therefore, present models largely adapt and apply single diagnosis methods to a more complex problem. Several models that are available to work with this client group have been developed and are outlined in Table 15.2.

Recognising existing engagement skills

Although reports into acute in-patient care (Sainsbury Centre for Mental Health, 1998a; Baker, 2000; Rose, 2001) are critical of the focus on medication management and control in these services, recipients of care valued aspects of their care including support and problem solving interventions delivered by mental health professionals (Sainsbury Centre for Mental Health, 1998a; Rose, 2001). Qualitative research identified interpersonal relationships and practical problem solving as highly valued by clients, although the service delivery process often prevents this kind of care occurring. 'Something always comes up' (Cleary & Edwards, 1999). These valued and prized engagement and practical skills need to be considered in terms of all patient populations in acute care areas.

Several developments in acute in-patient care, including the acute solutions project (Sainsbury Centre for Mental Health, 2002), the Tidal Model (Barker, 2001; Fletcher & Stevenson, 2001), the National Institute for Mental Health (NIMH) engagement project (NIMH, 2006); and a spectrum of psychosocial approaches address engagement, shared understanding and motivation for change. These skills are at the very centre of the Government's proposals for dual diagnosis working (Department of Health, 2002). Our aim should therefore be to recognise the best practice approaches that already exist in acute in-patient care and to apply these to our work with all clients, including those with dual diagnosis issues.

Barriers to treatment and engagement

On admission, some patients may also require stabilisation of one or both of their problems. For example, if a client has a drug or alcohol dependence, they made need medical intervention to minimise their withdrawal symptoms and correct any physical complications that have arisen as a result of their substance problem and associated lifestyle. Alternatively, they may need to have their mental health problems stabilised, which may involve medication. This can lead to conflicting information regarding these problems; nurses need to be clear about the distinction between prescribed and non-prescribed medication. The ethos of substance misuse work is of paramount importance, and is reflected in the attitude of the staff, which needs to be one of understanding and acceptance. Drake *et al.* (2001) states that nurses must have an empathic, non-judgemental approach, and endeavour to develop a therapeutic alliance, which is essential to the engagement stage of treatment (Drake *et al.*, 2001). Nurses need to learn and understand the benefits of harm reduction as part of the process in achieving abstinence, which may be the desired long-term goal. For example, patients with schizophrenia who misuse substances are generally unable to make and stand by definitive commitments to become abstinent. They need the ongoing support provided by programmes that extend over time and are tolerant of patients dropping in and out, sometimes trying to quit and sometimes not, abstaining for a while only to relapse. The goals of these programmes are to greatly increase durable levels of abstinence oriented motivation, rather than to demand abstinence as criteria for entering and remaining in treatment (Bellack *et al.*, 1999).

Staff may be able to develop this kind of approach if they can appreciate that treatment of dual diagnosis is a process that is likely to take years rather than months, and they can recognise that as with any chronic relapsing condition, relapse is a normal part of the recovery process as outlined in the Transtheoretical Model of Change (Prochaska & DiClemente, 1984). If staff can accept this approach they will be able to reframe relapse as an opportunity for further growth in the individual, by using it as a learning experience for both the patient and the client. By interpreting relapse in this manner, staff will reduce their sense of frustration and associated feelings of resentment towards those clients, which is a barrier to a therapeutic relationship, the focus of engagement. Clinical supervision offers a real opportunity to develop awareness and challenge our beliefs through introspection and feedback, if appropriately applied. It also provides an opportunity to reflect on practice, ventilate negative feelings and identify knowledge deficiencies, which require further education.

From the users' perspective, substance misuse meets a need. It is a coping strategy, and may not be simply hedonistic, pleasure seeking behaviour. An Alcoholic Anonymous member recalls from admission that 'nurses need to understand we are sick people who need to get well, not bad people who need to become good'. To overcome these blocks we always need to focus on the patient's story and through this identify areas for change, and assist the patient in exploring more constructive and healthy ways of meeting their needs without the assistance of substances.

Attempting to understand the patient's story is not a passive activity. Complex patterns of events that have led to the present crisis are difficult for both patients and us to begin to understand. This lack of understanding causes much of the distress we experience. Most therapeutic approaches suggest we need to act as a guide (Miller & Rollnick, 2002) or a co-voyager (Barker, 2001) and allow an evolving understanding to emerge (Fowler, 2000; Kinderman & Lobban, 2000). This is in contrast to a more treatment focused approach that attempts to identify and diagnose a set of signs and symptoms that may not have any meaning for the client. Thus, understanding the problem is about developing a shared understanding.

For treatment to lead to increased understanding the patient needs to be able to talk about and explore their own experiences or journey into ill health (Kovisto *et al.*, 2003). By exploring with a patient we can liberate ourselves from a pressured expert role and the patient from being a disempowered recipient of our knowledge (Kovisto *et al.*, 2003). Shared exploration and problem solving promote a more equal recognition of the present situation, scope of responsibility and a realistic recognition of our own scope of influence. This reduces our anxiety about cure and the patient's self-esteem may begin to grow. Within a psychosocial approach exploration ends in a flow diagram (schematic formulation) (Fowler, 2000). Both parties add their own unique contribution to the discussion and resulting formulation. Evolved formulations may begin simply but become complex, including family influence, internal patterns of behaviour (including substance misuse), thought (including illness and substance beliefs) and feeling, and social exclusion or inclusion issues.

True treatment can only begin when the behaviour that maintains the present health status has been understood and action plans have been agreed that allow the patient to begin investigating practical alternatives to the behaviour and coping that is maintained in their present difficulty. Diagnosis is the start of our understanding of the patient's problems; treatment can only begin when the patient understands the complex interactions between different elements of their problem themselves. Prochaska & DiClemente (1984) recognise that it is when we do not match our intervention to the client's understanding and recognition of a need to change (cycle of change) that engagement fails. Moving too quickly or too slowly for the client in terms of the recovery journey may both result in this occurring. Engagement and understanding form the foundation to change in mental health settings; however, change itself may need additional interventions. Particularly at this stage, a motivational interviewing approach may be of benefit in helping patients overcome competing motivations and moving towards recovery (Miller & Rollnick, 2002).

The transtheoretical model (Prochaska & DiClemente, 1984) helps us determine the patient's readiness for change. The aim of motivational interviewing (MI) is to facilitate the patient in moving to the action stage, where they understand, want and feel able to change, and are thus motivated to accept and commit themselves to the planned interventions aimed at facilitating the change. Due to its non-confrontational approach, MI may have a particular use with patients who have schizophrenia, who are less able to benefit from confrontational methods typical of traditional substance misuse treatment (Carey, 1996; Bellack & DiClemente, 1999). In acute in-patient settings this rapid mobilisation of the patient is essential and this makes a motivational approach a well matched in-patient approach. Although this approach builds on client strengths some other forms of intervention may also be necessary in dual diagnosis clients who may have difficulties accommodating to illness, relating to family members and coping with life stressors (Miller & Rollnick, 2002).

Interventions that are helpful in reducing interpersonal stress and developing alternative methods of coping with life stressors are behavioural family interventions to reduce the stress in the family situation (Barrowclough & Tarrier, 1997); cognitive behavioural interventions to help adaptation and accommodation to a new health status (Birchwood *et al.*, 2000), developing new adaptive patterns of thinking feeling and behaving including social skills and coping approaches. To continue the shared approach, however, it should be stated that selection from this range of treatment approaches should occur in consultation and collaboration rather than as a result of the nurse's preferred model of intervention.

All these components of treatment, including engagement, developing a shared formulation and motivation for change (MI) are brief focused approaches and are therefore well placed in settings such as acute wards, where we only have a short period of time to engage a client in collaborative effort. Overall, however, it is the continuity of care that is paramount in the treatment of relapse–recovery disorders such as substance misuse and schizophrenia.

Discharge planning and ongoing treatment

Recent research in in-patient care identified little benefit to offering brief motivational interviews when interventions were not actively followed up (Baker *et al.*, 2002). In this study, patient contact did not increase following discharge and remained very low, at 15%, which is comparable to a non-treatment group. This finding could relate to motivational deficits due to negative symptoms of schizophrenia (APA, 1994). An alternative explanation for the failure of this trial to reduce substance misuse in the group rests on the failure of a separate service model in treatment of all multiple conditions.

An integrated service approach is needed to patient care, offering continuity in a whole system approach (Department of Health, 2000). The need is to genuinely begin to dismantle boundaries between mental health and substance misuse services (Department of Health, 2002), and more importantly to provide integrated care in in-patient and community services (Department of Health, 2000). The approach would allow recovery through supported relapse learning, offering continuing hope, understanding and progress, whilst acknowledging the likelihood of relapse and potential benefit that can occur through careful handling of this process between a collaborative community and an in-patient care group. At present it is clear that an adequate whole system approach is only emerging and this means that client discharge planning is often ad hoc. In the future it is hoped pathways for these clients will emerge that allow a range of active initiatives including ward outreach, community in-reach and shared care.

Within the present service climate all that may be possible is a careful collaboration between the community and in-patient services that begins at the point of admission and plans towards a meaningful journey to recovery within a continuing care programming approach (Department of Health, 1999). Possibly, for those clients with the most serious dual problems, an assertive outreach approach that has dedicated (Maslin *et al.*, 2001) and even self-manned in-patient provision may be the ideal for a dual diagnosis client group (Sainsbury Centre for Mental Health, 1998b; Ho *et al.*, 1999).

Conclusion

Overall, within existing services, it is possible to offer an integrated treatment approach that maximises the potential to work alongside patients to help them begin to understand and to develop motivation to change their patterns of behaviour and thinking that perpetuate and continue both their substance abuse and their mental health problems. This work is a long-term undertaking and is likely to include periods of hospital admission and community intervention. To operate this to the best effect and the benefit of the patient it is necessary to consider new ways of managing the interface between ward and community. This suggests both optimism and challenge for the future.

References

American Psychiatric Association (1994) *Diagnostic and Statistical Manual of Mental Disorders*, 4th edn. American Psychiatric Association, Washington, DC.

Annath, J., Vandewater, S., Kamal, S., Broksky, A., Gamal, R. & Miller, M. (1989) Missed diagnosis of substance abuse in psychiatric patients. *Hospital and Community Psychiatry*, 40, 297–9.

Appleby, L., Dyson, V., Altman, E. & Lutchins, D.J. (1997) Assessing substance use in multi-problem patients: reliability and validity of the Addiction Severity Index in a mental hospital population. *The Journal of Nervous and Mental Disease*, 185 (3), 159–65.

Baker, A., Lewin, T., Reichler, H. *et al.* (2002) Evaluation of a motivational interview for substance use within psychiatric in-patient services. *Addiction*, 97, 1329–37.

Baker, J.A. (2000) Developing psychosocial care for acute psychiatric wards. *Journal of Psychiatric Mental Health Nursing*, 7, 95–100.

Barker, P. (1997) *Assessment in Psychiatric and Mental Health Nursing: in Search of the Whole Person*. Stanley Thornes, Cheltenham.

Barker, P. (2001) The Tidal Model: developing an empowering, person centred approach to recovery within psychiatric and mental health nursing. *Journal of Psychiatric and Mental Health Nursing*, 8 (3), 233–40.

Barnaby, B., Drummond, C., McCloud, A., Burns, T. & Omu, N. (2003) Substance misuse in psychiatric in-patients. Comparison of a screening questionnaire survey with case notes. *British Medical Journal*, 327 (Oct.), 783–4.

Barrowclough, C. & Tarrier, N. (1997) *Families of Schizophrenic Patients: Cognitive Behavioural Interventions*. Stanley Thorne Ltd, London.

Bellack, A.S. & DiClemente, C.C. (1999) Treating substance use among patients with schizophrenia. *Psychiatric Services*, 50, 75–80.

Birchwood, M., Fowler, D. & Jackson, C. (eds) (2000) *Early Interventions in Psychosis: a Guide to Concepts, Evidence and Interventions*. Wiley, Chichester.

Brooker, C. (2001) A decade of evidence based training for work with people with serious mental health problems: progress in the development of psychosocial interventions. *Journal of Mental Health*, 10 (1), 17–31.

Brunette, M.F., Mueser, K.T., Xie, H. & Drake, R.E. (1997) Relationship between symptoms of schizophrenia and substance abuse. *The Journal of Nervous and Mental Disease*, 185, 13–20.

Cantor-Graae, E., Nordstrom, L.G. & McNeil, T.F. (2001) Substance abuse in schizophrenia: a review of the literature and a study of correlates in Sweden. *Schizophrenia Research*, 48 (1), 69–82.

Cantwell, R., Brewing, J., Glazebrook, C. *et al.* (1999) Prevalence of substance misuse in first episode psychosis. *British Journal of Psychiatry*, 174 (2), 150–3.

Carey, K.B. (1996) Substance use reduction in the context of outpatient psychiatric treatment: a collaborative motivational harm reduction approach. *Community Mental Health Journal*, 32, 291–306.

Carey, K.B. & Correia, C.J. (1998) Severe mental illness and addictions assessment considerations. *Addictive Behaviors*, 23 (6), 735–48.

Chadwick, P., Birchwood, M. & Trower, P. (1996) *Cognitive Therapy for Delusion, Voices and Paranoia*. Wiley, London.

Chambers, M. (1998) Interpersonal mental health nursing: research issues and challenges. *Journal of Psychiatric and Mental Health Nursing*, 5, 203–11.

Chappel, J.N. (1993) Training of residents in the diagnosis and treatment of dual diagnosis patients. *Journal of Psychoactive Drugs*, 25, 293–300.

Chappel, J.N., Veach, T.J. & Krug, R.S. (1985) The substance abuse attitude survey: an instrument for measuring attitudes. *Journal of Studies on Alcohol*, 46, 48–52.

Cleary, M. & Edwards, C. (1999) Something always comes up: nurse-patient interaction in an acute psychiatric setting. *Journal of Psychiatric and Mental Health Nursing*, 6, 469–77.

Connors, G.J., Donovan, D.M. & DiClemente, C.C. (2001) *Substance Abuse Treatment and the Stages of Change*. The Guilford Press, London.

Department of Health (1996) *The Spectrum of Care. Local Services for People with Mental Health Problems*. NHSE LASSL (96)16/HSG(96)6.

Department of Health (1999) *National Service Framework for Mental Health: Modern Standards and Service Models*. Department of Health, London.

Department of Health (2000) *The NHS Plan*. Department of Health, London.

Department of Health (2002) *Mental Health Policy Implementation Guide: Dual Diagnosis Good Practice Guide*. Department of Health, London.

Drake, R.E., Osher, F.C., Noordsy, D.L., Hurlbut, S.C., Teague, G.B. & Beaudett, M.S. (1990) Diagnosis of alcohol use disorders in schizophrenia. *Schizophrenia Bulletin*, 16, 57–61.

Drake, R., Essock, S. & Shaner, A. (2001) Implementing dual diagnosis services for clients with severe mental illness. *Psychiatric Services*, 2, 469–76.

Dumaine, M.L. (2003) Meta-analysis of interventions with co-occurring disorders of severe mental illness and substance abuse: implications for social work practice. *Research on Social Work Practice*, 12 (2), 142–65.

English National Board (1996) *Substance Use Misuse. Guidelines for Good Practice in Education and Training of Nurses, Midwives and Health Visitors*. English National Board, Guilford.

Fletcher, E. & Stevenson, C. (2001) Launching the Tidal Model in an adult mental health programme. *Nursing Standard*, 15 (49), 33–6.

Fowler, D. (2000) Psychological formulation of early psychosis: a cognitive model. In: Birchwood, D.G., Fowler, G. & Jackson, C. (eds) *Early intervention in psychosis: a practical handbook*. Wiley, Chichester.

Gafoor, M. & Rassool, G.H. (1998) The coexistence of psychiatric disorders and substance misuse: working with dual diagnosis patients. *Journal of Advanced Nursing*, 27, 497–502.

Geller, G., Levine, D.M., Mamon, J.A., Moore, R.D., Bone, L.R. & Stokes, E.J. (1989) Knowledge, attitudes and reported practices of medical students and house staff regarding the diagnosis and treatment of alcoholism. *Journal of American Medical Association*, 261, 3115–20.

Graham, A.V., Christy, K., Emmitt-Meyers, S.E. & Zyzanski, S. (1997) Substance abuse education for clinical nurses: a controlled study. *Journal of Continuing Education in Nursing*, 28, 217–22.

Hambrecht, M. & Hafner, H. (2000) Cannabis, vulnerability and the onset of schizophrenia: an epidemiological perspective. *Australian and New Zealand Journal of Psychiatry*, 34, 468–75.

Hansen, S., Munk-Jorgensen, P., Guldback, B. *et al.* (2000) Psychoactive substance use diagnoses among psychiatric in-patients. *Acta Psychiatrica Scandinavica*, 102, 432–8.

Hawks, R.L. & Chiang, C.N. (eds) (1986) *Urine Testing for Drugs of Abuse* (DHSS Publication No. ADM 87-1481) US Government Printing Office, Washington, DC.

Ho, A., Tsuang, J., Liberman, R. *et al.* (1999) Achieving effective treatment of patients with chronic psychotic illness and co-morbid substance dependence. *The American Journal of Psychiatry*, 156 (11), 1765–70.

Kavanagh, D.J., Young, R., Boyce, L. *et al.* (1998) Substance treatment options in psychosis (STOP): a new intervention for dual diagnosis. *Journal of Mental Health*, 7 (2), 135–43.

Kinderman, P. & Lobban, F. (2000) Evolving formulations: sharing complex information with clients. *Behavioural and Cognitive Psychotherapy*, 28, 307–10.

Kovisto, K., Janhonen, S. & Vaisanen, L. (2003) Patients' experiences of psychosis in an in-patient setting. *Journal of Psychiatric and Mental Health Nursing*, 10, 221–9.

Krausz, M. (1996) Old problems – new perspectives. *European Addiction Research*, 2, 1–2.

McLellan, A.T., Luborsky, L., Woody, G.E. & O'Brien, C.P. (1980) An improved diagnostic evaluation instrument for substance abuse patients: the Addiction Severity Index. *Journal of Nervous and Mental Disease*, 168, 26–33.

Maslin, J., Graham, H.L., Cawley, M. *et al.* (2001) Combined severe mental health and substance use problems: what are the training and support needs of staff working with this client group? *Journal of Mental Health*, 10 (2), 131–40.

Mayfield, D., McCleod, G. & Hall, P. (1974) The CAGE questionnaire: validation of a new alcoholism screening questionnaire. *American Journal of Psychiatry*, 131, 1121–3.

Miller, W.R. & Rollnick, S. (1991) *Motivational Interviewing. Preparing People For Change*. Guilford Press, New York.

Miller, W.R. & Rollnick, S. (2002) *Motivational Interviewing. Preparing People For Change*, 2nd edn. Guilford Press, New York.

Milling, R.N., Faulkner, L.R. & Craig, J.M. (1994) Problems in the recognition and treatment of patients with dual diagnosis. *Journal of Substance Abuse Treatment*, 11, 267–71.

Moore, R.D., Bone, L.R., Geller, G., Mamon, J.A., Stokes, E.J. & Levine, D.M. (1989) Prevalence, detection, and treatment of alcoholism in hospitalised patients. *JAMA*, 261, 403–7.

NIMH (uploaded 12/04/06) http://kc.nimhe.org.uk/index.cfm?fuseaction=Item.viewResource&intItemID=48854

Pols, R.G., Sellman, D. & Jurd, S.A. (1996) What is the psychiatrist's role in drugs and alcohol? *Australian and New Zealand Journal of Psychiatry*, 30, 5540–9.

Prochaska, J.O. & DiClemente, C.C. (1984) *The Transtheoretical Approach: Crossing the Traditional Boundaries of Therapy*. DowJones, Pacific Grove, Calif.

Prochaska, J.O., DiClemente, C.C. & Norcross, J.C. (2002) *Systems of Psychotherapy: a Transtheoretical Analysis*, 4th edn. Brooks/Cole Publications, Pacific Grove, Calif.

Rassool, G.H. (2002) Substance use and dual diagnosis: concepts, theories and models. In: *Dual Diagnosis. Substance Misuse and Psychiatric Disorders* (Rassool, G.H., ed.), pp. 12–32. Blackwell Science, Oxford.

Regier, D.A., Farmer, M.E., Rae, D.S. *et al.* (1990) Co-morbidity of mental disorders with alcohol and other drug abuse: results from the Epidemiological Catchment Area (ECA) study. *Journal of the American Medical Association*, 21, 2511–18.

Richmond, I.C. & Foster, J.H. (2003) Negative attitudes towards people with co-morbid mental health and substance misuse problems: an investigation of mental health professionals. *Journal of Mental Health*, 12, Aug. (4), 393–403.

Ridgely, M.S. (1991) Creating integrated programmes for severely mentally ill persons with substance disorders. *New Direction for Mental Health Services*, 50, 29–41.

Roche, A.M., Parke, M.D., Campbell, J. & Saunders, J.B. (1995) Substance abuse disorders: psychiatric trainees' knowledge, diagnostic skills and attitudes. *Australian and New Zealand Journal of Psychiatry*, 29, 645–52.

Rose, D. (2001) *Users' Voices. The Perspectives of Mental Health Service Users on Community and Hospital Care*. Sainsbury Centre for Mental Health, London.

Rosenberg, S.D., Drake, R.E., Wolford, G.L. *et al.* (1998) Dartmouth Assessment of Lifestyle Instrument (DALI): a substance use disorder screen for people with severe mental illness. *American Journal of Psychiatry*, 155, 232–8.

Ryrie, I. & McGowan, J. (1998) Staff perceptions of substance use among acute in-patients. *Journal of Psychiatric and Mental Health Nursing*, 5, 137–42.

Sainsbury Centre For Mental Health (1998a) *Acute Problems: a Survey of the Quality of Care in Acute Psychiatric Wards*. The Sainsbury Centre for Mental Health Publications, London.

Sainsbury Centre for Mental Health (1998b) *Keys to Engagement*. Sainsbury Centre for Mental Health, London.

Sainsbury Centre for Mental Health (2002) *The Search for Acute Solutions Project*. www.scmh.org.uk

Sayce, L. (1999) *Outsiders Coming in: Achieving Social Inclusion for People with Mental Health Problems*. Mind Publications, London.

Sayce, L. (2000) *From Patient to Citizen*. Mind Publications, London.

Schuckit, M.A. (1983) Alcoholism and other psychiatric disorders. *Hospital and Community Psychiatry*, 341, 1022–6.

Schwartz, L.S. & Taylor, J.R. (1989) Attitudes of mental health professionals toward alcoholism recognition and treatment. *Medical Journal of Drug and Alcohol Abuse*, 15, 321–37.

Selzer, M.L., Vinokur, A. & VanRoojjen, L. (1975) A self-administered short Michigan Alcohol Screening Test (SMAST). *Journal of Studies of Alcohol*, 9, 27–38.

Sevy, S., Robinson, D.G., Solloway, S. *et al.* (2001) Correlation of substance misuse in patients with first episode schizophrenia and schizo-affective disorder. *Acta Psychiatrica Scandinavica*, 104, 367–74.

Shaner, A., Khalsam, P., Roberts, L., Wilkins, J., Anglia, D. & Hsieh, S. (1993) Unrecognised cocaine use among schizophrenic patients. *American Journal of Psychiatry*, 150, 758–62.

Siegfried, N., Ferguson, J., Cleary, M., Walter, G., Joseph, M. & Rey, M. (1999) Experience, knowledge and attitudes of mental health staff regarding patient's problematic drug and alcohol use. *Australian and New Zealand Journal of Psychiatry*, 33 (2), 267–73.

Skinner, H.A. (1982) The drug abuse screening test. *Addictive Behaviours*, 7, 363–71.

Smith, J. & Hucker, S. (1993) Dual diagnosis patients: substance abuse by the severely mentally ill. *British Journal of Hospital Medicine*, 50 (1), 650–4.

Stevenson, C. & Fletcher, E. (2002) The Tidal Model: the questions answered. *Health Practice*, 5 (8), 29–37.

Teesson, M., Hall, W., Lynskey, M. & Degenhardt, L. (2000) Alcohol and drug-use disorders in Australia: implications of the National Survey of Mental Health and Wellbeing. *Australian and New Zealand Journal of Psychiatry*, 34, 206–13.

Todd, F.C., Sellman, D. & Robertson, P.J. (2002) Barriers to optimal care for patients with coexisting substance use and mental health disorders. *Australian and New Zealand Journal of Psychiatry*, 36, 792–9.

Van Horn, D.H.A. & Bux, D.A. (2001) A pilot test of motivational interviewing groups for dually diagnosed inpatients. *Journal of Substance Abuse Treatment*, 20, 191–5.

Watkins, T.R., Lewellen, A. & Barrett, M.C. (2001) *Dual Diagnosis. An Integrated Approach to Treatment*. Sage, London.

Williams, R. & Cohen, J. (2000) Substance use and misuse in psychiatric wards. A model task for clinical governance? *Psychiatric Bulletin*, 24, 43–6.

16 Dual Diagnosis in a Forensic Setting

P. Ford & P. Woods

Introduction

The criminological literature clearly identifies intoxication, particularly with alcohol, as a risk factor for crimes of interpersonal violence (Williams, 1997). The psychiatric literature identifies intoxication, substance misuse and substance dependence as first rank risk indicators for violence by people with severe mental illness. It will come as no surprise, then, that a high proportion of mentally disordered offenders have significant histories of substance misuse. This group therefore is a major challenge for forensic mental health services.

Mullen (2000) defines forensic mental health as an area of specialisation that, in the criminal sphere, involves the assessment and treatment of those who are both mentally disordered and whose behaviour has led or could lead to offending. In the civil sphere forensic mental health has a more complex remit, not only being involved in the assessment and treatment of those who have potentially compensatable injuries, but also providing advice to courts and tribunals on competency and capacity. Users of forensic mental health services are usually referred to as mentally disordered offenders; a term that covers mentally disordered persons who have broken or who are alleged to have broken the law (Department of Health and Home Office, 1992).

Forensic mental health nurses are responsible for the day-to-day care and management of this population in a variety of assessment and treatment settings, which include prisons, high security hospitals, medium secure units, low secure units, acute mental health wards, specialised private hospitals, psychiatric intensive care units, court diversion schemes, and outpatient, community and rehabilitation services.

Dual diagnosis has frequently been associated with increased risk of crime, especially violent crime and therefore is of great importance for forensic mental health services and consequently for nurses that provide care and treatment in these services. Indeed McMurran (2002), in a recent review of dual diagnosis, highlighted that it is important that forensic mental health professionals understand the assessment and treatment of both substance misuse and mental disorder. According to Dale (2001) little research exists around substance misuse problems in forensic services. What there is has mainly concentrated on the problems of drug misuse in prisons, the community and local psychiatric hospitals. Furthermore, much of this body of work is concerned with drug misuse problems that are qualitatively and quantitatively different from those faced by staff and patients in forensic mental health services. This chapter will discuss the issue of substance misuse in forensic mental health care; whilst this includes outpatient work, the majority of research and practice relates to in-patient settings with people detained under the Mental Health Act (1983).

Demographics in forensic mental health services

Although there are abundant studies of dual diagnosis in general mental health settings, few studies have been undertaken within forensic mental health services (Phillips, 2000). Of those that have, Smith *et al.* (1994) studied 33 patients admitted to a UK medium secure hospital over a 12-month period, finding a prevalence rate of 54.5% for substance misuse or dependency history. Further, they found that 11 of the 15 patients who had a primary diagnosis of schizophrenia were dependent on drugs or alcohol, and that serious violence was associated with this dependence. Ford (2003) reported on a study of detained psychiatric inpatients undertaken within a medium secure psychiatric hospital. This random sample of 60 patients indicated the prevalence of dual diagnosis to be 58%, with rates of 13.3% for alcohol use disorder only, 28.3% drug use disorder only, and 16.7% for both drug and alcohol use disorders. Wheatley (1998) examined the prevalence and pattern of choice of substance misuse in a sample of schizophrenic patients detained in conditions of medium security. Sixty-three patients met his inclusion criteria. From these, 62% were considered to have a significant history of use as reflected in the extent of use or relevance to detention. Furthermore, 54% were considered to require special attention with respect to assessment of risk. Cannabis and alcohol were found to be the most commonly used substances. Moreover, 56% were described as poly-substance users (regular use of three or more substances). Users were found to be significantly younger and more likely to have forensic histories than non-users. Isherwood & Brooke (2001) examined the self-reported prevalence and severity of substance misuse among 146 of 209 consecutive referrals to a forensic service. Substance misuse diagnosis was found in 57% and dual diagnosis was found in 37%.

Some studies have also been undertaken within the high security hospitals. Norris (1984), when examining discharges from Broadmoor Hospital, found that over 20% had an alcohol problem and this group was more likely to reoffend. Taylor *et al.* (1998) surveyed all 1740 patients resident in Britain's high security hospitals and found that substance misuse before admission to hospital, which was probably under-recorded, had been most common amongst those with psychosis, together with an independent personality disorder. In this study and that of Corbett *et al.* (1998) rates of dual diagnosis among high security hospital patients were between 7.6% and 15%. More recently, D'Silva and Ferriter (2003) reported on substance use amongst the mentally disordered offenders admitted to high security hospitals in England and Wales. Data from 1972 to 1998 showed that 18.6% had taken substances at the time of their offence and 38.3% reported that they had regularly used substances during the 12 months prior to their offence. More importantly, though, their data showed that during the study period substance use had increased nearly three-fold, both at the time of the offence and for regular use during the 12 months prior to the offence. There is some evidence to suggest that the prevalence of substance misuse is increasing amongst forensic psychiatric patients.

There is relatively little research investigating possible differences in the prevalence of substance use disorder amongst different diagnostic groups within forensic psychiatric patients. This is due, in part, to the observed phenomenon that many detained patients have multiple psychiatric disorders such as combinations of mental illness, personality disorder and learning difficulty (Hughes & Thompson, 2001) over and above any co-morbid substance use disorder. However, clinical experience suggests that the findings from the Epidemiological Catchment Area (ECA) study data (Reiger *et al.*, 1990) that dual diagnosis is most prevalent amongst patients with a primary diagnosis of personality disordered and somewhat less so amongst the patients with a primary diagnosis of mental illness, applies to forensic psychiatric populations. In summary, all studies indicate higher levels of dual diagnosis within those considered as forensic patients than in both the general psychiatric population and the non-clinical population. Philips (2000) provides a useful literature review of substance misuse, offending and mental illness.

The relevance of the Mental Health Act (1983)

The Mental Health Act (1983) does not allow for the detention in hospital of a patient solely on the grounds of their substance use. It is invariably the case that the treatment of substance use disorders of patients detained in hospital under the Act will be the treatment of dual diagnosis. Detention in hospital for treatment requires the presence of mental illness, mental impairment or psychopathy of such a nature or degree that places the patient or another person at risk of harm. It is because of this high threshold of pathology that anxiety disorders and depressive illnesses rarely present to the forensic dual diagnosis worker. It is more common for the primary psychiatric diagnosis to be of schizophrenia or other psychotic disorder, personality disorder usually of the antisocial and borderline types, and mild to moderate learning difficulty. The nature and severity of these primary psychiatric disorders pose special challenges to the nurse assessing and treating such dually diagnosed persons.

Assessment

A successful assessment must give an integrated account of the patient's mental health difficulties, their past and current use of psychoactive substances and their criminal behaviour. This is no small task and requires the assessing nurse to be competent in each of these three domains. As a starting point for this assessment the nurse may wish to consider:

- The type of drugs used: the doses, frequency, duration and route of use
- In relation to alcohol abuse: the number of units per week, daily unit frequency, early morning drinking, how prolonged the abuse has been
- Family and social relationships, including social isolation
- Mental state, note any changes that co-vary with periods of intoxication
- Behaviour
- Insight, into both primary psychiatric diagnoses and substance use disorder
- Motivation to change substance use

Ford (2003) argues that screening instruments for drug and alcohol abuse, such as the Dartmouth assessment of lifestyle instrument (Rosenberg *et al.*, 1998) have reduced sensitivity among in-patients because the secure hospital environment reduces access to drugs and alcohol. An alternative approach to assessment is to play down the

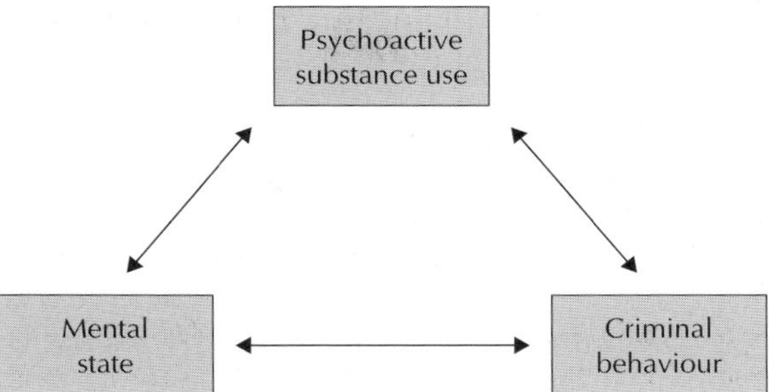

Figure 16.1 The dynamic interactions of psychoactive substance use, mental state and criminal behaviour.

significance of recent consumption of drugs and alcohol and to assess and give more weight to the underlying cognitive disposition towards dependent drug and alcohol use as described by Edwards *et al.* (1982). The Leeds dependence questionnaire (Raistrick *et al.*, 1994) is a useful self-report measure that has good reliability and validity with detained psychiatric patients.

We are of the opinion that the bi-directional interactions between these domains require a complex and dynamic understanding of the patient and their environment (see Figure 16.1). It is clear from animal models and clinical evidence that there are direct links between intoxication with various substances and changes in mental state, notably temporary effects such as reduction in cognitive functioning, disinhibition, excitation with increased motor activity and paranoia. Such transitory states should be considered as alternate or supplementary diagnoses to primary clinical hypotheses of major mental illness. There are also relatively permanent changes arising from chronic use of some substances, for example Korsakov's syndrome with chronic alcohol abuse. This disorder, in particular, should be considered as a possible explanation when faced with a patient presenting with paranoia and olfactory or tactile hallucinations.

In formulating a model of the interaction of substance use and criminal behaviour for a particular patient, the nurse might make use of two pathways, a direct causal link as described in the criminological literature as is established between heroin dependence and acquisitive crime, or an indirect pathway where intoxication leads to an alteration in mental state, such as disinhibition, which then leads to criminal behaviour. This indirect route is more likely to be suggested to account for violent acts that do not generate monetary gain for the perpetrator. This indirect model tends to be more readily applicable in the context of a primary diagnosis of paranoid schizophrenia complicated by cannabis use, central nervous system stimulant intoxication or alcohol intoxication. The assessing nurse should also be sensitive to the possibility that a patient's mental state might drive substance misuse. The patient may give an account of their use that can be understood as an attempt at self-medication. Although the empirical evidence does not support such an explanation (Mueser *et al.*, 1998), a patient with such cognition is likely to continue to use drugs to this end.

As we have discussed above, assessment is central for understanding the issues involved in a patient's history of substance misuse, but assessment also assists understanding of a patient's current substance use. The specific behaviours, timings and reasons for substance use by in-patients are crucial data for the assessing nurse who is attempting to formulate a treatment plan aimed at improving their patient's health, whilst simultaneously protecting the safety and security of the ward. The ideal forensic service would be able to eradicate all drugs from its premises. However, the demands of rehabilitation ensure that some members of this patient group will have access to the community. The admission of new and therefore untreated patients to a ward will ensure a variable but ever present demand for intoxicants on the ward. These factors pose two risks, the use of psychoactive substances by patients on leave, and bringing these substances back onto the forensic unit for personal use or distribution, perhaps for profit, to other patients. These are key areas where all nurses can actively contribute to the wider assessment of those either known or considered to be using illicit substances and the security of the ward. Observation and vigilance are the key issues here. Is the patient behaving in a different way, overtly or covertly? Are other patients taking more of an interest in this patient since they returned from community leave? Does a particular patient suddenly have a large disposable income? These are only examples of some of the things that nurses may assess.

The protective environment provided by a secure psychiatric hospital provides a special facility that assists with the particular problem of differentiating between the alternate diagnoses of drug induced psychosis and schizophrenia complicated by co-morbid substance misuse. The issue of differential diagnosis is particularly important for the nurse working with patients detained under the Mental Health Act (1983) because the legality of continued detention in hospital rests upon demonstrating that the patient is suffering from a mental illness. It is generally accepted that psychotic reactions to drug use, notably chronic amphetamine or cocaine abuse, chronic or acute use of cannabis or LSD, spontaneously remit after a period of days, or at most four weeks, of abstinence (Evans & Sullivan, 2001). It makes sense, given the gravity of the consequences of making an incorrect diagnosis, to apply a conservative cut-off of six weeks of abstinence, preferably confirmed by toxicology. If, after this time, the patient continues to display so-called first rank symptoms: auditory hallucinations, thought withdrawal insertion and interruption, thought broadcasting, somatic hallucinations, delusional perception feelings or actions experienced as made or influenced by external agents, or antipsychotic medication is required to moderate such symptoms, then it is reasonable to infer that the patient does have an underlying psychotic disorder that is worsened by drug use; that is a dual diagnosis of psychosis plus substance misuse. If on the other hand, after a period of six weeks' abstinence no such symptoms are evident and no antipsychotic medication is administered, then it is safe to infer that the previous psychotic symptoms were induced by substance misuse; the patient had a psychotic reaction.

Intervention

Whilst nurses working in forensic mental health services have a central role to play in the assessment process, either as part of the wider clinical team or specialist dual diagnosis services, they also have a clear role to play in the intervention or management of those identified with dual diagnosis. Some of these may involve clear therapeutic intervention, whilst others may be part of local policies or screening procedures.

Within the literature it is clearly suggested that cognitive behavioural interventions have had the most success with dual diagnosis, yet evidence is limited and what is there is often not transferable from one setting to another. Often, interventions include harm reduction and relapse prevention work, with realistic measures of success being behavioural changes in reduced amount and/or frequency of drug or alcohol use (Robertson *et al.*, 1989). Furthermore, according to Dale (2001) the different types of treatment that have been adapted for offenders with dual diagnosis disorders have typically involved use of integrated approaches through modification of traditional substance misuse or mental health approaches, such as therapeutic communities, cognitive behavioural interventions, relapse prevention and supportive psycho-educational approaches.

Brabbins & Poole (2000) suggest a harm reduction approach that provides a useful framework for nurses in forensic services to consider:

- Detection of substance misuse
- Shared recognition with the patient of the benefits and hazards of substance misuse
- Realistic goal setting
- Problem solving aimed at development of alternatives to substance use
- Planning of responses to relapse or escalation of substance misuse

McKeown (2000) discusses a relapse prevention programme running over 12 weeks. The main themes are providing accurate information about drug/alcohol use and its risks; developing skills appropriate to prevention of relapse; and promoting more helpful attitudes. Roberts *et al.* (1999) provide a detailed and comprehensive manual for relapse prevention and skills training that are adapted to the specific requirements of patients with a diagnosis of schizophrenia.

Clearly, these approaches have at the heart of them reducing risk, and abstinence from substance misuse is conceptualised as one means of achieving this. Furthermore, they suggest that the nurse should not only accurately assess substance misuse but also work in collaboration with the patient. This collaboration is crucial, as the patient has to recognise that there is a problem, perceive the need to reduce or alleviate their substance misuse, see how their substance misuse use is affecting both their mental state and offending behaviour, and how reduction in their substance misuse can work for them in the future to improve their quality of life. In summary, rapport, education and realism are at the heart of successful individual work.

The establishment of therapeutic rapport is particularly difficult with mentally disordered offenders detained in hospital, for two principal reasons. First, these patients tend to have a degree of psychopathology that is extreme and has a quality characterised as antisocial, paranoid or cognitively impaired. Any of these three characteristics are obstacles to the establishment of therapeutic rapport and so the nurse must invest more time and effort to achieve it. However, the second factor, the patient's detention against their will, compounds the problem. For the nurse, the solution is yet more time and effort combined with sensitivity to the reality of the circumstance that the patient, at least initially, wishes neither to be in hospital nor receiving treatment.

The nurse who successfully establishes rapport and embarks on the treatment of addiction in the context of the patient's chronic mental health problems should be aware of obstacles particular to schizophrenia and antisocial personality disorder. It is suggested that forensic in-patients with schizophrenia often have cognitive impairments that require modification of the usual pattern of treatment. Information processing is often impaired; processing speed is often reduced, requiring the therapist to reduce the pace of treatment; memory capacity may be poor, requiring the therapist to avoid long and convoluted explanations or homework tasks; and memory retrieval may be poor, requiring the therapist to repeat exercises. In addition, emotional recognition may be very limited, requiring the therapist to instruct the patient about emotions, and self-monitoring is often poor, requiring the therapist to teach this skill before setting any tasks aiming to link emotions to behaviours such as keeping a thought diary. The nurse treating addiction in the context of a patient's antisocial personality disorder is likely to see the motivating factors for abstinence as being at odds with those of other patients (Evans & Sullivan, 2001). It may be difficult for a nurse to work collaboratively with a patient who wants to get sober because then he will be more powerful and more able to control other people.

The nurse who engages a patient in longer-term treatment of substance misuse problems ought to be prepared to address, during the course of the treatment, two likely eventualities. The first is the manifestation of psychopathologies previously obscured by the dependence on drugs. For those patients with a primary diagnosis of personality disorder, it is quite likely that detoxification and treatment for addiction will unearth emotional disorders such as generalised anxiety disorder, post-traumatic stress disorder and social phobia. This does not mean to say that the nurse therapist should immediately treat these presenting problems, but they should be ready to make a preliminary assessment and refer on to other members of the multidisciplinary team.

The second issue arises for those patients whose substance misuse has functioned as a defining feature of their self-image. For such patients, their drug or alcohol use has been for many years an existential feature, the removal of such a role defining activity, if not replaced, will sooner rather than later lead to relapse to dependence. For some patients this may not mean a return to their previous drug of choice, rather the nurse may see substance substitution, possibly a transference of the chemical dependency onto prescribed drugs. Longer-term treatment can address this dilemma in two ways: first, through careful activity scheduling that will provide novel and meaningful structure to the patient's day-to-day existence; second, the nurse therapist can spend time in sessions directly addressing the patient's self-image and assist the patient in redefining themselves without reference to drug or alcohol use. Clearly, access to self-help groups such as Alcoholics Anonymous is a possibility, but creative solutions can be achieved by close working with occupational therapy, adult education and vocational schemes. As the care programme approach pays increasingly close attention to the spiritual and cultural needs of patients, these avenues can be explored profitably in filling the potential existential void left by successful addiction treatment.

Training issues

Above, we have discussed many issues for nurses working in forensic mental health services when assessing and intervening with patients with dual diagnosis. Therefore, it is inevitable that there are many related training issues that need to be tackled. This list is not exhaustive and is merely meant to reflect how many training issues there are.

- Awareness and understanding of reasons for problematic substance misuse
- Awareness of the relationships between substance misuse and offending behaviour
- Legalisation issues
- The effect on mental state, other patients, ward environment, security
- Awareness of the complex cultural issues
- How to recognise when patients are dealing or misusing substances; the related manipulation and taking advantage of other patients that can occur
- Awareness of one's own value base
- How do you intervene with problems?
- Awareness of the high prevalence of recidivism

Future challenges for forensic mental health services

The challenges for forensic mental health services in relation to dual diagnosis are not dissimilar to those of their mainstream mental health service partners. These have also been discussed by Dale (2001). First, develop dedicated services to work with people with problems of substance misuse. Second, reduce the supply of illicit drugs. Third, introduce harm reduction measures, which are truly multidisciplinary in approach. Fourth, improve staff training in identification, screening, assessment and intervention.

McMurran (2002), in a recent expert paper on dual diagnosis of mental disorder and substance misuse for the NHS National Programme on Forensic Mental Health Research and Development, highlighted three pressing research questions. First, we need to know how to assess co-morbid mental disorder and substance abuse, to avoid misdiagnosis and gain a better clinical picture. Second, we need to develop and test effective treatments. Third, we need longitudinal studies. None of these points will come as any surprise, but without information about them services for the mentally disordered offender with dual diagnosis will only develop in a haphazard fashion.

Conclusions

Forensic mental health services, and consequently nurses who choose to work in them, will undoubtedly always have patients with dual diagnosis. The complexities of their treatment will always be difficult for nursing intervention. Nurses need to use structured and evidence based programmes of individualised care to intervene with this patient group. They need to consider not only the complexities of the substance misuse and the mental disorder, but also the offending behaviour that brought them into the forensic services. Education has to be the first step to achieving more structured treatment programmes where nurses contribute not only to the specialised services that are developing but also to the multidisciplinary care that also exists. The currently high recidivism rates of dually diagnosed mentally disordered offenders means that they continue to be a significant challenge for forensic mental health in-patient and community services and worthy of increased nurse led interventions.

References

Brabbins, C. & Poole, R. (2000) Substance misuse complicating mental illness. In: *Forensic Mental Health Care: A Case Study Approach* (Mercer, D., Mason, T., McKeown, M. & McCann, G., eds), pp. 191–7. Churchill Livingstone, Edinburgh.

Corbett, M., Duggan, C. & Larkin, E. (1998) Substance misuse and violence: a comparison of special hospital in-patients diagnosed with either schizophrenia or personality disorder. *Criminal Behaviour and Mental Health*, 8, 311–21.

Dale, C. (2001) Dual Diagnosis. In: *Forensic Mental Health: Issues in Practice* (Dale, C., Thompson, T. & Woods, P., eds), Chapter 18, pp. 189–202. Harcourt Publishers Limited, London.

Department of Health and Home Office (1992) *Review of Health and Social Services for Mentally Disordered Offenders and Others Requiring Similar Services, Final Summary Report*. Cm. 2088. HMSO, London.

D'Silva, K. & Ferriter, M. (2003) Substance use by the mentally disordered committing serious offences – a high-security hospital study. *Journal of Forensic Psychiatry and Psychology*, 14 (1), 178–93.

Edwards, G., Arif, A. & Hodgson, R. (1982) Nomenclature and classification of drug and alcohol problems: a shortened version of a WHO memorandum. *British Journal of Addiction*, 77, 3–20.

Evans, K. & Sullivan, J.M. (2001) *Dual Diagnosis: Counselling the Mentally Ill Substance Abuser*, 2nd edn. Guilford Press, New York.

Ford, P. (2003) An evaluation of the Dartmouth assessment of lifestyle inventory and the Leeds dependence questionnaire for use among detained psychiatric in-patients. *Addiction*, 98, 111–18.

Hughes, G.V.H. & Thompson, K. (2001) Violence, substance abuse and pathology: characteristics of psychiatric patients detained in medium security. Paper presented at XXVIIth Congress of the International Academy of Law and Mental Health, Amsterdam.

Isherwood, S. & Brooke, D. (2001) Prevalence and severity of substance misuse among referrals to a local forensic service. *Journal of Forensic Psychiatry*, 12 (2), 446–54.

McKeown, M. (2000) Relapse prevention for problematic alcohol use. In: *Forensic Mental Health Care: A Case Study Approach* (Mercer, D., Mason, T., McKeown, M. & McCann, G., eds), pp. 205–12. Churchill Livingstone, Edinburgh.

McMurran, M. (2002) *Dual Diagnosis of Mental Disorder and Substance Misuse*. NHS National Programme on Forensic Mental Health Research and Development, Liverpool.

Mueser, K.T., Drake, R.E. & Wallach, M.A. (1998) Dual diagnosis: a review of etiological theories. *Addictive Behaviors*, 23, 717–34.

Mullen, P.E. (2000) Forensic mental health. *British Journal of Psychiatry*, 176, 307–11.

Norris, N. (1984) *Integration of Special Hospital Patients into the Community*. Gower, Aldershot.

Phillips, P. (2000) Substance misuse, offending and mental illness: a review. *Journal of Psychiatric and Mental Health Nursing*, 7 (6), 483–9.

Raistrick, D., Bradshaw, J., Tober, G., Weiner, J., Allison, J. & Healy, C. (1994) Development of the Leeds dependence questionnaire (LDQ): a questionnaire to measure alcohol and drug dependence in the context of a treatment evaluation package. *Addiction*, 89, 563–72.

Reiger, D.A., Farmer, M.E., Rae, D.S. *et al.* (1990) Comorbidity of mental disorders with alcohol and other drug abuse: results from the epidemiological catchment area (ECA) study. *Journal of the American Medical Association*, 264, 2511–18.

Roberts, L.J., Shaner, A. & Eckman, T.A. (1999) *Overcoming Addictions: Skills Training for People with Schizophrenia*. Norton and Company, New York.

Robertson, J.R., Bucknall, A.B.V., Skidmore, C.A., Roberts, J.J.K. & Smith, J.H. (1989) Remission and relapse in heroin users and implications for management: treatment control or risk reduction. *International Journal of Addiction*, 24, 229–46.

Rosenberg, S.D., Drake, R.E., Wolford, G.L. *et al.* (1998) Dartmouth assessment of lifestyle instrument (DALI):

a substance use disorder screen for people with severe mental illness. *American Journal of Psychiatry*, 155, 232–8.

Smith, J., Frazer, S., Boer, H. & Donavan, M. (1994) Dual diagnosis in the UK. *Hospital and Community Psychiatry*, 45 (3), 280–1.

Taylor, P.J., Leese, M., Willis, D., Butwell, M., Daly, R. & Larkin, E. (1998) Mental disorder and violence: a special hospital study. *British Journal of Psychiatry*, 172 (3), 218–26.

Wheatley, M. (1998) The prevalence and relevance of substance use in detained schizophrenic patients. *Journal of Forensic Psychiatry*, 9 (1), 114–29.

Williams, K.S. (1997) *Textbook on Criminology*, 3rd edn. Blackstone, London.

17 Models of Care and Dual Diagnosis

D. Gallivan

Introduction

The National Treatment Agency (NTA) is a special health authority, created by the Government on 1 April 2001, with a remit to increase the availability, capacity and effectiveness of treatment for drug misuse in England. The overall purpose of the NTA is to double the number of people in effective, well managed treatment and to increase the proportion of people completing or appropriately continuing treatment, year on year. The NTA works closely with regional drug alcohol action teams (DAATs) that implement the national drug treatment policies and strategies on a regional and local level. The DAATs are multi-agency Government funded teams responsible for the effective management and commissioning of drug treatment services. Representatives from the police, the county council, probation, Customs and Excise, local NHS services and voluntary groups make up the partnership board of the DAATs. This chapter provides an overview of models of care and its relevance and appropriateness to dual diagnosis. It is based on *Models of Care Parts 1 and 2* (National Treatment Agency, 2002).

Legal framework: Mental Health Act and dual diagnosis

The Mental Health Act defines mental disorder as 'mental illness, arrested or incomplete development of mind, psychopathic disorder and any other disorder or disability of mind' (Mental Health Act Commission, 1999). Diagnosis of substance misuse disorder is not specified under the categories and therefore patients cannot be subject to detention for treatment under the Mental Health Act. However, the management difficulties associated with this patient group who have psychiatric co-morbidity (dual diagnosis) include increased violence, non-compliance with treatment and disengagement from services. Due to the nature of psychiatric co-morbidity and the relative uncertainty, these patients should be subject to the care programme approach (CPA). Some patients who pose a risk to themselves and others may need to be considered for the supervision register under Section 117.

Why do we need models of care?

The prevalence of substance misuse in Britain is a changing picture, which is difficult to assess. The British crime survey research indicates that around one third of those aged 16 to 59 have taken illegal drugs at some time in their lives, with 11% having used in the previous year and 6% describing themselves as regular users. Most drug use is cannabis use, with only 1% of the population reporting the use of heroin and crack cocaine. Estimating the number of people who require drug treatment is highly problematic. The national drug treatment monitoring system (NDTMS) reflects those seeking help and existing biases in drug treatment. The Audit Commission (2002) reports that 0.5% of the population of Britain may be dependent upon psychoactive substances, that is, 226 000 people.

Whilst substance misuse can affect rich and poor alike, deprivation and social exclusion are likely to make a significant contribution to the causes, complications and intractability of drug misuse. Deprivation relates statistically to the types and intensities of substance misuse that are problematic. Similarly, poor housing, or lack of access to affordable housing, is another contributory factor in drug misuse. Other important factors include educational disadvantage, criminal involvement, unemployment and low income (ACMD, 1998). Recent research indicates that many substance misusers are also offenders, although the relationship between drugs and crime is complex. The criminal justice system is increasingly a referral source and venue for the provision of substance misuse treatment. Substance misuse has been called a chronic relapsing condition. Whilst many substance misusers do successfully recover from drug dependence or addiction, most make several attempts to do so, lapsing or relapsing into drug misuse in intervening periods.

Typical drugs of misuse include: opiates (for example heroin and illicit methadone); stimulants (for example amphetamines, cocaine and crack cocaine); and alcohol. Many substance misusers, however, take a cocktail of drugs and alcohol, including hallucinogens, cannabis and prescribed drugs such as benzodiazepines. The use of heroin together with cocaine or crack cocaine is also becoming increasingly common. Substance misusers present with a myriad of other health and social problems, particularly in relation to physical and psychiatric co-morbidity (dual diagnosis) and social care needs:

- Physical health problems, for example thrombosis, abscesses, overdose, hepatitis B and C, HIV, weight loss, respiratory problems
- Mental health problems, for example depression, anxiety, paranoia, suicidal thoughts
- Social problems, for example relationship problems, unemployment, homelessness
- Criminal problems, including legal and financial issues

Therefore, a wide range of health, social care and other responses is required. *Models of Care* guidelines provide a framework for various agencies to work together to provide a multidisciplinary intervention for substance misuse clients that require this approach.

Models of care: what works best for drug misusers?

Over the years, the attitude towards treatment of substance misusers has changed from dealing with people considered to be part of the criminal community, to treating an underprivileged sector of society that needs help, support, and therapeutic and clinical interventions. The *Models of Care* guidelines were developed in order to provide a consistent, multi-agency approach to treatment for clients presenting with substance misuse issues, underpinned by a range of social, financial and emotional problems that require an integrated treatment approach. *Models of Care* is based upon current evidence, guidance, quality standards and good practice in drug treatment in England. It sets out a national framework and guidelines for the commissioning of adult treatment for drug misuse (drug treatment) expected to be available in every part of England to meet the needs of diverse local populations. All guidance is in line with the recommendations contained in *Drug Misuse and Dependence: Guidelines on Clinical Management* (Department of Health, 1999a) and other current guidance and legislation.

Models of Care provides the framework required to achieve equity, parity and consistency in the commissioning and provision of substance misuse treatment and care in England. It will support drug and alcohol action teams (DAATs), joint commissioners and treatment providers in the development of an efficient and effective treatment and care system for drug misusers. *Models of Care* also provides specific guidance to support the coordination of drug and alcohol treatment and the effective management of care across drug misuse treatment services and general health, social and other care. *Models of Care* advocates a systems approach to meeting the multiple needs of drug and alcohol misusers. This is achieved through the development of local systems that maximise the gains achieved through drug and alcohol treatment by having explicit links to the other generic health, social care and criminal justice services, including through-care and aftercare. *Models of Care* reflects professional consensus of 'what works best' for drug misusers, resulting from an extensive consultative process that was used for its development. It is also consistent with the *NHS Plan* (Department of Health, 2000) and agendas to modernise health and social care services.

What is the scope of *Models of Care*?

Models of Care addresses all drug and alcohol misuse including hallucinogens, nicotine and cannabis. However, it does not address detailed consideration of the misuse of prescribed drugs (particularly benzodiazepines), volatile substances (or solvents), or steroid misuse. *Models of Care* focuses on commissioning drug treatment for adults (for example, those aged 18 years and older). The provision of drug and alcohol treatment for adolescents and young people is extensively covered elsewhere (Health Advisory Service, 1996). *Models of Care* does have great relevance to the development of alcohol service provision, but it does not provide specific guidance on the commissioning or implementation of this framework for alcohol treatment generally. The quality standards cover both drugs and alcohol in substance misuse services, for example Quality in Alcohol and Drugs Services (QuADS) and the Drugs and Alcohol National Occupational Standards (DANOS).

Four tiers system of *Models of Care*

The following section describes the *Models of Care* four-tiered treatment framework for drug treatment services. A specific description relating to dual diagnosis considerations is given further on in this chapter.

Tier 1: non-substance misuse specific services requiring interface with drug and alcohol treatment

Tier 1 services work with a wide range of clients, including drug and alcohol misusers, but their sole purpose is not drug or alcohol treatment. The role of tier 1 services, in this context, includes the provision of their own services plus, as a minimum, screening and referral to local drug and alcohol treatment services in tiers 2 and 3. Tier 1 provision for drug and alcohol misusers may also include assessment, services to reduce drug-related harm and liaison or joint working with tiers 2 and 3 specialist drug and alcohol treatment services. Tier 1 services are crucial to providing services in conjunction with more specialised drug and alcohol services (for example general medical care for drug misusers in community based or residential substance misuse treatment units, or housing support and aftercare for drug misusers leaving residential care or prison). The wide range of professionals involved at this level, including primary care or general medical services, social workers, teachers, community pharmacists, probation officers, housing officers and homeless persons units, need to be sufficiently trained and supported to work with drug and alcohol misusers. There may be a need for a specialised drug treatment or 'addiction' liaison service to provide a coordinated response with tier 1 where there is a high prevalence rate of substance misuse.

Tier 2: open access drug and alcohol treatment services

The aim of the treatment in tier 2 is to engage drug and alcohol misusers in drug treatment and reduce drug-related harm. This tier is defined by having a low threshold to access services, and limited requirements on drug and alcohol misusers to receive services, and includes needle exchange, drug and alcohol advice and information services, and ad hoc support not delivered in the context of a care plan. Specialist substance misuse social workers can provide services within this tier, including the provision of access to social work advice, childcare/parenting assessment and assessment of social care needs. Tier 2 can also include low-threshold prescribing programmes aimed at engaging opioid misusers with limited motivation, whilst offering an opportunity to undertake motivational work and reduce drug-related harm.

Tier 3: structured community-based drug treatment services

Tier 3 services are provided solely for drug and alcohol misusers in structured programmes of care. Tier 3 structured services include psychotherapeutic interventions, such as cognitive behavioural therapy, motivational interventions, structured counselling, methadone maintenance programmes, community detoxification or day care provided either as a drug and alcohol-free programme or as an adjunct to methadone treatment. Community based aftercare programmes for drug and alcohol misusers leaving residential rehabilitation or prison are also included in tier 3 services. Tier 3 services require the drug and alcohol misuser to receive a drug assessment and to have a care plan, which is agreed between the service provider and client. For clients whose needs cross several domains, there should be a key worker, responsible for coordination of that individual's care on behalf of all the agencies and services involved. Changes to the care plan would take place in consultation with the drug and alcohol misusers. Tier 3 services may be required to work closely with other specialist services to meet the needs of specific client groups. For example, tier 3 services and mental health services should work closely together to meet the needs of drug misusers with dual diagnosis. In this instance, providers should have access to medical clinical supervision and/or advice from mental health specialists in line with good practice guidelines (Department of Health, 2002).

Tier 4a: residential drug and alcohol misuse specific services

Tier 4 services are aimed at individuals with a high level of presenting need. Services in this tier include in-patient drug and alcohol detoxification or stabilisation services; drug and alcohol residential rehabilitation units; and residential drug crisis intervention centres. Referral is usually from tiers 2 or 3 services or via community care assessment. Tier 4a services may be abstinence oriented programmes, detoxification services or services that stabilise clients (for example on substitute drugs). Access to tier 4a requires careful assessment, detoxification prior to placement in a drug and alcohol free residential programme, and preparation of the client in order to maximise readiness, compliance and the programme's effectiveness. Drug and alcohol misusers receiving tier 4 services will require a designated care coordinator, allocated before entry to this tier.

Tier 4b: highly specialist non-substance misuse specific services

Note that Tier 4b services are highly specialised and will have close links with services in other tiers, but they are, like tier 1, non-substance misuse specific. Examples include specialist liver units that treat the complications of alcohol-related and infectious liver diseases, and forensic services for mentally ill offenders. Some highly specialist tier 4b services also provide specialist liaison services to tiers 1–4a services, for example specialist hepatitis nurses, HIV liaison clinics, genitourinary medicine.

Dual diagnosis: care management and pathways for clients

A number of organisations and agencies will be faced with the issues of dual diagnosis as a result of the complex needs of those with this diagnosis. This service will include health and social services, voluntary organisations, probation services, housing departments and the police. The care and management of patients with co-morbidity therefore needs to be multidisciplinary in approach. It is recommended that services involved in the treatment of those with dual diagnosis need to:

- Adopt a common language
- Operate common referral criteria and processes
- Be in a position to provide a comprehensive multidisciplinary assessment procedure
- Have equal access to a range of treatment modalities (access to outreach, community treatment, home visits, outpatient treatment, in-patient treatment, and day care provision, including therapeutic interventions)
- Involve the GP in the care and management of the patient and be included in all correspondence on all aspects of care

Good systems of care planning and care coordination will ensure that service provision is client centred and aid continuity between care pathways. It is important that the care pathway addresses the key role and contribution of each local provider agency concerned. The Health Advisory Service (2001) recommends the following for the care management of dual diagnosis clients:

- Mental health services should have treatment protocols for those with alcohol and drug problems.
- Clients with co-morbidity should have access to the range of tiers 1 to 4 substance misuse treatment interventions.
- Combined pharmacological and psychological treatments should be provided to clients (where appropriate) including those who are receiving shared care between mental health services and substance misuse services.
- Clients with co-morbidity should be given help in developing better support systems within the community.
- There should be clear policies for the follow-up of clients who are discharged, either planned or unplanned, from in-patient psychiatric care.
- Clients with co-morbidity should have access to residential and community rehabilitation services that are able to meet their complex needs.

Groups with special needs

The Health Advisory Service (2001) recommends that attention is given to special populations in relation to co-morbidity. Mental health services for older people should explicitly tackle the misuse of alcohol and tranquillisers. The needs of young people with co-morbidity must be addressed by child centred services. Strategies should be in place to work with homeless people in the care and management of those with mental health and substance misuse co-morbidity. Commissioners and providers should ensure that all local services are able to meet the diverse needs of the local populations, and that the services are accessible to black and ethnic minority groups and effective at meeting their needs. Mental health professionals should consider post-traumatic stress amongst clients with co-morbidity and amongst refugees and asylum seekers in particular. The assessment and care of women should take into account gender specific issues. The care of parents with co-morbidity needs to focus on the needs of their children, assessing the need for support and interventions to prevent harm.

Implications for nursing

Models of Care has several implications for addiction and mental health nurses. The provision of adequate training and continuing professional development for both addiction and mental health nurses should be based on local training audit of addiction and mental health service teams. It is recommended that mental health services should appoint staff who have formal training in mental health and substance misuse. Mental health services should have a substance misuse training strategy that pertains to all staff and professional groups and which is monitored and evaluated (Health Advisory Service, 2001). For staff working within substance misuse services, training should be provided that includes the recognition and care of service users with mental illness and collaborative working with mental health services. Training of staff should incorporate three main elements: inter-agency collaboration and information exchange through inter-agency training; theoretical and skills-based training; and practice development and supervision (Department of Health, 2002).

References

Advisory Council on the Misuse of Drugs (1998) *Drug Misuse and the Environment*. HMSO, London.

Audit Commission (2002) *Changing Habits*. Audit Commission, London.

Department of Health (1999a) *Drug Misuse and Dependence: Guidelines on Clinical Management*. The Stationery Office, London.

Department of Health (1999b) *Clinical Governance in the New NHS, Health Service Circular 1999/065*. Department of Health, London.

Department of Health (2000) *The NHS Plan*. Department of Health, London.

Department of Health (2002) *Policy Implementation Guide. Dual Diagnosis Good Practice Guide*. Department of Health, London.

Health Advisory Service (1996) *Children and Young People: Substance Misuse Services: the Substance of Young Need*. HMSO, London.

Health Advisory Service (2001) *The Substance of Young Needs Review 2000*. Health Advisory Service, London.

Mental Health Act Commission (1999) *Mental Health Act Commission Eighth Biennial Report*. HMSO, London.

National Treatment Agency (2002) *Models of Care Parts 1 and 2*, NTA Publications, London.

Part 4

Intervention and Treatment Strategies

Chapter 18 Framework for Multidimensional Assessment

Chapter 19 Dealing with Intoxication, Overdose, Withdrawal and Detoxification: Nursing Assessment and Interventions

Chapter 20 Prescribing Authority and Medication Management in Mental Health and Addiction Nursing

Chapter 21 Spiritual and Cultural Needs: Integration in Dual Diagnosis Care

Chapter 22 Dual Diagnosis: Interventions with Carers

Chapter 23 Psychological Approaches in the Treatment of Dual Diagnosis

Chapter 24 A Person Centred Approach to Understanding and Helping People with a Dual Diagnosis

Chapter 25 Motivational Interviewing

Chapter 26 Relapse Prevention in Dual Diagnosis

18 Framework for Multidimensional Assessment

G.H. Rassool & J. Winnington

Introduction

Assessment is a continuing process and a foundation of good clinical practice. It is a fundamental component within the framework of the systematic approach to nursing care and interventions. Because substance misuse and psychiatric problems are complex, assessment must be comprehensive and multi-professional to plan effective care and treatment. Nursing assessment is a comprehensive analysis of an individual's needs and related problems that is based on the collection of data of the physical/medical, psychosocial and spiritual needs of the individual. Its aim is to facilitate, in the context of dual diagnosis, the identification and recognition of substance misuse and/or mental health problems and should be needs led. Assessment takes the form of interviewing in the taking and recording of a medical/nursing and psychosocial history. Detection and screening can be conducted through self-report methods, laboratory tests and from collateral data sources. Rapid and effective assessment are necessary for individuals in crisis or those who wish to engage with treatment or rehabilitation substance misuse services. Through the assessment process, there is a window of opportunity to promote health education and harm reduction strategies.

Many individuals with dual diagnosis remain unnoticed in both drug and alcohol services and mental health services. The lack of integration or segregation of mental health and drug and alcohol services perpetuates this problem, as staff from different service domains often focus on observation and assessment that are part of their repertoire of knowledge and skills. Mental health workers may identify mental health problems but overlook drug and alcohol problems, whereas workers in drug and alcohol services focus on substance misuse and fail to recognise mental health problems. It is argued that individuals with dual diagnosis can become system misfits when they do not conform to the expectations established with drug and alcohol and mental health care systems (Bachrach, 1986).

The provision of care and treatment should be needs led across different care settings, and reflected in the capacity to assess needs, diagnose, formulate care plans, and implement and evaluate care. The emphasis is on collaborative working or shared care with other members of the team. The empowerment of individuals and their carers to actively participate in the planning, delivery and evaluation of care is also part of the strategy of good practice. The aims of the chapter are to provide an overview of assessment and screening of individuals with a dual diagnosis and the challenges faced. An examination of the factors that are important when assessing mental health status and substance misuse in individuals with dual diagnosis is given. An outline of screening tools and risk assessment is also presented.

Barriers in the assessment process

Individuals with dual diagnosis often have complex or multiple needs, which are often difficult to assess comprehensively. The lack of knowledge and skills in assessing mental health or taking a drug and alcohol history and the attitudes towards substance misusers or individuals with drug and alcohol problems may influence the assessment process and subsequent interventions. Social prejudice, negative attitudes and stereotyped perceptions of substance misusers (Hanna, 1991; Carroll, 1996; Rassool, 1998a; Selleck & Redding, 1998) and dual diagnosis patients (Williams, 1999) are widely held amongst health care professionals and this may lead to poor assessment and minimal care being given to those individuals. The assessment and diagnosis of a 'primary problem' of substance misuse or mental health problems by respective services may result in poor intervention strategies and treatment outcomes. It is suggested that drug services will generally screen out of their service individuals who display a primary mental health problem, whilst mental health services will generally screen out individuals who present with a primary substance use problem. Assessment may therefore become focused on the need to establish primacy rather than the pursuit of meeting the individual's needs (Banerjee *et al.*, 2002).

Clinical assessment for dual diagnosis is difficult because substance misuse can mask psychiatric symptoms or distort diagnosis. The inability to distinguish the effects of psychoactive substances on the individual's mental state from symptoms of mental health problems add to the complexities of assessing an individual with dual diagnosis, since many psychiatric symptoms are a temporary result of substance misuse withdrawal or drug or alcohol intoxication rather than dual diagnosis. It would be sensible for workers to manage the immediate symptoms until the individual has had time to recover from drug intoxication or drug withdrawal state. That is why it is unlikely that a comprehensive assessment can be completed at first contact with individuals.

Substance misusers do not often admit to being physically or psychologically dependent on drugs and alcohol and may go to great lengths in concealing their substance misuse from mental health staff. Some nurses may lack the confidence to ask patients about their substance misuse or may have pessimistic views regarding treatment. The mental state of the patient may act as a barrier to recognition as some patients may not be able to understand the nature of the symptoms they experience or adequately describe them in a way that enables clinical staff to make an accurate assessment (Gafoor & Rassool, 1998). The task of diagnosis is further compounded if the patient is a polydrug user and is taking a combination of psychoactive substances at the same time. There are other factors that can have an impact on an adequate and comprehensive assessment process and a summary is presented in Table 18.1.

Table 18.1 Some of the factors that can impact on dual diagnosis assessment.

System barriers	Clinical barriers	Process barriers
• Parrallel vs. sequential vs. integrated approaches • Philosophical issues • Lack of training • Debate over focus of care • Transcultural issues • Protocols, procedures and policies	• Understand the nature of the symptoms and presentation • Assessment tools (reliability, validity) • Client's mental state • Reliance on self-report • Client's motivation • Perception of risk	• Setting • Confidentiality • Access • Timeframe • Trust • Poor previous experience (staff and client) • Interview skills • Consent • Collateral informants • Laboratory investigations

Source: Banerjee *et al.* (2002).

Assessment and screening

The purpose of screening and assessment is to collect data on the individual's substance use and misuse and mental health problems with a view to having a better understanding of the relationship between the two disorders. The identification of both disorders requires a team approach, which may include family, friends, caseworkers, doctors, nurses, laboratory investigations, and alcohol and drug screening. However, before undertaking a full and comprehensive assessment, there are some observations that may indicate substance misuse and/or mental health problem(s). This may warrant further investigation in the process of assessment and diagnosis. Table 18.2 presents the indicators for assessment.

The art of completing a dual diagnosis assessment relies on incorporating the following essential elements:

- Assessment of history and current nature of the type and frequency of psychoactive substances used
- Assessment of mental health history and current symptoms
- Assessment of current physical health
- Assessment of level and nature of risks in evidence
- Assessment of social needs (housing, employment, social networks)
- Assessment of self-awareness of diversity issues and cultural competence

Table 18.2 Indicators for further assessment.

- Use of psychoactive substances to control thoughts and feelings
- Self-medication of psychoactive substances for alleviating mental health problems
- Use of psychoactive substances to balance or reduce side effects of prescribed medications
- Misuse of prescription and over-the-counter drugs
- Expression of feelings of sadness
- Frequency of mood swings
- Showing anger and impulsiveness
- Self-harm
- Lack of interest or activities
- Strange thoughts and speech
- Over suspiciousness
- Unable to reduce alcohol and/or drug use
- Recent weight gain or loss of more than 15% body weight
- Previous detoxification and/or rehabilitation
- Symptoms of withdrawal
- High tolerance of psychoactive substances
- Drug seeking behaviour

Central to the aspect of working in dual diagnosis is the ability to provide a comprehensive assessment of mental health history and current symptoms, current and historical substance use and misuse, current physical health, social needs and the awareness of diversity amongst those individuals with dual diagnosis and how these major aspects impact on the current presentation or baseline behaviour. One feature of a dual diagnosis assessment is the use of 'time lines', by recording the sequence of events for both substance misuse and mental health problems over a given time period. Time lines can provide invaluable information, particularly in relation to which event occurs first, substance misuse or mental health; additionally, they can be used to help indicate priority for treatment actions (Moore & Rassool, 2002).

Assessment of mental health problems

The main focus in the assessment of dual diagnosis is to identify primary issues that may be associated with mental health and substance misuse. It is crucial that all patients are routinely screened to detect mental health problems in those presenting to substance misuse services. The aims of a mental health assessment are to gather data on the neurobiological, psychological and social factors. The assessment should include a statement of the presenting problem, development and educational history, family history, drug and alcohol assessment, a mental health assessment, medical examination, strengths and resources, and a risk assessment. An aspect of the mental health examination is the examination of the mental/psychological functioning of the individual. The mental/psychological examination, usually conducted by a mental health specialist, is based on an interview focusing on the cognitive, affective and behavioural factors (appearance, thoughts, feelings, insight, etc.) and observation over a period of time. Taken all together, a psychiatric diagnosis is made and a plan of care and intervention strategies are developed and implemented. The mental health assessment (incorporating the mental state examination, see Davies, 1997) is presented in Tables 18.3 and 18.4.

It is important to identify and manage symptoms before arriving at a definitive diagnosis. The individual immediate needs and problems should be met, dealing with physical, social or psychological problems. Support and harm reduction strategies should be implemented, depending on the holistic needs of the individual. For example, a homeless person is likely to need help with housing, irrespective of whether he has depression or is using alcohol in a harmful way.

Table 18.3 Mental health assessment.

- Initial data (if the individual has case notes, review previous assessments, issues and summaries)
- The presenting issue/problem(s)
- Personal history (health, childhood, schooling, current interests, employment, relationship history, pre-morbid personality)
- Ethnicity, culture and spiritual belief
- Past psychiatric history (mental health problems, past admissions treatment, relapse)
- Past medical history
- Risk assessment
- Current medication
- Family psychiatric and substance use history
- Alcohol and other substance use (current levels, history, pattern of use, drug-free period, tolerance, withdrawal symptoms, relapse, medical and psychological complications, coping strategies)
- Social support system
- Legal status
- Physical/medical examination
- Individual's strengths and limitations

Table 18.4 Mental state examination.

- Appearance: attire, cleanliness, posture and gait
- Behaviour: facial expression, cooperation or aggression, activity, agitation, level of arousal (including physiological signs)
- Speech: form and pattern, volume and rate, is it coherent, logical and congruent with questioning?
- Mood: apathetic, irritable, labile, optimistic or pessimistic, thoughts of suicide, do reported experience and observable mood agree?
- Thought: particular preoccupations, ideas and beliefs, are they rational, fixed or delusional? Do they concern the safety of the patient or other people?
- Perception: abnormalities including hallucinations occurring in any modality (auditory, visual, olfactory, gustatory, tactile)
- Intellect: brief note of cognitive and intellectual function; is the patient oriented in time, place and person? Is the patient able to function intellectually at the level expected from his or her history?
- Insight: how does the patient explain or attribute his or her symptoms?

Source: Davies (1997).

Assessment of substance use

Taking a drug and alcohol history is a detailed assessment of the current presentation of an individual's drug and alcohol taking pattern of use. One of the initial tasks of the assessment is to discern the individual's views of their drug and/or alcohol consumption. The assessment should then focus on the current pattern of substance misuse, the type of drug used, quantities of substances used, level of dependence, risk behaviours, associated problems, sources of help, sources of access to psychoactive substance(s) and periods of abstinence and relapse. In order to ascertain the level of dependency, it is important to ask about experiences of withdrawal symptoms or any medical complications.

Assessment all too often focuses only on the individual's negative aspects of substance misuse such as an individual's weakness, risks and problems. The inclusion of an assessment of positive aspects of the individual regarding substance misuse may highlight and enhance the self-efficacy and self-esteem of the individual. This positive approach may enable the individual to engage with the service with less resistance and also influence the individual's coping strategies and treatment outcomes. The position of strengths should focus on strategies that the individual has 'successfully' used in previous attempts to manage substance misuse and psychiatric symptoms, for example previous coping strategies used to be drug or alcohol free. An outline of the assessment of substance use in individuals with dual diagnosis is shown in Table 18.5.

A good practice suggestion for assessment (Rethink & Turning Point, 2004) includes the following:

- Consider the client's concerns
- Consider a range of needs
- Avoid assumptions and keep an open mind
- Timelines can be a useful tool (Moore & Rassool, 2001)

Table 18.5 Assessment of substance use.

• Statement of the need/problem	Consider the individual's concerns, issues, needs or problems
• Current drug and alcohol use	Type, quantity, frequency and route of administration (drug)
• Pattern of drug or alcohol use	Details of drug/alcohol taking for past week/month
• Current use of other substances	Prescribed, illicit or over-the-counter drugs
• Level of dependence	Any withdrawal symptoms Evidence of increasing tolerance
• Associated problems	Any medical, psychiatric, social or legal problems
• Risk behaviours	Source of injecting equipment Sharing of equipment Knowledge about sterilisation and needle exchange services Sexual behaviour when intoxicated
• Periods of abstinence/relapse	Duration, periods of abstinence, voluntary or enforced Reasons for lapse or relapse
• Sources of help	Social support systems Statutory agencies, local authorities, voluntary agencies, self-help groups
• Coping strategies and strengths	Previous strategies in coping with use of alcohol and drugs Achievements, strengths and positive aspects of the individual

- Monitor regularly
- Recognise positive achievements

The use of self-report or a checklist in the assessment of the levels of substance misuse is limited. Additional and independent collateral data and laboratory investigations would provide confirmation of the presence or absence of substance use. A number of screening instruments have been introduced to assess dual diagnosis. Table 18.6 presents a summary of the screening tools in the detection of dual diagnosis.

Table 18.6 Screening tools to assess co-morbidity.

AUDIT: The alcohol use disorders identification test	Brief self-report questionnaire (World Health Organization) to identify people whose alcohol consumption has become hazardous or harmful to their health.	Babor *et al.*, 1992
CUAD: The chemical use, abuse and dependence scale	Brief (20 minutes to administer), reliable and validated tool for the identification of substance use disorders in severely mentally ill in-patients.	Appleby *et al.*, 1996
DAST–10: The drug abuse screening test	Self-report questionnaire for measuring the severity of drug (not alcohol) dependence.	Skinner, 1982
DALI: The Dartmouth assessment of lifestyle instrument	An 18-item interviewer administered tool (on average six minutes to complete). It was developed primarily to detect alcohol, cannabis and cocaine use disorders.	Rosenberg *et al.*, 1998
MMSE: Mini-mental state examination	Brief, quantitative measure to screen for cognitive impairment, to estimate its severity, to follow cognitive changes over time and to document response to treatment.	Folstein *et al.*, 1975
PRISM: The psychiatric research interview for substance and mental disorders	Diagnostic interview based on DSM-IV. More reliable for assessing psychiatric disorders in those who have co-morbid substance use disorders.	Hasin *et al.*, 1996
SATS: The substance abuse treatment scale	To evaluate treatment progress or as an outcome measure. The scale is intended for assessing a person's stage of substance misuse treatment.	McHugo *et al.*, 1995

Source: adapted from Crawford & Crome (2001).

Testing for current drug and alcohol use

If self-reported assessment indicates current use of drugs and/or alcohol, laboratory investigations may be undertaken to aid early identification and diagnosis. The investigations are also helpful in contributing objective information to the overall assessment. Drugs and alcohol can be measured directly in serum, urine, exhaled air and hair. Urine analysis is widely undertaken to measure or assess drug use.

There are two main methods for testing a urine sample. Special immunological procedures called immunoassay tests are based on detecting antibodies to ingested drugs but gas chromatography is more accurate. Hair testing can be used to detect drugs laid down within the growing hair follicle, but is more expensive than urine testing. However, hair analysis carries a major advantage over urine testing in that it covers much longer periods than a single urine test (McPhillips *et al.*, 1997). Serum saliva tests are currently under evaluation. These tests only estimate whether drugs are present or absent and do not measure the amount of drugs in the body. The detection periods for urine drug screening are presented in Table 18.7.

A number of blood tests can be undertaken to assess the presence of drugs or alcohol. Essential investigations include liver function tests (LFT), gamma-glutamyl transferase (GGT), aspartate transaminase (AST) and mean corpusclar volume (MCV). A summary of those special blood tests for drugs and alcohol is provided in Table 18.8. When injecting drug users share needles, syringes or other paraphernalia, cross infections are likely to occur. Blood tests can also be carried out to determine HIV and hepatitis B and C. These tests must always be accompanied by pre-test and post-test counselling. A guidance on hepatitis C (Department of Health, 2001) is available for those working with drug users.

Table 18.7 Detection periods for urine drug screening.

Substance	Maximum range (hours and days)
Amphetamine	48 hours
Methamphetamine	48 hours
Barbiturates:	
• Short-acting	24 hours
• Intermediate-acting	48–72 hours
• Long-acting	7 days or more
Benzodiazepines:	
• Therapeutic dose	3 days
• Ultra-short-acting (e.g. midazolam)	12 hours
• Short-acting (e.g. triazolam)	24 hours
• Intermediate-acting (e.g. temazepam/chlordiazepoxide)	40–80 hours
• Long-acting (e.g. diazepam/nitrazepam)	7 days
Cannabinoids (marijuana):	
• Single use	3 days
• Moderate use (four times per week)	4 days
• Heavy use (daily)	10 days
• Chronic heavy use	21–27 days
Cocaine metabolites	2–3 days
Codeine/morphine/propoxyphene (Heroin is detected in urine as the 48 hours metabolite morphine)	48 hours
Methaqualone	7 days or more
Methadone (maintenance dosing)	7–9 days (approximate)
Norpropoxyphene	6–48 hours
Phencyclidine (PCP)	8 days (approximate)

Source: Department of Health (1999).

Risk assessment and management

There has been a greater awareness recently of the need for risk assessment and management. This interest appears to be in response to perceived failings in the policy of community care, criticisms of current practice following inquiries into tragedies involving people with serious mental illness, Government initiatives to reduce self-harm and improve community management of people with mental illness, and the need for mental health providers to reduce the increasing costs associated with litigation and complaints (Doyle, 1999). The aim of risk assessment is to identify risk factors that can be used to determine the likelihood of 'harm' to self and others and then to use the information acquired to intervene as part of the care plan. It has been suggested that the severity of substance

Table 18.8 Special laboratory alcohol and drug tests.

Tests	Detected substance(s)	Observations
Gamma-glutamyl transferase (GGT)	Alcohol	Elevated before liver damage, more likely to have liver damage at higher readings
Liver function tests (LFT)	Alcohol and drug	Liver damage due to alcohol
Full blood count	Alcohol	Mean red blood cells raised in heavy chronic drinkers
Aspartate transaminase (AST)	Alcohol	Suggest alcohol-related liver damage
Uric acid	Alcohol	Increase of urates and possibly gout
Haemoglobin	Drug and Alcohol	Anaemia due to poor nutrition or vitamin deficiencies
Tests for HIV, hepatitis B and C	Drug	History of injecting

misuse, including the combination of substances used, is related to the risk of overdose and/or suicide. Exploration of the possible association between substance misuse and increased risk of aggressive or antisocial behaviour forms an integral part of the risk assessment, and should be explicitly documented if present (Department of Health, 2002).

The risk management process should enable the optimum level of care to be given to an individual with dual diagnosis. Risk assessment should fully involve the individual being assessed, relevant professionals and any informal carer or significant other. It is also important to seek information from other sources such as carers, or significant others, as an individual may not disclose 'risky behaviours' or self-harm. However, this may be more apparent from their feelings, moods and behaviours. Risk assessment is an ongoing process and there are several critical points when practitioners need to conduct further assessment of 'risky behaviours'. For example, before individuals are discharged from hospital, referred to any agency or service provision, or return to be looked after by their informal carers.

The principal elements of risk assessment and management are:

- Suicide or self-harm: ideas, plans and intentions
- Ideas, thoughts and actions of harming others
- Self-neglect
- Risk of unintentional harm to self, or exploitation

Individuals with dual diagnosis are more likely to pose a risk to themselves than to others. However, it is critical to assess the risk of self-harm and attempted suicide to determine the appropriate intervention strategies. This will include an examination of previous self-harm and its frequency and seriousness, whether the previous attempt(s) was accidental or intended, previous coping or intervention strategies, current intentions and plans, and the ability to carry out those plans. This assessment should be conducted with a sensitive approach and in a non-judgemental manner despite the difficulties that the practitioner may face in asking about such 'risky behaviours'. It is a myth that raising the subject of 'risky behaviours' or self-harm is likely to encourage the individual to engage in them. By acknowledging the thoughts and feelings relating to the 'risk' behaviour, practitioners can work through with them, using techniques such as anger management, individual therapy and group work (Rethink & Turning Point, 2004).

An examination of the 'risky behaviours' should include the following questions:

- Does the individual have a suicide plan or serious intentions?
- How specific is the plan?
- What method will be used?
- Does the individual have the means to carry out the plan?
- When will the 'risky behaviour' happen?

There is no specific method of predicting 'risky behaviours', but there are several factors that have been reported in the literature to be associated with an increasing probability of risk behaviours. There may be patterns of past and current factors of psychosocial and physical problems that may be indicative of risk behaviours. A summary of the predisposing and precipitating risk factors is presented in Table 18.9.

Assessment of a risk of violence to others should be notified to informal carers and all agencies and key people involved in the care and support of the patient. Where there is such a risk, it is crucial that adequate personal care, supervision and treatment are provided. Special consideration should be given regarding the assessment of harm or violence to others. It is worth exploring the issues of the likely victims and whether the victims are aware of the risks posed to them and to others. Another element of risk assessment that requires attention from practitioners includes the individual's vulnerability to dangers or exploitations such as sexual, financial, occupational and familial, particularly when their judgement or cognitive functioning is seriously impaired.

Finally, it is stated that effective risk management should not disempower people but should minimise risk through open discussion, standardised assessment and the use of up-to-date, jointly owned care plans and the key to all these is greater collaboration and communication (O'Rourke & Bird, 2001). Equally, it is important that risk assessment is based on an appropriate evidence base and the management of risk is reached in a systematic way by the multidisciplinary team to enable more effective interventions. Consultations and communications between members of the multidisciplinary team and appropriate personnel from other agencies or services about risk assessment and management of the individual are good clinical practice. The importance of documentation, records and information sharing is fundamental when assessing the future potential risk of an individual.

Table 18.9 Predictors of risk.

Predisposing risk factors	Precipitating factors
• Previous history of harm to self or others • Family history of harm or mental illness • Borderline or impulsive personality • Social exclusion • Lack of support network • Past sexual or physical abuse • Depression • Schizophrenia • Substance misuse	• Specific plan • Neurological (organic disorders) • Continuing high suicidal and behavioural intent • Hopelessness • Hallucinations • Persecutory delusions • Social isolation • Recent loss or separation • Recent psychiatric hospitalisation • Relationship breakdown • Unemployment • Imprisonment or threat of imprisonment • Homelessness • Cultural and diversity issues (for example shame) • Intoxication with alcohol or drugs • Poor compliance with medication or treatment programmes • Poor communication between professionals

Source: adapted from Evans & Sullivan (2001).

Conclusion

- Assessment for dual diagnosis is based on a multidimensional approach. It is everyone's business.
- Assessment of an individual with dual diagnosis is broader than assessment of substance misuse or mental health.
- Assessment of an individual with dual diagnosis should be 'person specific' in meeting their physical, social, psychological and spiritual needs.
- Assessment of substance misuse, mental health and associated risk factors are derived from data collection through observation, interview, examination, screening tools and collateral sources.
- Critical to effective care planning and interventions is good screening and assessment.
- Observation for the reappearance of mental health problems after a period of abstinence from substance use is important.
- Symptoms of intoxication and withdrawal from psychoactive substances may be masked by, or blurred with, symptoms of mental health problems.
- When assessing individuals with relapsing mental health problems (high prevalence rate

of dual diagnosis), indicators associated with substance misuse and dependence should be examined.

- Assessment is the time when therapeutic relationships can be enhanced to enable the individual with dual diagnosis to engage with the service.
- Assessment of complex needs of the individual with dual diagnosis should be part of a care pathway or care plan for subsequent interventions.
- A good practice in assessment is to consider the client's concerns and needs, and to recognise positive achievements.

References

Bachrach, L. (1986) The context of care for the chronic mental patient with substance abuse. *Psychiatric Quarterly*, 87 (58), 3–14.

Banerjee, S., Clancy, C. & Crome, I. (2002) *Coexisting Problems of Mental Disorder and Substance Misuse (Dual Diagnosis)*, p. 32. An information manual. The Royal College of Psychiatrists' Research Unit, London.

Carroll, J. (1996) Attitudes to drug users according to staff grade. *Professional Nurse*, 11, 718–20.

Crawford, V. & Crome, I. (2001) *Coexisting Problems of Mental Health and Substance Misuse (Dual Diagnosis): a Review of Relevant Literature*. Royal College of Psychiatrists, London.

Davies, T. (1997) ABC of mental health: mental health assessment. *British Medical Journal*, 314, 1536.

Department of Health (1999) *Drug Misuse and Dependence – Guidelines on Clinical Management*. Her Majesty's Stationery Office, Norwich.

Department of Health (2001) *Hepatitis C – Guidance for those working with drug users*. Department of Health, London.
www.drugs.gov.uk

Department of Health (2002) *Mental Health Policy Implementation Guide: Dual Diagnosis Good Practice Guide*. Department of Health, London.

Doyle, M. (1999) Organisational responses to crisis and risk: issues and implications for mental health nurses. In: *Managing Crisis and Risk in Mental Health Nursing* (Ryan, T., ed.), pp. 40–56. Nelson Thornes, Cheltenham.

Evans, K. & Sullivan, J.M. (2001) *Dual diagnosis. Counselling the Mentally Ill Substance Abuser*, 2nd edn. Guilford Press, New York.

Gafoor, M. & Rassool, G.H. (1998) The coexistence of psychiatric disorders and substance misuse: working with dual diagnosis patients. *Journal of Advanced Nursing*, 27, 497–502.

Hanna, Z.E. (1991) Attitudes towards problem drinkers revisited: patient-therapist factors contributing to the differential treatment of patients with alcohol problems. *Alcoholism: Clinical and Experimental Research*, 15 (6), 927–31.

McPhillips, M.A., Kelly, F.J., Barnes, T.R.E., Duke, P.J., Gene-Cos, N. & Clark, K. (1997) Detecting co-morbid substance misuse among people with schizophrenia in the community: a study comparing the results of questionnaires with analysis of hair and urine. *Schizophrenia Research*, 25, 141–8.

Moore, K. & Rassool, G.H. (2002) Synthesis of addiction and mental health nursing: an approach to community interventions. In: *Dual Diagnosis: Substance Misuse and Psychiatric Disorders* (Rassool, G.H., ed.). Blackwell Publishing, Oxford.

O'Rourke, M. & Bird, L. (2001) *Risk Management in Mental Health. A Practical Guide to Individual Care and Community Safety*. Mental Health Foundation Publications, London.

Rassool, G.H. (1998a) Contemporary issues in addiction nursing. Chapter 23. In: *Substance Use and Misuse: Nature, Context and Clinical interventions* (Rassool, G.H., ed.). Blackwell Science, Oxford.

Rassool, G.H. (1998b) Working with Dual Diagnosis Clients. Chapter 24. In: *Substance Use and Misuse: Nature, Context and Clinical Interventions* (Rassool, G.H., ed.). Blackwell Science, Oxford.

Rethink & Turning Point (2004) *Dual Diagnosis Toolkit. Mental Health and Substance Misuse. A Practical Guide for Professionals and Practitioners*. Rethink & Turning Point, London.

Selleck, C.S. & Redding, B.A. (1998) Knowledge and attitudes of registered nurses towards perinatal substance abuse. *Journal of Obstetric, Gynaecologic and Neonatal Nursing*, 27, 70–8.

Williams, K. (1999) Attitudes of mental health professionals to co-morbidity between mental health problems and substance misuse. *Journal of Mental Health*, 8 (6), 606–13.

19 Dealing with Intoxication, Overdose, Withdrawal and Detoxification: Nursing Assessment and Interventions

G.H. Rassool & J. Winnington

Introduction

Emergency medical attention is often required by those misusing psychoactive substances as a result of toxic or adverse effects of the substance, the route of administration (injecting may lead to blood poisoning and deep vein thrombosis), lifestyle behaviours (poor nutrition, dehydration) and risk taking whilst under the influence of psychoactive substances (accidents, self-harm). Intoxication, overdose and withdrawal are the potential consequences of substance misuse, whether the psychoactive substance is illicit, prescribed or purchased over the counter. Drugs taken in combination with alcohol or other psychoactive substances increase the risk of death by overdose and can have serious long-term consequences. Nurses in both hospital and community settings have a vital role to play in the provision of nursing interventions during the withdrawal phase of psychoactive substances, detoxification, acute states of intoxication and in the reduction of drug-related deaths. This chapter covers four aspects of substance misuse: intoxication, overdose, withdrawal and detoxification, and relevant nursing interventions are discussed.

Acute intoxication

Acute intoxication frequently occurs in people who have persistent alcohol or drug-related problems. It is a transient condition following the administration of alcohol or other psychoactive substance, resulting in disturbances in level of consciousness, cognition, perception, affect or behaviour, or other psychophysiological functions and responses (WHO, 2005). Intoxication is highly dependent on the type and dose of drug ingested and is influenced by an individual's level of tolerance and other factors. In alcohol intoxication, for example, the level of intoxication will largely be influenced by body weight, tolerance, the volume of alcohol consumed, alcohol percentage in the drinks consumed and the period over which the alcohol was taken. The cultural and personal expectations regarding the effects of the drug will also influence the level of intoxication. Symptoms of intoxication do not always reflect the desired or expected effects of the psychoactive substance. For instance, depressant drugs (alcohol or GHB) may lead to symptoms of agitation or hyperactivity, and stimulant drugs (amphetamines or cocaine) may lead to socially withdrawn and introverted behaviour.

Most psychoactive substances will have an effect upon the central nervous and the cardiopulmonary systems. The common features of psychoactive intoxication include disinhibition, euphoria, lack of coordination and impaired judgement. Alcohol and drug intoxication may influence a person's mental health problem and may imitate or mask symptoms of an underlying mental or physical disorder. The resulting lack of inhibition and the depressant effect on the central nervous system may increase the risk of harm to self and others and exacerbate the risk of suicide.

People in an acute stage of intoxication of alcohol are most frequently seen in accident and emergency departments. It is extremely common for an intoxicated individual to vomit once or twice. However, continued vomiting may be a sign of head injury or other serious illness. Alcohol affects coordination and reactions, so individuals are prone to accidents. Trauma and head injuries caused by poor coordination and judgement when intoxicated are common. Head injury also increases the risk of seizures. It is possible for an individual who has acute alcohol poisoning to go into respiratory arrest whilst they are asleep and they can also choke to death on their vomit. Hypothermia is also a high risk factor for homeless problem drinkers. The individual may become belligerent, paranoid and even violent, necessitating caution and sensitivity when approaching them. Information on the use of, desired effects of and acute intoxication with psychoactive substances is found in Chapter 4.

Nursing interventions

When an individual is acutely intoxicated, the following actions must be taken.

Medical/physical needs

- Place in recovery position – if appropriate
- Assessment of airway, breathing and circulation
- Assess level of consciousness (Glasgow coma scale)
- Monitor vital signs
- Implement seizure safety precautions
- Monitor fluid intake and output
- Implement interventions to decrease systemic absorption of drugs such as use of absorbents (activated charcoal), induced diarrhoea, induced vomiting, gastric lavage, if appropriate
- Administration of antidote, if appropriate

Psychosocial needs

- Orientation
- 'Being there'
- Non-judgemental approach in interactions
- Create a supportive environment
- Assess for 'risk behaviours' (self-harm, potential for violence)
- Contact relatives/friends who are best able to support and reassure the patient

Additional interventions

- Monitor withdrawal syndrome and treat as necessary
- Screening for drug and alcohol problems (assessment, urine/saliva testing)
- Referral to an appropriate service to meet these needs
- Contact point for further help (self-help groups)
- Harm reduction (advice to reduce the harm caused by drug use, such as safer modes of use or how to access sterile injecting equipment)
- Provision of information literature on overdose prevention, viral transmission and local drug services
- Developing close liaison with drug treatment providers facilitates better access to treatment

Overdose

Drug-related deaths are defined as 'deaths where the underlying cause is poisoning, drug abuse, or drug dependence and where any of the substances are controlled under the Misuse of Drugs Act (1971) (ONS, 2003). There has been concern about the high prevalence of mortality amongst substance misusers. According to the Advisory Council on the Misuse of Drugs (2000), a report on *Reducing Drug-related Deaths* highlighted their concern about this issue and acknowledged that the prevention of drug-related deaths is a matter of pressing urgency. The report indicated that the number of such deaths must be substantially reduced. In England and Wales, there were more than 2300 drug-related deaths due to accidental or intentional overdose during 1998 and the trend is rising. Following the recommendations of the Advisory Council on the Misuse of Drugs report (2000), and the report *Action Plan to Prevent Drug-related Deaths* (Department of Health, 2001) the Government's *Updated Drug Strategy* (Home Office, 2002) has given a higher profile to a range of harm reduction measures to reduce premature death associated with fatal and non-fatal overdoses amongst drug users.

According to the National Treatment Agency (2002) an overdose is:

> 'an event in which a person intentionally or accidentally ingests one or more psychoactive substances at unsafe levels, leading to physical trauma, which may require immediate medical care to reverse and manage symptoms and other complications.'

Whilst many victims of drug overdose recover without long-term consequences, there can be serious implications for health due to the failure of the respiratory or circulatory systems or major organs such as the kidneys or liver. The pattern of the type of drug taken in overdose has changed in recent years, largely with changes in their availability and accessibility.

Substance misusers are at higher risk of suicide than the general population, and prescribed drugs, notably antidepressants and methadone, heighten that risk. Drug overdose is the most common method of suicide amongst substance misusers and the likelihood of overdose is increased when drugs are taken by injection, and fatal overdose (immediate death) is particularly associated with injecting opioid users. (Oyefeso *et al.*, 1999; National Treatment Agency, 2002). There is evidence to suggest that about 80% of people who present to A & E departments following self-harm will have taken an overdose of prescribed or over-the-counter medication and most will meet criteria for at least one psychiatric diagnosis at the time they are assessed (Haw *et al.*, 2001; Horrocks *et al.*, 2003). About one third of those who self-harm will be misusing drugs or alcohol on a regular basis (Merrill *et al.*, 1992; Haw *et al.*, 2001). The misuse of a combination of psychoactive substances such as benzodiazepines and alcohol with opiates, or combining heroin with cocaine as a 'speedball' can increase the chances of an overdose. In a prospective study of mortality amongst drug misusers, Gossop *et al.* (2002) found that the majority of deaths (68%) were associated with drug overdoses. Opiates were the drugs most commonly detected during post-mortem examinations. In the majority of cases, more than one drug was detected. Polydrug use and, specifically, heavy drinking, and use of benzodiazepines and amphetamines, were identified as risk factors for mortality. The use of antidepressants amongst polysubstance users has also been found to heighten the risk of fatality (Oyefeso *et al.*, 2000).

The are several risk factors that are reported to be associated with an increased likelihood of overdose. The multiple risk factors include administration by injection; concomitant use of other depressant drugs; loss of tolerance after a period of abstinence; injecting in public places (which may be associated with the use of untested drugs) or solitary drug use; a long history of opiate dependence; older age; and possibly unexpected changes in purity (EMCDDA, 2003). A summary of risk factors associated with incidence of overdose is presented in Table 19.1.

Nursing interventions with overdose

Drug overdose amongst substance misusers is a relatively common phenomenon and an acute life-threatening emergency. For many substance misusers, the first or only point of contact with health services is the accident and emergency

Table 19.1 Predictors of risk associated with overdose.

- Injecting drugs (heroin users, high level of dependence)
- Combinations of drugs (depressant drugs such as heroin, methadone, alcohol and benzodiazepines)
- High tolerance levels (users who have experienced non-fatal overdoses recently)
- Low tolerance levels (using opiates when tolerance is low, particularly after a break in use following imprisonment or detoxification)
- Cocaine and crack (cocaine and crack use amongst heroin users can play a role in fatal overdoses, as they can temporarily mask the sedative effects of heroin and other depressant type drugs)
- Poor mental health, depression, hopelessness and suicidal thoughts
- Not being in treatment (heroin injectors not in methadone treatment are around four times more likely to die in comparison to those in treatment)
- Premature termination of treatment (loss of tolerance, increased polydrug use after detoxification)
- Solitary drug use (using drugs alone, especially injecting, places a person at increased risk)

Source: adapted from Roberts & McVeigh (2004).

department due to overdoses, accidents or psychological crises. There are some general principles that define interventions of individuals with drug overdose, and in any setting emergency treatment should begin immediately. The priority is treating life-threatening problems such as respiratory depression, airway obstruction, cardiovascular collapse and convulsions (epileptic form seizures), alongside specific measures to treat the overdose.

Emergency nursing interventions include:

- Establishing a patent airway
- Providing ventilation support (artificial respiration, respirator)
- Maintaining adequate circulatory status (chest compressions, defibrillator, intravenous line)
- Controlling seizures (safety measures, intravenous diazepam)
- Administration of naloxone, if appropriate

After implementing acute interventions to stabilise the individual, a thorough history and physical examination are completed. Obtain information about the substance: name, route of administration, amount taken, when and period of time taken. If the individual is unable to participate in the assessment process, collateral information should be obtained whenever possible, from family members or significant others or past medical notes. Investigations for routine blood count and chemistry, urinalysis and toxicological screens of blood and urine will provide further evidence about the overdose. Monitor vital signs including temperature. Perform electrocardiogram and continue to monitor. The level of consciousness should be checked and should continue to be monitored at 15-minute intervals using the Glasgow coma scale (Teasdale & Jennett, 1974). Maintaining hydration and monitoring fluid intake and output are important. Safety precautions must be maintained during acute interventions as the individual may show signs of varying levels of consciousness, hallucinations and seizures. Reassurance and support should be provided. Measures to decrease systemic absorption of the substance such as gastric lavage, induced emesis (vomiting), absorbents (activated charcoal) or induced diarrhoea (magnesium) should be used as appropriate. An antidote may be administered depending upon the type of substance used.

Opiate and other drugs overdose

The treatment of overdose from opiates is the antidote naloxone hydrochloride (naloxone). A dose at 0.8–2 mg by intravenous injection should be administered, repeated at intervals of 2–3 minutes to a maximum of 10 mg. If respiratory function does not improve, other diagnostic options such as other drug intoxication, or other organic causes of loss of consciousness, including hypoglycaemia, should be considered (Department of Health, 1999). If an intravenous route is not accessible due to vein collapse, subcutaneous or intramuscular injection routes should be used. Naloxone is short-acting, and repeated injections or intravenous infusion may be needed if a longer acting opiate such as methadone has been taken. Naloxone can be given as a continuous intravenous infusion of 2 mg diluted in a 500 ml intravenous solution titrated at a rate determined by the clinical response (Department of Health, 1999). In methadone overdose, the effects can persist for up to 72 hours. Even in circumstances where patients have been resuscitated, depending on the magnitude of the overdose, they should be observed as an in-patient for a period of up to 72 hours. For high dose intoxication, naloxone infusion should be considered.

No antidote exists for the treatment of overdose from other drugs such as amphetamines, cocaine, cannabis, LSD and ecstasy. Treatment should therefore be aimed at the presenting symptoms and may include:

- Management of the unconscious patient.
- Management of hypothermia.
- Management of acute psychosis.

For a more comprehensive guideline on the clinical management of drug users see *Drug Misuse and Dependence: Guidelines on Clinical Management*, Department of Health (1999), and for accident and emergency staff, see *Guidance for A & E Staff on Reducing Deaths Caused by Illicit Drugs* (NTA, 2004a). For helplines, see *Drug Overdose: Prevention and Response Guidance for Helplines* (NTA, 2004b).

Detoxification

Detoxification means the withdrawal of a substance from the body, and the substance may be alcohol, heroin or benzodiazepine. It is also a process of treatment designed to control both medical and psychological complications of psychoactive substances. It may be carried out in hospital or in a community setting such as the individual's home, or at a day care agency. However, detoxification from drugs or alcohol can be potentially harmful and should be done under nursing and medical supervision only. The length of time required for detoxification from alcohol or drugs depends on the process being utilised and the substance being withdrawn. In general, alcohol detoxification can take anywhere from three to ten days and for drugs such as heroin, opiates, methadone or benzodiazepines the time can range from five to twenty-eight days of medically supervised detoxification. Home detoxification from alcohol lasts approximately seven to ten days. However, home detoxification can take months or even years to allow the dependent individual to gradually adjust to reduced doses, make withdrawal symptoms manageable and enable them to make appropriate lifestyle changes to sustain lasting changes in their drug-taking behaviour. The medical process of detoxification from alcohol or drugs usually includes administering a variety of substances to relieve the withdrawal symptoms and minimise the potentially harmful consequences.

Detoxification is the first step in rehabilitation and treatment of drug and/or alcohol misuse and also allows an individual an opportunity to reflect upon the negative consequences associated with their drug and alcohol misuse and to take up additional offers of interventions. In this context, detoxification can be regarded as a prelude to further social and psychological help, aimed at influencing and motivating the problem drinkers or problem drug users to modify or change their behaviour (Gafoor & Rassool, 1998).

Withdrawal or abstinence syndrome

Withdrawal syndrome is the physiological and psychological response to the sudden absence of a drug on which the individual had become dependent. Withdrawal syndrome differs greatly across the different categories of psychoactive substances. The duration and severity of withdrawal symptoms vary according to the drug, the dose and the length of time the drug was used. Withdrawal symptoms from all psychoactive substances tend to be the opposite of the desired or sought after effects of the substances and produce similar symptoms of anxiety and depression. Alcohol, stimulants, opiates and hypno-sedatives will produce withdrawal syndromes when the individual no longer has access to the substance. Table 19.2 presents the withdrawal syndrome and effects of toxic/overdose states.

Alcohol withdrawal syndrome

Alcohol withdrawal syndrome is a set of symptoms that individuals have when they suddenly stop drinking alcohol, following continuous and heavy consumption. Withdrawal symptoms rarely occur in individuals who are recreational drinkers. Problem drinkers who have gone through withdrawal before are more likely to have withdrawal symptoms each time they stop drinking. Some individuals have the forms of the syndrome including tremors, seizures and hallucinations, typically occurring within 6–48 hours after the last drink. The worst form of alcohol withdrawal is delirium tremens (DTs), which involves profound confusion, hallucinations, agitations, tachycardia, dilated pupils, typically beginning between three to four days after the last drink. The signs and symptoms of alcohol withdrawal are summarised in Table 19.3.

Nursing interventions

Alcohol

The early recognition and clinical assessment of alcohol withdrawal syndrome is important, as severe alcohol withdrawal can be life threatening. Individuals with a history of withdrawal seizures, delirium tremens, medical problems and risk of self-harm should be considered for hospital admission rather than having home detoxification. The approach to the safe management of alcohol withdrawal will include pharmacological, physical and psychological treatments. The provision of a quiet and safe environment is important for those individuals experiencing anxiety, agitation, thought disturbances and epileptiform seizures. Precautions need to be taken for the potential risk of

Table 19.2 Withdrawal syndrome and effects of toxic/overdose states.

Drug	Withdrawal Syndrome	Effects of Toxic/Overdose State
Cannabis Marijuana Hashish	Insomnia, hyperactivity (rare syndrome)	Fatigue, paranoia, hallucinogen like psychotic state (high dose), depersonalisation
Depressants Alcohol GHB	Tremors, clouding of consciousness, disorientation of time and place, visual or tactile hallucinations, paranoid delusions, anxiety, fear, suspicion and anger, suicidal behaviour, withdrawal fits (approximately 12 hours after abstinence)	Decreased alertness, exaggerated emotions, shock, confusion, coma, possible death
Hallucinogens Ecstasy LSD Ketamine Mushrooms[1]	No clinical syndrome	Tiredness, confusion, anxiety, depression, paranoia, more prolonged episodes, possibly mimic psychotic episodes
Opiates and opioids Heroin Methadone Morphine Codeine	Watery eyes, runny nose, yawning, loss of appetite, tremors, panic, sweating, nausea, cramps, hypertension, back or muscle aches, gooseflesh, diarrhoea	Slow and shallow breathing, clammy skin, constricted pupils, coma, possible death
Stimulants Amphetamines Anabolic steroids Cocaine Khat[2]	Severely depressed mood and feelings, excessive sleep, apathy, irritability, disorientation, craving	Agitation, high body temperature, hallucinations, convulsions, tachycardia, cardiac arrest, cerebral stroke
Sedative-hypnotics Benzodiazepines Barbiturates	Anxiety, insomnia, tremors, delirium tremens, convulsions, possible death	Repiratory depression, shallow respirations, cold and clammy skin, weak and rapid pulse, amnesia, coma, possible death
Volatile substances Alkyl nitrites[3] Solvents	No clinical syndrome	Anxiety, mental impairment, depressed respiration, cardiac dysrhythmias, self-harm, sudden death

[1] fatal overdose rare, unless poisonous mushrooms
[2] no fatal overdose
[3] swallowing liquid may be fatal but rare

Table 19.3 Withdrawal syndrome of alcohol.

- Anorexia, nausea, vomiting
- Delusions
- Elevated temperature
- Increased heart rate and blood pressure
- Grand mal seizures
- Hallucinations
- Impaired concentration, memory and judgement
- Insomnia and nightmares
- Restlessness, irritability, anxiety and agitation
- Tremor

suicide and the management of grand mal seizures. The standard pharmacological treatment for alcohol withdrawal is a reducing dose of cross-tolerant drugs, such as benzodiazepines with thiamine. The dose during detoxification with benzodiazepines (chlordiazepoxide or diazepam) will be influenced by the individual's health, the severity of the symptoms and level of alcohol use. The severity of the withdrawal, especially epileptiform seizures, should be monitored and the dose of benzodiazepines administered accordingly. Anti-emetics may also be given to reduce vomiting. Problem drinkers would also need attention given to their nutritional requirements as they are frequently malnourished due both to poor nutritional intake as a result of their lifestyle, and because alcohol affects the absorption of certain vitamins and minerals, as the majority of their calories are derived from alcohol. Folic acid, thiamine, vitamin B-complex, given intramuscularly or intravenously, will be needed to prevent irreversible cognitive impairment. The individual response to medications, vital signs, the severity of withdrawal, degree of comfort and risk behaviours need to be monitored.

Although the medical consequences of alcohol withdrawal must be the priority goal of treatment, any underlying psychiatric co-morbidity must also be managed. Failure to intervene in those secondary conditions would ultimately increase risk behaviours or relapse. Other interventions such as harm reduction, health education and referral to a specialist unit should be initiated once the management of acute withdrawal is under control.

Opiates

Opiate users can have detoxification in hospital settings or without medical assistance by 'do-it-yourself' withdrawal. Heroin, morphine, codeine and methadone will produce similar withdrawal signs and symptoms but withdrawal symptoms from shorter acting opiates will appear and abate sooner. The time of onset and the duration of the withdrawal syndrome will depend on the drug itself, the total intake of the drug, the duration of use and the health of the individual. The signs and symptoms of heroin or morphine withdrawal begin 8–12 hours after the last dose of the drug and they become less over a period of five to seven days. The signs and symptoms from methadone begin 12 hours after the last dose and the peak intensity occurs on the third day of abstinence. Symptoms usually subside after 2–3 weeks. The common signs and symptoms of opiate withdrawal syndrome are summarised in Table 19.4.

Methadone

Methadone can be used in the treatment of withdrawal syndrome and it is long-acting, which allows for symptoms to be controlled over a period of time. For certain individuals with a history of relapse and treatment dropout, methadone is the treatment of choice. Methadone has many advantages (Department of Health, 1999) such as:

Table 19.4 Withdrawal syndrome of opiate.

Anxiety	Nausea and vomiting
Insomnia	Diarrhoea
Increased respiratory rate	Weakness
Sweating	Abdominal cramps
Yawning	Tachycardia
Runny nose	Hypertension
Restlessness	Muscle spasms
Anorexia	Muscle and bone pain
Irritability	Lachrymation
Dilated pupils	

- It is licensed for the treatment of opiate dependence.
- It is longer acting (typically 24–48 hours) making stability from daily dosing easier to achieve.
- It is straightforward to titrate in order to achieve the correct dose.
- It is less likely to be diverted than shorter-acting drugs.
- It is less likely to be injected.
- Its clinical effectiveness is supported by research.

The baseline dose of methadone aims to minimise the severity of the withdrawal, produce a degree of comfort and lessen the risk of overdose. Dose reduction of methadone can be undertaken depending on the results of the assessment and treatment plan. The most rapid regime can be carried out by incremental cuts in dose over 7–21 days and slower regimes may take several months to complete. When there are complex social or other needs, slow reductions of methadone are prescribed. The general principle being that at higher dose levels a greater reduction is possible, as it represents a smaller percentage of the total. As the dose falls, reduction should be more gradual (Department of Health, 1999). This gradual reduction of methadone can occur at any time interval, for example daily, alternate days or weekly. In order to decrease the individual's anxiety and increase their sense of control, it may be necessary to hold the reduction steady at a given dose over a few days. Delays in the rate of reduction should be accompanied by psychological support. Progress should be monitored at intervals and the individual's progress should be discussed with the multidisciplinary team.

Buprenorphine

Buprenorphine is licensed in the UK for the treatment of drug dependence. This drug has an effective duration of at least 24 hours and is taken as a sublingual tablet daily. It is reported to have low euphoric effects at higher doses compared with methadone. There is interest in its use as an alternative to methadone maintenance and also in the management of opiate withdrawal as its mixed agonist-antagonist properties make it a potentially good agent for the management of opiate withdrawal (Department of Health, 1999). However, because of its double action, it can paradoxically aggravate withdrawal symptoms if used in combination with methadone or other opiates. Buprenorphine needs to be administered at least 24 hours after the last dose of methadone and at least four hours after the use of heroin. It is also reported to have lower overdose potential, which makes it more suitable than methadone.

Non-opiates

There are now satisfactory non-opiate treatments (such as lofexidine) for opiate withdrawal. These non-opiate drugs are effective in alleviating opiate withdrawal symptoms and are not liable to, or less open to, misuse by the patient and less likely to be diverted onto the black market (Department of Health, 1999). Lofexidine, a fully licensed drug in the UK for the management of the symptoms of opiate withdrawal, can be used with supervision in in-patient, residential and community settings. There is evidence to suggest that it is equally as efficacious as methadone in withdrawal and has a role in the treatment of opiate dependent individuals seeking abstinence and whose drug use is already well controlled. Clonidine is not licensed for the treatment of opiate withdrawal symptoms but is useful as a non-opiate treatment for opiate withdrawal. Because of its substantial hypotensive effect there is a need to monitor blood pressure and to modify or withdraw the treatment if symptomatic hypotension occurs.

Table 19.5 Withdrawal syndrome of benzodiazepines.

Anxiety symptoms	• Anxiety • Sweating • Insomnia • Headache • Tremor • Nausea
Disordered perceptions	• Feelings of unreality • Abnormal body sensations • Abnormal sensation of movement • Hypersensitivity to stimuli
Major complications	• Psychosis • Epileptic seizures

Benzodiazepines

Benzodiazepines have their own addictive potential and are often taken in combination with opiates. Sudden cessation in the use of benzodiazepines can lead to a recognised withdrawal state. Many opiate users use benzodiazepines as part of polydrug use. Table 19.5 summarises withdrawal states associated with use of benzodiazepines. The discontinuation of benzodiazepine dependence should be done under nursing and medical supervision. There are different strategies in the management of benzodiazepine withdrawal, such as the use of decreasing doses of the drug of dependence or the substitution of a long-acting benzodiazepine. Withdrawal prescribing should only be initiated where there is clear evidence that the individual is dependent on benzodiazepines. A comprehensive assessment, followed by laboratory investigations such as urine drug sceens, would confirm the need to instigate withdrawal prescribing. The management of withdrawal from benzodiazepines involves the gradual tapering of the dose, and this may be extended over the course of several weeks depending on the length of use and severity of symptoms.

Stimulants

Amphetamines, cocaine and ecstasy are the most commonly abused stimulants and they do not produce a major physiological withdrawal syndrome. Although the withdrawal syndrome is similar, the withdrawal symptoms differ between intermittent binge users and chronic users. After cessation regular users of stimulants may experience exhaustion, insomnia, intense dreaming and depressed mood. These symptoms tend to subside over a period of two to four days of abstinence from the drug. Antidepressant drugs are sometimes used, but occasional toxic reactions have been described when selective serotonin re-uptake inhibitors (SSRIs) are prescribed and stimulants continue to be taken. In some individuals with a dual diagnosis abrupt cessation of stimulants may trigger a profound transient depression with suicidal thoughts necessitating hospitalisation or close monitoring (Banerjee *et al.*, 2002). Antidepressants, such as fluoxetine, can be effective in the management of major depressive episodes associated with stimulant use. There is no indication for the prescription of cocaine or methylamphetamine in the treatment of stimulant withdrawal, and it is not recommended that other stimulants, such as methylphenidate or phentermine, are prescribed (Department of Health, 1999). There may be a limited place for the prescription of dexamphetamine sulphate 5 mg (five) in the treatment of amphetamine misuse.

GHB

A GHB withdrawal syndrome that has aspects of alcohol and benzodiazepine withdrawal has been reported. The syndrome appears to manifest itself in individuals who have self-administered GHB every 2–3 hours and are at increased risk for the emergence of severe symptoms. GHB withdrawal can occur after several months of regular use. Management of the withdrawal syndrome has necessitated the use of high dosages of sedative-hypnotic and physical restraints to control the confusion, delirium, psychosis and resultant agitation.

Cannabis/hallucinogens/phencyclidine

There is no acute abstinence syndrome associated with withdrawal from cannabis. Some individuals are irritable and have difficulty sleeping for a few days after chronic use. Where agitation and severe insomnia are prominent short-term low dose of antipsychotics is sometimes the appropriate measure. There are also no acute withdrawal syndromes with hallucinogens and phencyclidine (PCP), although chronic use of PCP may lead to a toxic psychosis.

References

Advisory Council on the Misuse of Drugs (2000) *Reducing Drug-related Deaths. A report by the Advisory Council on the Misuse of Drugs*. The Stationery Office, London.

Banerjee, S., Clancy, C. & Crome, I. (2002) *Coexisting Problems of Mental Disorder and Substance Misuse (Dual Diagnosis)*. Royal College of Psychiatrist's Research Unit, London.

Department of Health (1999) *Drug Misuse and Dependence: Guidelines on Clinical Management*. The Stationery Office, London.

Department of Health (2001) *Action Plan to Prevent Drug-related Deaths*. Department of Health, London. www.doh.gov.uk

Department of Health (2003). *The Models of Care for the Treatment of Adult Drug Misusers, Parts 1 and 2*. National Treatment Agency, London.

European Monitoring Centre for Drugs and Drug Addiction (2003) *Annual Report 2003: The State of the Drugs Problem in the European Union and Norway*. European Monitoring Centre for Drugs, and Drugs Addiction, Lisbon.

Gafoor, M. & Rassool, G.H. (1998) Alcohol: community detoxification and clinical care. In: *Substance Use and Misuse: Nature, Context and Clinical Interventions* (Rassool, G.H., ed.). Blackwell Science, Oxford.

Gossop, M., Stewart, D., Treacy, S. & Marsden, J. (2002) A prospective study of mortality among drug misusers during a four-year period after seeking treatment. *Addiction*, 97 (1), 39–47.

Haw, C., Hawton, K., Houston, K. & Townsend, E. (2001) Psychiatric and personality disorders in deliberate self-harm patients. *British Journal of Psychiatry*, 178, 48–54.

Home Office (2002) *Updated Strategy 2002*. www.drugs.gov.uk

Horrocks, J., Price, S., House, A. & Owens, D. (2003) Self-injury attendances in the accident and emergency department. *British Journal of Psychiatry*, 183, 34–9.

Merrill, J., Milner, G., Owens, D. & Vale, A. (1992) Alcohol and attempted suicide. *British Journal of Addictions*, 87, 83–9.

Miotto, K. & Roth, B. (2001) *Patients with a History of Around-the Clock use of Gamma-hydroxybutyrate may Present as Disturbing and Difficult to Manage*. UCLA

Integrated UTSW Toxicology Substance Abuse Program Training Service.
www.tcada.state.tx.us

National Treatment Agency (2002) *Models of Care for Treatment of Adult Drug Misusers*. National Treatment Agency, London.

National Treatment Agency (2004a) *Guidance for A & E Staff on Reducing Deaths Caused by Illicit Drugs*. National Treatment Agency, London.

National Treatment Agency (2004b) *Drug Overdose: Prevention and Response Guidance for Helplines*. National Treatment Agency, London.

Office for National Statistics (2003) Deaths related to drug poisoning: results for England and Wales, 1993 to 2001. *Health Statistics Quarterly* (Spring), London.

Oyefeso, A., Ghodse, A.H., Clancy, C. & Corkery, J.M. (1999) Suicide among drug addicts in the UK. *British Journal of Psychiatry*, 175, 277–82.

Oyefeso, A., Valmana, A., Clancy, C., Ghodse, A.H. & Williams, H. (2000) Fatal antidepressant overdose among drug abusers and non-drug abusers. *Acta Psychiatrica Scandinavica*, 102, 295–9.

Roberts, L. & McVeigh, J. (2004) *Lifeguard: Act Fast Save A Life. An Evaluation of a Multi-component Information Campaign Targeted at Reducing Drug-related Deaths in Cheshire and Merseyside*. Centre for Public Health, Faculty of Health & Applied Social Sciences, Liverpool John Moores University, Liverpool.

Teasdale, G. & Jennett, B. (1974) Assessment of coma and impaired consciousness. A practical scale. *Lancet*, 2, 81–4.

World Health Organization (2005) *The ICD-10 Classification of Mental and Behavioural Disorders: Diagnostic Criteria for Research*. WHO, Geneva.

20 Prescribing Authority and Medication Management in Mental Health and Addiction Nursing

G.H. Rassool & J. Winnington

Introduction

The prescribing of medication plays a more significant therapeutic intervention in mental health treatment than in substance misuse treatment. In England, nurse prescribing is seen as part of the NHS modernisation plans and is on the agenda for the nursing profession (Department of Health, 1999, 2000a, 2000b). The Health and Social Care Act 2001, Section 63, allows Ministers, by order, to designate new categories of prescribers of medications and to set conditions for their prescribing. This legislation allows nurses, pharmacists or other health professionals to prescribe prescription only medicines (POMs) (Office of Public Sector Information, 2001). The prescribing legislation has passed to devolved governments in the UK and nurse prescribing (extended and supplementary prescribing) is similar in Scotland, England and Northern Ireland. Recent implementation guidance has been to broaden the range of medications and increase the autonomy that nurse prescribers have in supplementary prescribing (Department of Health, 2003). The guidelines include the general principles of supplementary prescribing, such as the roles and responsibilities of doctors and nurses/pharmacists, how a process of supplementary prescribing should occur and the types of forms used to record the clinical management plan. This prescribing initiative has been extended to controlled drugs. Diamorphine, morphine and naloxone hydrochloride have been included in the range of medications that can be administered by practicing midwives without a specific prescription (NMC, 2004). Six controlled drugs are included – three for pain relief and three that are restricted for use in palliative care. At present, nurses cannot prescribe controlled drugs independently for substance misuse (National Treatment Agency, 2005). Medication for acute alcohol withdrawal may be added, but any controlled drug would first need further changes to Home Office regulations.

The National Treatment Agency for Substance Misusers' (2005) review outlines the current situation in relation to nurses prescribing for substance misuse and supplies information to commissioners, treatment providers and health professionals on the potential role of nurse prescribing in service development, thus supporting the development of clinical practice in this area. A recent addition is a good practice guide on implementing supplementary prescribing for mental health nurses (National Prescribing Centre, the National Institute for Mental Health in England and the Department of Health, 2005). This guidance has been helpful in refocusing the agenda for mental health nurses to prescribe and supply medication in new ways in order to improve services for people with mental health problems. The guidance also points to a broadened outlook for mental health nursing interventions and emphasises combining medication management together with psychological approaches to care. This good practice guide provides information about these opportunities, what potential benefits can come from their introduction and how organisations might go about implementing them.

This change in legislation would have a profound effect on the role of addiction and mental health nurses, and would provide them with a more autonomous therapeutic role in both community and residential settings (health, social care and criminal justice systems). In addition, the process and outcome of this prescribing initiative could transform the dynamics of the multi-professional team and have the potential to radically change the service provision and delivery in both mental health and substance misuse services. The aim of this chapter is to provide some perspectives on aspects of nurse prescribing with reference to addiction nursing and mental health nursing in the UK, with selected literature reviews on nurse prescribing. In addition, the issues, problems and implications of nurse prescribing and medication management are presented.

Context of nurse prescribing

Nurse prescribing has been in existence in the USA for about 30 years and is now contributing to the management and treatment of conditions such as cancer, cardiac disease, multiple sclerosis and severe mental illness (Nolan *et al.*, 2004). In a survey of psychiatric clinical nurse specialists in the USA, Nolan *et al.* (2004) concluded that nurse prescribing has advantages for both nurses and patients, including enhanced career development opportunities and better quality of patient care. However, issues of concerns were identified regarding the relationship between nurse prescribers and non-prescribers, and the relationship between nurse prescribers and medical supervisors. Four types of prescribing initiatives are currently in practice: patient group directions (PGDs), nurse prescribers' formulary, independent nurse prescribers and supplementary prescribers. More explanation on the four types of prescribing is presented in Table 20.1.

Table 20.1 Types of nurse prescribing.

Patient group directions (PGDs)
- Written instructions for the supply and administration of specified medicines; also known as prescribing under protocol
- No limit on clinical focus and cover a wide range of situations from vaccination to emergency care
- Nurses and other health care professionals are eligible to prescribe

Nurse prescribers formulary
- Limited to a few prescription only medicines
- Mainly consists of wound dressings and non-drug items designed to meet needs of housebound patients
- District nurses and health visitors are eligible

Independent nurse prescribers
- Uses the nurse prescribers' extended formulary
- Consists of 180 prescription only drugs, plus licensed products for general and pharmacy sales
- Focuses on minor illness, minor injuries, health promotion and palliative care
- Nurses with three years of clinical experience are eligible

Supplementary prescribers
- Legally allowed to prescribe from a wide range of medicines
- All prescribable medicines except unlicensed drugs outside clinical trials and controlled drugs (under review)
- Before prescribing, a clinical management plan must be agreed upon with the doctor, nurse or pharmacist and the patient
- Individual clinical management plan for each patient
- Nurses and pharmacists are eligible

Source: Department of Health (2003).

Over the past two decades, the growing demand for increased access to health care for substance misusers has resulted in some innovations in service provision. With the massive expansion of community services for substance misusers, such as the development of community drug/alcohol teams, drug and alcohol liaison teams, day care programmes, street agencies, outreach work, needle exchange schemes, smoking cessation clinics, mobile methadone clinics, satellite clinics for homeless drinkers and residential rehabilitation, the development of addiction nursing as a community specialty has true potential (Rassool & Gafoor, 1997). Addiction nurses are now working in a range of agencies in health, social and criminal justice systems. Many of these innovations in substance abuse services have been nurse led. There has also been educational development of multi-professional certificate and postgraduate programmes in substance misuse and addictive behaviour (Rassool,

2000, 2004a), and the provision of clinical guidelines aimed at nurses, midwives and health visitors from the Association of Nurses in Substance Abuse (1997).

In mental health, there has been a 'cultural shift' of the traditional medication role of mental health nurses from a task oriented to a more person centred approach since the early 1990s. In addition to the checking of prescriptions and safe administration of medication, the focus now includes health information about the benefits and the risks of treatment, checking the service user has given informed consent, monitoring effects and adverse effects, and communicating with the prescriber. Taken together with psychosocial interventions, medication is a central part of the treatment of individuals with mental health problems. Nurse prescribing represents an important change in the way services are delivered to individuals with mental health problems and reflects an emphasis on user choice and making services more responsive to service user needs (National Prescribing Centre, the National Institute for Mental Health in England and the Department of Health, 2005).

Rationale for nurse prescribing

Nurse prescribing, in addition to medication management, is seen as a positive development with regard to the care and treatment responses in meeting the holistic needs of individuals with substance misuse and mental health problems. Nurse prescribing, in general, has been found to enhance career development of nurses and also to promote job satisfaction (Jordan & Griffiths, 2004; Nolan *et al.*, 2004). The strengths of addiction nurses are that they are able to deliver high quality nursing care as well as other biopsychosocial interventions. In substance misuse services, expanding the role of the nurse to include prescribing would result in increased access to treatment for the service users, increased partnership with pharmacists and other stakeholders, increased capacity to provide a wide range of intervention strategies and, it is hoped, increased effectiveness of treatment programmes with substance abusers (health, social functioning and crime reduction) (Rassool, 2004b). Mental health nurses who can prescribe, supply and administer medications via patient group directions may confer many benefits, which include allowing service users quicker access to medication, providing services more efficiently and effectively, and increasing service user choice (National Prescribing Centre, the National Institute for Mental Health in England and the Department of Health, 2005). With regard to service innovations, it would enhance the provision of a more comprehensive and streamlined service and improve the quality of care (Mundinger, 2000; Wilhelmsson & Foldevi, 2003). A study (Gray *et al.*, 2005) looking at mental health nurse supplementary prescribing one year after its implementation showed that nurse supplementary prescribing was an important means for improving patient care and treatment, particularly in community settings. It also indicated that directors of nursing perceived nurse supplementary prescribing as positive. The findings also showed that psychiatrists were generally not opposed to its introduction.

Guidance on prescribing for mental health nurses has already been proposed (National Prescribing Centre, the National Institute for Mental Health in England and the Department of Health, 2005). There is, as yet, no clarification of how the new prescribing authority will extend the role of addiction nurses into a new dimension. However, they are already taking a major role in prescribing in substance abuse services. Addiction nurses have made significant contributions in decision making with medical practitioners, and they have provided advice and medication management to junior medical practitioners. In general health care practice, nurse prescribing is not a new development since nurses have been involved in decision making about medications for some time (Department of Health, 2002). This is put succinctly by Rodden (2001) who stated that 'nurse prescribing therefore not only formalises what is currently happening in practice, but also allows the nurse to take full responsibility for prescribing decisions.'

In the context and nature of dual diagnosis and the role of addiction, future prescribing directions would include prescribing for minor injuries, pain, nutritional supplements, antibiotics, emergency contraceptives, medications for detoxification and psychotropic substances. This is subject to an adequate preparation for those prescribers. It is acknowledged that nurses are already prescribing for smoking cessation regimens. Nurse prescribing, such as methadone for opiate dependence would significantly reduce the waiting time for service users to gain access to appropriate services, based on the *Model of Care* (National Treatment Agency, 2002). The National Treatment Agency has issued maximum acceptable waiting time targets so that substance misusers should not have to wait for more than two weeks to access a community based prescribing service. It is argued that setting waiting times at three weeks for referral to drugs services provides another convincing reason to extend methadone prescribing by nurses, leading to more nurse led services. The NTA's *Research into Practice* series (National Treatment Agency, 2004) on the effectiveness of methadone maintenance treatment examines the key factors that can assist practitioners in achieving optimal methadone maintenance treatment and improved outcomes. The briefing concludes that good practice can lead to higher retention rates and reduce illicit drug use. It is worth reiterating that diamorphine, morphine and naloxone hydrochloride can be administered by practicing midwives without a specific prescription. Both the NTA and the Advisory Council on the Misuse of Drugs agree that supplementary prescribing provides a robust and safe structure to enable nurses to prescribe controlled drugs used in substance dependence (National Treatment Agency, 2005).

Following changes to regulations for controlled drugs, it is envisaged that supplementary prescribing would be carried out by a psychiatrist or a GP with a special interest. They would undertake an initial patient assessment and then agree a clinical management plan with a nurse, who would then be able to initiate, titrate, continue and adjust doses (for example methadone and buprenorphine) (National Treatment Agency, 2005). Furthermore, supplementary prescribing has been identified as particularly appropriate for the management of long-term conditions. This added value would be for nurses and, potentially, pharmacists to jointly manage prescribing responsibility with doctors for individuals on long-term maintenance regimes. It may also provide the opportunity for addiction nurses to take on prescribing for longer-term detoxification and stabilisation regimens within the parameters of the clinical management plan (National Treatment Agency, 2005). It has been suggested that patient group directions (PGDs) may have potential for use in ensuring greater access to medication to prevent drug overdoses, for example in supplying take home naloxone, for other management of symptomatic relief of opiate withdrawal, and enabling greater access to hepatitis A and B immunisation (National Treatment Agency, 2005).

The contributions of nurse prescribing to improving the quality of care offered to service users are beyond dispute. Findings from several small-scale studies indicate that patients were highly satisfied with nurse prescribers and valued their advice on self-care. Prescribing nurses offered more choice for service users and carers, reduced the side effects of medication, promoted better health promotion activities, reduced the health care costs, improved service user education and improved concordance with medication regimens (Luker *et al.*, 1998; Brooks *et al.*, 2001; Nolan *et al.*, 2001; Aldridge, 2002; Hay *et al.*, 2004).

The involvement of service users as part of the process of care and self-care approaches would enhance the quality and continuity of care. It is suggested that nurse prescribing fosters continuity of care, accelerates access to care and enhances the involvement of service users in the formulation of their care plan in identifying the most appropriate treatment (Brooks *et al.*, 2001). The new therapeutic alliance could benefit from information about service users' experiences of their needs and health related problems. This new working paradigm would enable addiction and mental health nurses to assume total responsibility for the holistic care and management of individuals with coexisting substance misuse and mental health problems, in partnership with other health, social and criminal justice services, and to increase the availability and effectiveness of intervention strategies.

New approach, new dangers

A new prescribing dimension added to the clinical medication practices of addiction and mental health nurses would undoubtedly distort the professional boundaries in the multidisciplinary team. This would result in the erosion of the traditional role boundary of medical practitioners and the acceptance of new roles by other health care professionals. However, it has been reported that there is a lack of clarity and some misgivings about the role of supplementary subscribers.

Nurse prescribers reported the lack of acceptance by other disciplines and potential for professional envy (Hay *et al.*, 2004). In a study of specialist psychiatric nurses in the USA, the respondents commented that medical practitioners felt threatened by nurse prescribers and that nurses are attacked on the grounds of insufficient knowledge and clinical experience (Nolan *et al.*, 2004). In a focus group study (Hay *et al.*, 2004) of a multiprofessional group of health care professionals, the authors concluded that a considerable amount of preparation would be required to ensure that nurse prescribers have the organisational and team support to adapt to their new roles. However, issues of concerns were identified regarding the relationship between nurse prescribers and non-prescribers, and the relationships amongst nurse prescribers and medical supervisors. Communication systems need to be improved across teams to enable nurses to share and have access to medical information to support nurse prescribers (Hay *et al.*, 2004).

Introducing supplementary prescribing may have an impact on nursing workloads and may require role redesign and a reduction in caseload management (National Treatment Agency, 2005). A clear operational role for addiction nurses within a defined framework of prescribing parameters needs to be implemented. Clear practice guidelines within this prescribing framework and continuing professional development would minimise the harm done by role conflict and role adequacy in clinical practice.

It is beyond the scope of this chapter to examine all the relevant risk factors about nurse prescribing. A number of issues and problems that need to be examined and reflected on are presented in Table 20.2.

Table 20.2 Risk factors associated with nurse prescribing.

- Poor clinical judgement (lack of diagnostic skills)
- Medication errors
- Poor assessment of side effects of medication
- Lack of competence in dealing with minor physical problems
- Failure to communicate information about medication benefits and risks
- Need for increased clinical supervision
- 'Postcode' lottery of prescribing
- Disregard of the right to informed consent
- Ethical responsibilities (relationship with pharmaceutical companies)
- Increased workload and risk of burn-out
- Therapeutic alliance diluted due to the role of a 'script machine'
- Lack of comprehensive knowledge about medication management
- Clinical liability, responsibility, fear of litigation
- Spillage of controlled drug
- Increased record keeping and monitoring
- Dangers of using generic prescriptions
- Access to service-users' information

Source: Rassool (2005).

Rational use of psychoactive substances

It is well known that over-prescribing of controlled medicines can lead to dependence and abuse (Ghodse & Khan, 1988). A proper understanding of the definition of substance use and misuse and dependence, in the context of appropriate prescribing and rational use of psychoactive substances, is required (see Rassool, 2002). The 'Conference of experts on the rational use of drugs' (WHO, 1989) stated that the:

> 'rational use of drugs requires that patients receive medications appropriate to their clinical needs, in doses that meet their own individual requirements for an adequate period of time, and the lowest cost to them and their community.'

This definition is medically oriented and focuses on the prescribing process. When prescribing patterns do not always conform to the criteria set in the definition they can be classified as inappropriate or irrational prescribing. However, the definition does not make it explicit that there is an alternative to prescribing in the use of complementary or alternative therapies. The meaning of rational use also implies that the right drug is taken by the right patient, in the right dose and for the right duration of therapy, that the risks of therapy are acceptable (WHO, 1989; Rassool & Winnington, 1993; Rassool, 2005).

Irrational use is the use of psychoactive substances that does not conform to good clinical practice. Irrational prescribing may be regarded as 'pathological' prescribing, where the criteria in the process of prescribing are not fulfilled (WHO, 2004), for example extravagant prescribing, over-prescribing, incorrect prescribing, multiple prescribing, indiscriminate use of injections and under-prescribing of medication of sedative-hypnotic drugs and

Table 20.3 Common patterns of irrational prescribing.

	Examples
Use of drugs when no drug therapy is indicated	Antibiotics, benzodiazepines, amphetamine-type stimulants
Use of the wrong drug for a specific condition requiring drug therapy	Tetracycline in childhood diarrhoea
Use of drugs with limited evidence of efficacy	Anti-motility agents in acute diarrhoea
Use of drugs of uncertain safety status	Cytotoxic drugs
Failure to provide available, safe and effective drugs	Failure to vaccinate against measles or tetanus
Use of correct drugs with incorrect administration, dosages and duration	Use of IV when suppositories or oral formulations would be appropriate
Use of unnecessarily expensive drugs	Use of a third-generation, broad spectrum anti-microbial when a first-line, narrow spectrum agent is indicated

Source: adapted from WHO (2004).

antibiotics. The patterns of irrational drug use and irrational prescribing are shown in Table 20.3.

Some medications used in general health care are inherently unsafe and these are manifested through cases of adverse drug reactions (ADRs), which may result in serious harm, increased hospitalisations and consume a proportion of the health budgets. In a study by Pirmohamed *et al.* (2004) the drugs most commonly implicated in causing in-patient admissions included low dose aspirin, diuretics, warfarin and non-steroidal anti-inflammatory drugs other than aspirin, the most common reaction being gastrointestinal bleeding. The impact of this irrational use of drugs may lead to increased morbidity and mortality. Studies show that as much as 18% of serious, preventable adverse drug events occur because health care practitioners do not know enough about the patient before prescribing, dispensing and administering medications. (Smetzer & Cohen, 2001, Smetzer *et al.*, 2003). The incidence of adverse drug reactions would increase because of the increased availability of, and exposure to, psychoactive and non-psychoactive substances.

Factors underlying the irrational use of medication

There are many different perceptions and factors that affect the irrational use of psychoactive substances and other drugs. The variations from culture to culture can affect the way drugs are prescribed and used. The underlying irrational use of drugs can be categorised as those deriving from patients, prescribers, the workplace; the supply system, including industry influences; regulation; drug information and misinformation; and combinations of these factors (WHO, 2004). In Figure 20.1 the major factors underlying irrational use of drugs are outlined.

Some of the underlying problems that are associated with medication errors include: inadequate communication; lack of competencies among health care professionals; the number of drugs and complexity of medication per patient; wrong diagnosis; lack of disclosure of information on self-medication of non-prescribed drugs; and the process of prescribing, dispensing and administering drugs. Currently, medication errors are being addressed by the Government (Department of Health, 2004). The impact of inappropriate use of drugs or psychoactive substances is shown in Figure 20.2.

Medication management

Medication is essential for those with serious and enduring mental health problems. A whole range of psychotropic medication is prescribed to this population: antipsychotics, antidepressants, anxiolytics and mood stabilisers. Antipsychotic and/or mood stabilising medication is most likely to be the main prescription of medication over the short term to treat acute episodes and over the long

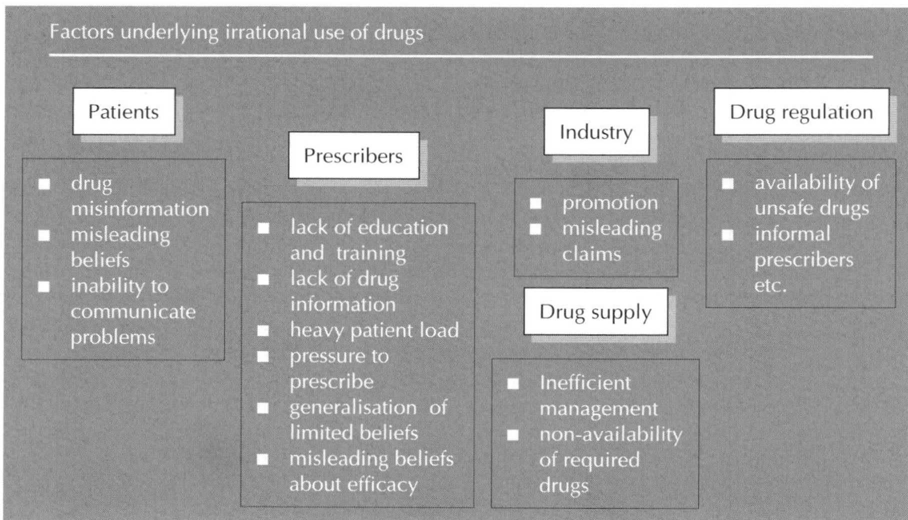

Figure 20.1 Factors underlying irrational use of drugs.
Source: WHO (2004) Promotional rational drug use.

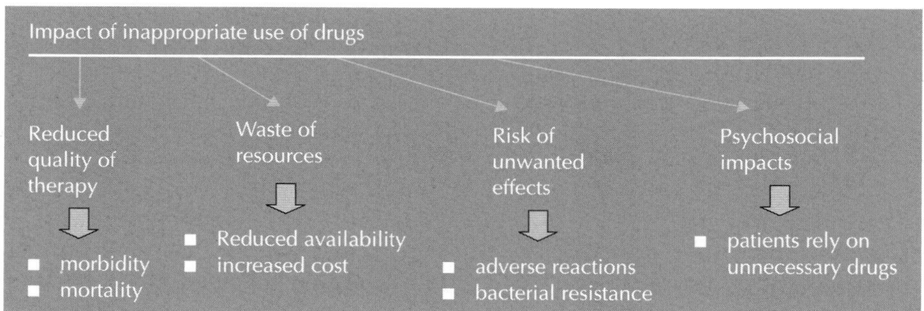

Figure 20.2 Impact of inappropriate use of drugs.
Source: WHO (2004) Promotional rational drug use.

term to prevent relapse. Medication management can include all aspects of supply and therapeutic use of medicines, from individual service user level to the organisational delivery of an entire service (National Prescribing Centre and National Primary Care Research and Development Centre, 2002).

A report by The Standing Nursing and Midwifery Advisory Committee (1999) highlighted that the skills of acute mental health nurses need to be improved through research, training and the development of evidence based policies and guidelines. One of the recommendations includes the management of medication, including detection and alleviation of side effects. Medication management has been defined as the facilitation of safe and effective use of prescription and over-the-counter medicinal products (Bulechek & McCloskey, 1999). This definition embraces the notion of the dangers inherent in both prescribed and over-the-counter medications that can cause serious harm, as well as dependence. Medication management has also been described as a process of promoting and involving service users in treatment decisions, exchanging information and monitoring, evaluating and providing feedback about treatment (Gray *et al.*, 2002). This broad definition is more focused on the active participation of service users in medication management and in enabling the service users to achieve the greatest benefit and best outcomes involving medications. In the context of this chapter, medication management refers to the prescribing, administration and associated health interventions of medications.

Implications for nursing practice

Managing patients' medications involves more than the task of administering medications (Jordan & Reid, 1997; Jordan & Hughes, 1998; Jordan & Griffiths, 2004). The process of rational prescribing and the rational use of drugs includes assessing the health care needs of the patient (making a nursing diagnosis); planning and setting goals for care; administering and monitoring the effects of medications; providing patient education and discharge planning; interdisciplinary collaboration; evaluating desired and adverse effects of medications and documenting the process (Latter *et al.*, 2000; Manias & Street, 2000). Intervention strategies to promote self-medication and harm reduction skills would be an added value of the component of medication management. The rules for medication management are presented in Table 20.4.

Table 20.4 Rules for medication management.

- Engage service users in a comprehensive assessment of their physical and mental health
- Take a drug and alcohol history
- Inform and educate service users and carers of the purpose of medication
- Give information on benefits and risks of proposed medication (orally and in writing)
- Facilitate concordance by agreeing a care/treatment plan with the service user
- Prescribe safely and appropriately within the scope of current evidence and guidelines
- Make sure informed consent has been given and is ongoing
- Administer safely
- Monitor outcomes systematically
- Initiate regular reviews
- Maintain clear communication with service users and their carers
- Maintain clear communication across service interfaces and between practitioners
- Teach self-medication skills
- Promote harm reduction strategies
- Maintain professional competence

Source: adapted from White (2004).

Good practice in medication management requires interpersonal and process skills (National Prescribing Centre, the National Institute for Mental Health in England and the Department of Health, 2005). The use of interpersonal skills includes use of open-ended questions, reflective listening, and eliciting, summarising and responding to feedback. The process skills include working collaboratively, agreeing a clear agenda in meeting service users and emphasising personal choice and responsibility. A number of techniques have been shown to be useful in medication management. These techniques enable service users to explore and discuss their medications. A summary of the skills and techniques is presented in Table 20.5.

Part of the nursing assessment process is the inclusion of a comprehensive history taking of prescribed and non-prescribed psychoactive substances (including drugs and alcohol) and over-the-counter medications. The goals of accurate history taking are to identify current and previous use of psychoactive substances and other medications, the potential risks for adverse drug reactions and the provision of health education in the rational use of drugs. In addition, nurses will be involved in making an informed choice in defining effective and safe treatments (drugs and non-drugs), in selecting appropriate drugs, dosage and duration, and in writing a prescription in consultation with the multidisciplinary team.

The *Guide to Good Prescribing* (De Vries *et al.*, 1994) provides a series of steps in rational prescribing. These include defining the patient's problem, specifying the therapeutic objective, verifying whether treatment is suitable for the patient, starting the treatment, giving information, instructions and warnings and monitoring (stopping) the treatment. The prescription process often makes for irrational and inconsistent use of psychoactive drugs in clinical practice. In Table 20.6, the criteria underlying rational use and rational prescribing are presented.

The skills and techniques of problem solving,

Table 20.5 Medication management key skills.

Key Skills	Examples
Problem solving	Dealing with practical problems with medication • What is the problem? • How would you like things to be different? • What are the possible solutions to the problem? • Action plan
Looking back	Facilitating discussion about past medications • Examine situations and look at what has helped • Examine situations and look at what has not helped • Develop a new action plan
Exploring ambivalence	Having ambivalence about taking medication • Explore the positive aspects of taking and not taking medications • Explore the negative aspects of taking and not taking medications
Beliefs and concerns	Some beliefs and concerns about medication • Examine beliefs and concerns about taking medication
Looking forward	Medication has a negative connotation • Reframe medication as a positive strategy • Identify realistic goals to achieve • Explore how medications may enable service users to achieve the goals
Advanced directives	A plan can be made regarding the type of treatment to prescribe and treatment to be avoided • Copy of plan to service users and carers • Copy of plan in case notes • Awareness of plan by the multidisciplinary team

Source: adapted from National Prescribing Centre, the National Institute for Mental Health in England and the Department of Health (2005).

looking back, exploring ambivalence, exploring beliefs and concerns, looking forward and advancing directives would form part of the ongoing assessment and be included in the care plan.

Table 20.6 Criteria underlying rational use and rational prescribing.

Appropriateness	Decision making
Appropriate indication	The decision to prescribe drug(s) is entirely based on medical rationale and the fact that drug therapy is an effective and safe treatment.
Appropriate drug	The selection of drugs is based on efficacy, safety, suitability and cost considerations.
Appropriate patient	No contraindications exist and the likelihood of adverse reactions is minimal, and the drug is acceptable to the patient.
Appropriate information	Patients should be provided with relevant, accurate, important and clear information regarding their condition and the medication(s) that are prescribed.
Appropriate monitoring	The anticipated and unexpected effects of medications should be appropriately monitored.

Source: WHO (2004).

Addiction and mental health nurses should be aware that there may be an alternative to prescribing and avoid the irrational (unnecessary) use of psychoactive substances. Nursing interventions and non-pharmacological therapies such as counselling, cognitive behavioural therapies, relaxation and other complementary therapies may be used as an alternative to the prescribing of psychoactive substances. Several studies have shown that educating patients in the art of relaxation reduces the need to use hypno-sedatives and tranquillisers (Tilly & Weighillk, 1986; Gournay, 1988). There is consistent data to suggest that individual psycho-educational interventions, cognitive behaviour therapy and family interventions can decrease the risk of relapse in patients with severe mental health problems and may also improve the patient's mental state, at least in the short term (NHS Centre for Reviews and Dissemination, 2000). It is recommended that health authorities should promote the use of culturally relevant and proven complementary or alternative treatment modalities (WHO, 2004). It is argued that whilst focusing on the irrational use of psychoactive drugs, consideration must also be given to the proper use of therapeutic medications (Rassool & Winnington, 1993).

In summary, nurses have important responsibilities for medication management and also for assessing the use and abuse of psychoactive medications. Pain management can be a complex problem in mental health, substance misuse and emergency services because of self-medication. This requires a different set of intervention strategies in dealing with a growing drug seeking population of controlled psychoactive substances (Roscoe, 2004). By effective goal planning and having adequate knowledge and competencies, nurses can plan interventions for preventing and identifying adverse drug reactions, ensuring therapeutic effectiveness of medications and the use of psychoactive substances in a rational way. There is evidence to suggest that good medication management complements and reinforces good prescribing practices and will promote treatment adherence and improve health related clinical outcomes for service users (Gray *et al.*, 2005).

Continuing professional development

With the broadening of prescribing authority that mental health and addiction nurses now have, an added dimension requires nurses to have complex knowledge of psychopharmacology and the nature of psychoactive drug selections. This new prescribing authority also creates demands for the continuing education and professional development of addiction and mental health nurses in order to match service needs. The educational and training programmes based on the competencies identified by the National Prescribing Centre (NPC, 2001), have already commenced for nurse prescribers. With the current focus on medication errors (Department of Health, 2003) and its related costs, the supplementary prescribers must demonstrate these competencies before they will be allowed to prescribe. They will need to meet the 25 competencies stipulated by the Nursing and Midwifery Council (2004). The NPC has developed competency frameworks for both nurse and pharmacist supplementary prescribers (NPC, 2001). The educational programmes consist of 26 to 27 taught days plus 12 days with a designated medical practitioner over 3–6 months in higher educational institutions. Some commentators have remarked that no competencies exist to use as a basis for training or assessing the prescribing ability of undergraduate medical students and medical practitioners. Medical practitioners will be required to act as trainers and supervisors of supplementary prescribers. The NPC's (2001; 2003) key principles that should underpin educational programmes in supplementary prescribing emphasise the:

- Importance of communication between the prescribing partners
- Need for access to shared patient records
- Patient is treated as a partner, involved at all stages in decision making

Several concerns have been raised regarding the quality of training for nurse prescribers, their supervision, ongoing professional support and the identification of the limited knowledge of psychopharmacology (Maslen *et al.*, 1996; Gournay & Gray, 2001; Hay *et al.*, 2004). There is a limited time devoted to psychopharmacology, let alone substance abuse, in the overcrowded undergraduate nursing curriculum. King (2004) used a qualitative approach to explore nurses' pharmacology knowledge on a general emergency admissions ward and noted a gap between theory and practice. It was suggested that greater attention should be paid to pharmacology at the undergraduate level, particularly on groups of drugs and on drug updates following registration. The curricula for undergraduate nursing and health care sciences should also devote more time to exploring medication management and the rational use of psychoactive substances. In general, similar conclusions can be made regarding mental health nurses. It is indicated that medication management training needs to go beyond 'preceptorship' and prepare nurse prescribers for their new responsibilities (Jones & Jones, 2005)

For prescribers in addiction nursing, there is no clarity on the type of training they require. Instead, training is influenced by the extent and scope of their roles. Currently, the competencies set by the NMC (2004) include the principles of prescribing, the practice of prescribing, the accountability and responsibility. The principles of prescribing are holistic assessment, strategy and choice of product; concordance; review of prescription; record keeping; and reflection (NPC, 1999). A supplementary programme in the areas of administration of detoxification medications, side effects of both substances of abuse and prescribed medications, and additional information on substance misuse would meet the training and learning needs of addiction nurses. A training needs analysis is of paramount importance, due to the nature and context of prescribing in-service provisions.

Evidence based practice and research

Evidence based practice and the dissemination of knowledge would further enhance the prescribing authority of addiction and mental health nurses. There is limited literature on the practice of mental health prescribing nurses in the UK and a dearth of research in addiction nursing. To bridge this practice research gap nurses must implement more nursing oriented studies and be proactive in multi-professional and multi-centre studies. Nurse prescribing opens up new opportunities for research that cross the divide between medically and caring oriented studies (Nolan *et al.*, 2004). It is through research that new knowledge can be obtained in order to implement good quality care in clinical practice. However, even when new knowledge is gained, it is difficult to make practicing nurses use research. Implementing research or evidenced based practice is not an individual process but a collective process through partnerships of stakeholders.

Conclusion

This is a selected review of the literature and caution must be exercised because of its limited nature, and also when extrapolating from small studies undertaken with different health care disciplines in different health care systems and contexts. The chapter is meant to set an agenda and illustrate problems that could contribute to the current debate on nurse prescribing in addiction nursing. Nolan *et al.* (2004) suggested that valuable lessons can be learnt from the USA's experiences and hoped that UK nurses are sufficiently astute to incorporate these into their deliberations and learn from them. The implementation of research findings requires more than the dissemination of information. In order to make changes from ritualistic procedures to evidenced based practice, there is a need to create an organisational climate that supports the use of research evidence and establishes the opportunities and processes to apply research. However, it is argued that individual nurses' knowledge about research may not be as important as the process by which organisations implement research (McCleary & Brown, 2003). Addiction nurses in the UK are emerging as a significant specialist partner in providing services that are responsive to health care demands, but they need a specialist identity to meet the divergent and complex health needs (psychiatric disorders and substance abuse) of the service users (Rassool, 2001).

The need for advocacy by nurses is required to promote understanding amongst health care professionals, service users and the public about the potential dangers in the misuse of psychoactive substances and the rational use of prescribed and non-prescribed medications (Rassool, 2004b). Education and training of potential nurse prescribers in specialised service provision in reaching the level of professional competencies are of paramount importance. The main challenge, in the context of rational use of psychoactive substances, is that educational preparation in line with the Nursing and Midwifery Council competencies (2004) would be part of the process of change. Other complementary measures, such as increased clinical supervision, professional support, quality assurance, good practice guidance and policy, increase in the professional development of nurses, improved labelling of medicines and public health education in a socio-cultural context are also part of the fabric of change in improving the quality of life of our patients. Research and evaluative studies are required to assess the competency and effectiveness of nurse prescribing in different specialties.

We need to develop an 'upstream' approach to avoid the pitfalls of the medical profession in producing more iatrogenic disease with the irrational use of prescribing and to commit ourselves in promoting the rational use of psychoactive substances (Rassool, 2005) and good practice in nurse prescribing.

References

Aldridge, S. (2002) Nurse practitioners are a hit with patients. *British Medical Journal*, 324, 819–23.

Association of Nurses in Substance Abuse (1997) *Working with Alcohol and Drug Users*. ANSA, London.

Brooks, N., Otway, C., Rashid, C., Kilty, L. & Maggs, C. (2001) Nurse prescribing: what do patients think? *Nursing Standard*, 15 (17), 33–8.

Bulechek, G.M. & McCloskey, J.C. (1999) *Nursing Interventions: Effective Nursing Treatments*, 3rd edn. W.B. Saunders Company, Philadelphia.

Department of Health (1999) *Making a Difference: Strengthening the Nursing, Midwifery and Health Visiting Contribution to Health Care*. The Stationery Office, London.

Department of Health (2000a) *The NHS Plan: a Plan for Investment, a Plan for Reform*. The Stationery Office, London.

Department of Health (2000b) *A Health Service of all Talents: Developing the NHS Workforce*. The Stationery Office, London.

Department of Health (2002). *Pharmacist to Prescribe for the First Time. Nurses will Prescribe for Chronic Illness*. Press Release 2002/0488, November. Department of Health, London.

Department of Health (2003) *Forms of Nurse and Pharmacist Prescribing and Supply of Medicines*. The Stationery Office, London.

Department of Health (2004) *Building a Safer NHS for Patients: Improving Medication Safety*. The Stationery Office, London.

Department of Health and the Royal College of Nursing (1994) *Good Practice in the Administration of Depot Neuroleptics: a Guidance Document for Mental Health and Practice Nurses*. Department of Health, London.

De Vries, T.P.G.M., Henning, R.H. & Fresle, D.A. (1994) *Guide to Good Prescribing. A Practical Manual*. WHO/DAP/94.11. World Health Organization, Geneva.

Ghodse, A.H. & Khan, I. (1988) *Psychoactive Drugs: Improving Prescribing Practices*, pp. 22–35. World Health Organization, Geneva.

Gournay, K. (1988) Sleeping without drugs. *Nursing Times*, March, 16, 22, 46–9.

Gournay, K. & Gray, R. (2001) *Should Mental Health Nurses Prescribe*? Maudsley Discussion Paper Series No. 11. Institute of Psychiatry, London.

Gray, R., Wykes, T. & Gournay, K. (2002) From compliance to concordance: a review of the literature on interventions to enhance compliance with antipsychotic medication. *Journal of Psychiatric and Mental Health Nursing*, 9 (3), 277–84.

Gray, R., Wykes, T., Edmonds, M., Leese, M. & Gournay, K. (2004) Effect of a medication management training package for nurses on clinical outcomes for patients with schizophrenia. Cluster randomised controlled trial. *The British Journal of Psychiatry*, 185, 157–62.

Gray, R., Parr, A.M. & Brimblecombe, N. (2005) Mental health nurse supplementary prescribing: mapping progress one year after implementation. *Psychiatric Bulletin*, 29 (8), 295–7.

Hay, A., Bradley, E. & Nolan, P. (2004) Supplementary nurse prescribing. *Nursing Standard*, 18 (41), 33–9.

Jones, A. & Jones, M. (2005) Mental health nurse prescribing: issues for the UK. *Journal of Psychiatric and Mental Health Nursing*, 12, 527–35.

Jordan, S. & Reid, K. (1997) The biological sciences in nursing: an empirical paper reporting on the applications of physiology to nursing care. *Journal of Advanced Nursing*, 26, 169–79.

Jordan, S. & Hughes, D. (1998) Using bioscience knowledge in nursing: actions, interactions and reactions. *Journal of Advanced Nursing*, 27, 1060–8.

Jordan, S. & Griffiths, H. (2004) Nurse prescribing: developing the evaluation agenda. *Nursing Standard*, 18 (29), 40–4.

King, R.L. (2004) Nurses' perceptions of their pharmacology educational needs. *Journal of Advanced Nursing*, 45, 392–400.

Latter, S., Rycroft-Malone, J., Yerrell, P. & Shaw, D. (2000) Evaluating educational preparation for a health education role in practice: the case of medication education. *Journal of Advanced Nursing*, 32, 1282–90.

Luker, K., Hogg, C., Austin, L., Ferguson, B. & Smith, K. (1998) Decision making: the context of nurse prescribing. *Journal of Advanced Nursing*, 27, 657–65.

McCleary, L. & Brown, G.T. (2003) Barriers to pediatric nurses' research utilisation. *Journal of Advanced Nursing*, 42 (4), 364–72.

Manias, E. & Street, A. (2000) Legitimation of nurses' knowledge through policies and protocols in clinical practice. *Journal of Advanced Nursing*, 32, 1467–75.

Maslen, C., Rees, L. & Redfern, P. (1996) Role of community pharmacist in the care of patients with chronic schizophrenia in the community. *International Journal of Pharmacy Practice*, 4, 187–95.

Mundinger, M. (2000) Primary care outcomes in patients treated by nurse practitioners or physicians: a randomised controlled trial. *Journal of American Medical Association*, 83, 59–68.

National Prescribing Centre (1999) Signposts for prescribing nurses. *Prescribing Nurse Bulletin*, 1, 1–4.

National Prescribing Centre (2001) *Maintaining Competency in Prescribing. An Outline Framework to Help Nurse Prescribers*. National Prescribing Centre, Liverpool.

National Prescribing Centre (2003) *Supplementary Prescribing: a Resource for Health Care Professionals to Understand the Framework and Opportunities*. National Prescribing Centre, NHS, Liverpool. http://www.npc.co.uk/publications/healthcare resource

National Prescribing Centre and National Primary Care Research and Development Centre (2002) *Modernising*

Medicines Management: a Guide to Achieving Benefits for Patients, Professionals and the NHS: Books 1 and 2. National Prescribing Centre, Liverpool.

National Prescribing Centre, the National Institute for Mental Health in England and the Department of Health (2005) *Improving Mental Health Services by Extending the Role of Nurses in Prescribing and Supplying Medication: Good Practice Guide*. Department of Health, London.

National Treatment Agency for Substance Abusers (2002) *Models of Care for Treatment of Adult Drug Misusers*. National Treatment Agency, London. www.nta.nhs.uk

National Treatment Agency for Substance Abusers (2004) *Research into Practice Series*. National Treatment Agency, London. www.nta.nhs.uk

National Treatment Agency (2005) *Nurse Prescribing in Substance Misuse*. National Treatment Agency for Substance Misusers, London.

NHS Centre for Reviews and Dissemination (2000) Psychosocial interventions for schizophrenia. *Effective Health Care*, 6 (3) University of York, England.

Nolan, P., Sayeed, H.M., Badger, F., Dyke, R. & Khan, I. (2001) Mental health nurses' perceptions of prescribing. *Journal of Advanced Nursing*, 36, 527–34.

Nolan, P., Carr, N. & Doran, M. (2004) Nurse prescribing: the experiences of psychiatric nurses in the United States. *Nursing Standard*, 10 (18), 33–8.

Nursing and Midwifery Council (2004) Diamorphine added to midwives' medicines. *NMC News*, April, p. 16. NMC, London.

Office of Public Sector Information (2001) *Prescription Only Medicines. Order 1997*. HMSO, London. www.opsi.gov.uk

Pirmohamed, M., James, S., Meakin, S. *et al.* (2004) Adverse drug reactions as cause of admission to hospital: prospective analysis of 18 820 patients. *British Medical Journal*, 329 (3 July), 15–19.

Rassool, G.H. (2000) Editorial. Addiction: global problem and global response. Complacency or commitment? *Journal of Advanced Nursing*, 32, 505–8.

Rassool, G.H. (ed.) (2002) Dual diagnosis: substance misuse and psychiatric disorders. Blackwell Science, Oxford.

Rassool, G.H. (2002) Substance misuse and mental health: an overview. *Nursing Standard*, 16 (50), 46–52.

Rassool, G.H. (2004a) Curriculum model, course development and evaluation of substance misuse education for health care professionals. *Journal of Addictions Nursing*, 15, 85–90.

Rassool, G.H. (2004b) Prescription for change: perspectives on prescribing authority for addiction nurses in the United Kingdom. *Journal of Addictions Nursing*, 15, 1–5.

Rassool, G.H. (2005) Nursing prescription: the rational use of psychoactive substances. *Nursing Standard*, 19 (21), 45–51.

Rassool, G.H. & Winnington, J. (1993) Using psychoactive substances. *Nursing Times*, 89 (47), 38–40.

Rassool, G.H. & Gafoor, M. (1997) Themes in addiction nursing. In: *Addiction Nursing: Perspectives on Professional and Clinical Practice* (Rassool, G.H. & Gafoor, M., eds). Stanley Thornes, Cheltenham.

Rodden, C. (2001) Nurse prescribing: views and autonomy and independence. *British Journal of Community Nursing*, 6 (7), 350–5.

Roscoe, M.S. (2004) The drug-seeking patient: undertreated pain or underhanded motives? *Clinician Reviews*, 14 (2), 51–8.

Smetzer, J. & Cohen, M.R. (2001) Instilling a measure of safety into those 'whispering down the lane' verbal orders. The Institute for Safe Medication Practices (ISMP). *Medication Safety Alert!*, 6, 1–2.

Smetzer, J.L., Vaida, A.J., Cohen, M.R., Tranum, D., Pittman, M.A. & Armstrong, C.W. (2003) Findings from the ISMP Medication Safety Self-Assessment® for Hospitals. *Joint Commission on Quality and Safety Journal*, November, 29, 11.

The Standing Nursing and Midwifery Advisory Committee (1999) *Mental Health Nursing: 'Addressing Acute Concerns'*. Department of Health, London.

Tilly, S. & Weighillk, V.E. (1986) How nurse therapists assess and contribute to the management of alcohol and sedative drug use among anxious patients. *Journal of Advanced Nursing*, 11, 499–503.

White, J. (2004) Medication management. In: *Good Practice in Adult Mental Health* (Ryan, T. & Pritchard, J., eds), p. 95. Jessica Kingsley Publishers, London.

Wilhelmsson, S. & Foldevi, M. (2003) Exploring views on Swedish district nurses' prescribing: a focus group study in primary health care. *Journal of Clinical Nursing*, 12, 643–50.

World Health Organization (1989) *Report of the WHO Meeting on Nursing/Midwifery Education in the Rational use of Psychoactive Drugs*. DMP/PND/89.5. WHO, Geneva.

World Health Organization (2004) *Promoting Rational Drug Use. A CD–Rom Training Programme in collaboration with Boston University School of Public and International Health*. WHO, Geneva.

21 Spiritual and Cultural Needs: Integration in Dual Diagnosis Care

A. Hammond & G.H. Rassool

Introduction

The ideology behind the modernisation of the National Health Service in the UK is the provision and delivery of effective and accessible health care services to all, regardless of race, ethnicity, religion, sex or national origin. *National Service Framework, The NHS Plan* and *Your Guide to the NHS* (Department of Health, 1999, 2000, 2001) provide national standards for respect for privacy and dignity, religious beliefs and people's spirituality. These are the shared values of all the UK health care regulatory bodies. The Human Rights Act, introduced in October 2000, enshrines in law the right of the individual to religious observance. This underlines the need for NHS trusts to provide appropriate world faith representatives and worship spaces for faith communities within the health care population. The National Institute for Mental Health in England (NIMHE) is working on a project with the Mental Health Foundation to produce a report on the 'Importance of spirituality in a whole person approach to mental health'. The aim is to provide a framework of good practice to encourage mental health professionals to engage with the spiritual dimension of client groups. The *Good Practice Guide* (Department of Health, 2002a) on meeting the religious and spiritual needs of patients sets a framework for the context and provision of chaplaincy spiritual care services throughout the NHS and offers guidance about providing spiritual care that is equal, just, humane and respectful.

The total care concept or holistic approach is also emphasised within the guidelines of the international and national nursing bodies for nurses and other health care professionals, to recognise and respect the uniqueness and dignity of each patient or client, respect the patient or client as an individual and respond to their need for care (ICN, 1973; UKCC, 1992; NMC, 2002). A holistic approach to care recognises spirituality as the thread that joins the biological, physical and psychological together; one cannot be treated without the other. A biopsychosocial approach to care is recommended when working with those with a dual diagnosis (Checinski, 2002); this includes the spiritual dimension (Hammond, 2003).

Most nursing models of care advocate the need to meet the total or holistic care of the individual, but have not incorporated the spiritual dimension into their theoretical frameworks (Rassool, 2000). The holistic approach involves meeting the physical, social, psychological and spiritual needs of the patient. In addition, the 'legal need' is also of importance for some substance misusers or those with dual diagnosis. In clinical practice, this frequently means catering for the physical and psychological needs of patients, to the exclusion of the spiritual needs (Oldnall, 1996). There is evidence to suggest that spiritual care is often poor, infrequent or non-existent (Granstrom, 1995; Taylor *et al.*, 1995; Oldnall, 1996). Nurses are reluctant to include the spiritual dimension within their practice as a result of inadequate preparation, lack of self-spiritual awareness, problems with the assessment of spiritual need, fear of imposing personal beliefs on the client, uncertainty about personal, spiritual and religious beliefs/values and believe that spirituality does not lie within the domain of nursing (Carson, 1989; Taylor *et al.*, 1995; Oldnall, 1996; Pullen *et al.*, 1996; Swinton, 2001).

It has been acknowledged that patients' psychosocial, spiritual and cultural values affect how they respond to their care (JCAHO, 2003). Research suggests that those who practice a religion have less than average substance misuse problems, marriage breakdown, loneliness, sexual promiscuity, and mental and physical health problems (Fontana, 2003; Miller & Thoresen, 2003). A study by McDowell *et al.* (1996), exploring spirituality and the dually diagnosed, surveyed 101 patients in an in-patient dual diagnosis unit. The authors reported that the clients believed spirituality to be an essential part of their recovery and they wanted more groups focused on spirituality and more access to religious services.

Historical background

Before the enlightenment, it was generally thought that a person's fate was determined by the gods; that psychoactive substances had supernatural powers and that mental illness as other illnesses was a punishment by the gods or bad spirits (Escohotado, 1999; Porter, 2002). Psychoactive substances were used as medicine and shamans and medicine men used them to help people enter a trance-like state that they believed allowed them to intercede and expel the bad spirits thought to be causing the illness. They were also used in religious ceremonies and also for pleasure (Escohotado, 1999). The early Greeks warned of the dangers of the use of drugs. Escohotado (1999) quoted from an old Greek text Hist. Pant. IX 11.6 on the prescribing of *Datura metal*, a solanaceous plant:

> 'One administers one drachma, if the patient must only be animated and made to think well of himself; double that, if he must enter delirium and see hallucinations; triple it, if he must become permanently deranged; give a quadruple dose if he is to die' (p. 13).

He also cited from a first-century Chinese medical text that warns:

> 'Hemp taken in excess makes one see monsters, but if used over a long time it can establish contact with spirits and lighten the body' (p. 7).

It seems, therefore, not surprising that the coexistence of substance misuse and mental health problems (dual diagnosis) is not a new phenomenon. Like nowadays, it was probably difficult to distinguish whether a person had a mental illness before their use of drugs, as a result of drug use or had a combined mental illness and substance misuse problem. An example of someone experiencing a mental illness and combined substance misuse can be seen in the following example. It is difficult to determine which problem came first, which highlights the difficulty of making a diagnosis then as now. Porter (2002) describes a gentleman who woke after a heavy drinking session to find he was hearing voices, one of which was telling him to cut off his hair. The gentleman first believed it to be God commanding him to do this, then he decided it was the Devil. He described how his mental state worsened as he continued to experience voices and have visions. Today many clients who are physically dependent on alcohol and in a state of withdrawal will describe similar symptoms.

Despite the enlightenment, there were still many who continued to believe in the power of the supernatural. This was evident in the Inquisition and the witch trials. Many who were mentally ill and/or using drugs and behaving in a way that was not thought to be normal, but heretic, were often thought to be witches and burned at the stake. As the enlightenment grew, the belief in the supernatural was taken out of mental illness and drugs, which gradually brought the witch hunts to an end (Escohotado, 1999; Porter, 2002). Descartes' philosophy, which gave impetus to the enlightenment, separated the mind from the body and became known as Cartesian Dualism (Porter, 2002). As Descartes' followers developed these ideas, Newtonian mechanistic physics and reductionist psychology was born. Scientists and physicians deserted God in favour of the measured, controlled and tested;

therefore, predictive and seen (Whittemore, 1999). Problems in the human body, including mental illness, were thought to be caused by a mechanical breakdown in need of repair (Porter, 2002). Religion and its partner, spirituality, became increasingly divorced from health care. This is in contrast to the East that did not follow this path but continued as they do today to have a holistic view of society and health (Fernando, 2002).

The twentieth century brought the discovery of quantum physics, and scientists are now catching up with those who study spirituality and mysticism as they realise that just because something cannot be seen it does not mean it does not exist; that particles can affect other particles at a distance, and that time and space is relative to the person observing it (Capra, 1982). This more holistic view of the universe has again allowed medicine to develop a more holistic framework, and gives room for the study of spirituality (Capra, 1982) as we become what Beesley (1980) describes as spiritual scientists. The next sections will examine the concepts of spirituality and religion and how these concepts can be integrated into the community care plans of those with a dual diagnosis.

Spirituality, religion and holism

There are a host of critical analyses and definitions of the concept of spirituality in the nursing literature. Spirituality refers to 'that aspect of human existence that gives it its "humanness"'. It concerns the structures of significance that give meaning and direction to a person's life and help them to deal with the vicissitudes of existence. As such, it includes such vital dimensions as the quest for meaning, purpose, self-transcending knowledge, meaningful relationships, love and commitment, as well as the sense of the holy amongst us. A person's spirituality is that part of them which drives them on towards their particular goals, be they temporal or transcendent (Swinton, 2000). This is a broad definition focusing on a number of dimensions of spirituality, but although it includes the religious element, it is not defined by religion, though there are some common elements such as meaning and purpose, a belief in a god, higher power or transcendent dimension, feeling connected to and interconnected with self, others, the environment and the universe (Elkins *et al.*, 1988; Burkhardt, 1989; Goldberg, 1998; McSherry, 2000; Swinton, 2001). When these are well integrated the person may be said to be experiencing spiritual well-being (McSherry, 2000). These experiences and feelings may lead to what Abraham Maslow described as high peak experiences. Such feelings may be described as 'moments of rapture' (Hurding, 1986). Some writers prefer to compartmentalise spirituality, such as Miller (1998, 2002). The characteristics of spirituality (Miller & Thoresen, 2003) are summarised in Table 21.1.

Table 21.1 Characteristics of spirituality.

Behaviours	• Worship attendance • Prayer and meditation
Beliefs	• A belief in God/higher power • Interconnectedness • Life after death
Spiritual values and motivations	• Karma • Love of others • Duty to God
Experiences that might be described as mystical	• Feeling near to God

Source: Miller & Thoresen (2003).

Other writers such as Elkins *et al.* (1988) take a phenomenological approach to the understanding of spirituality that identifies nine dimensions:

(1) Transcendent dimension such as God or higher consciousness
(2) Meaning and purpose
(3) Mission to life such as a sense of vocation or calling
(4) Life is sacred
(5) Appreciate material values but do not believe they are all that matters
(6) Altruism
(7) Idealism
(8) Awareness of the tragic
(9) The fruits of spirituality show in the person's relationship with self, others, nature and whatever is considered the ultimate

Religion and spirituality

The message of all the great religious prophets such as Muhammad, Moses and Jesus (may peace be upon them), was for their followers to lead a spiritual life. From this message social groups gradually rose that engaged in worship, ceremonies, rituals, laws and rites of passage that formed the new religions of the time. These religious groups, then as now, may offer a sense of belonging, support, a common purpose and a moral code.

Religion, as a concept, is perceived by many (in the West) as not being interchangeable with spirituality (Rassool, 2000). In this context, the concept of spirituality has a broader meaning than religion and encompasses philosophical ideas about life, its meaning and purpose (Stoll & Stoll, 1989; Harrison, 1993, Dyson *et al.*, 1997). In the West, it is acknowledged that not every individual who seeks self-awareness, self-empowerment and self-actualisation pursues a particular religious belief or faith (Rassool, 2000). Coyle (2002) differentiates between those who draw their spirituality from the transcendent approach that is based on a belief in God or a transcendent dimension; those who draw their understanding of spirituality from religious beliefs and practices (structural behaviourists); and those who draw their spirituality from personal values that give meaning and purpose to life (value guidance). Spiritual needs may not always be expressed within a religious framework. It is important to be aware that all human beings are spiritual beings who have spiritual needs at different times of their lives. Although spiritual care is not necessarily religious care, religious care, at its best, should always be spiritual (Association of Hospice and Palliative Care Chaplains, 2003). Other writers such as Bradshaw (1994) writing from the Judaeo-Christian perspective and Rassool (2000) writing from the Islam perspective believe religion and spirituality are a way of life and therefore not possible to separate. Information about the major faiths is presented in Table 21.2.

Spirituality/psychology

Swinton (2002) has suggested that there are four central themes that encapsulate the spirituality functions in the process of mental health development and maintenance: interpretative framework, emotional support, source of coping strategies and a sense of community. To explore the difference between the spiritual and the psychological further we need to go back in time and explore the ponderings of the early philosophers and theologians. The following is drawn from Kurtz (2003) who has written that the ancients, as people do now, debated such issues as what leads to a healthy state of mind or wholeness. These early philosophers and theologians agreed that certain behaviours were good and healthy, such as having a sense of responsibility for the community and society.

The early Christians recognised spiritual distress in terms of the 'logismos', which were thought to be ways of thinking that were bad for the health, unwholesome and 'arch enemies of the soul' (Kurtz, 2003). They included feelings of unresolved anger, fear of the future, preoccupation with the past, depression and self pity. Today, such problems are the mainstay of therapeutic work. Also, then, as now, there were and are those who looked outside the self for spiritual or esoteric help and those, such as Protagaras, who thought 'man is the measure of all things' (Kurtz, 2003). Kurtz (2003) comments that the ancients recognised these concepts in terms of 'bad thinking' or 'wrong vision', which was translated as 'seeing things from fear and fantasy rather than as they really are'. The reader will recognise these as what are now known as cognitive distortions and negative thinking (Kurtz, 2003).

People then, as now, sought help from a variety of practitioners, some spiritual, some medicinal (Kurtz, 2003). Today, as we move full circle into a more holistic approach to health, complementary therapies are coming into mainstream treatment and people are using them alongside mainstream medicine. Some experiences cannot be measured, and psychologists such as Carl Jung, Abraham Masow, Stanislav Groff and Ken Wilber developed the transpersonal approach to psychology that recognises that some experiences cannot be explained and go beyond the individual into the super consciousness, the higher self and the metaphysical (Hurding, 1986). It is suggested that there are four ways to psychological and spiritual well-being, depending on an individual's philosophy and belief system; that found in organised religion; medical science; a belief in a god or higher power outside religious affiliation; and those who draw on the self or higher consciousness for their spiritual well-being. With or without a belief in God an

Table 21.2 Religious faiths.

	Belief	Prophet/teacher	Followers	Holy book	Spiritual leader	Place of worship	Festivals	Ceremonies/practices	Diet	Birth	Marriage	Death
Judaism	One God, life after death	Moses	Jews, orthodox, non-orthodox, different movements	The Hebrew bible: Torah	Rabbi	Synagogue (Sabbath: Friday)	Yom Kippur (day of atonement and fasting)	Bar mitzvah (boy, 13yrs), bat mitzvah (girl, 12yrs)	Kosher: meat prepared in a certain way, different utensils for meat and dairy produce	Circumcised eight days after birth, maternal line of descent	Synagogue or open air by Rabbi	Buried within 24 hrs, non-orthodox Jews may cremate
Christianity	One God, life after death	Jesus (Mother of Jesus, the Virgin Mary)	Christians, Catholics, Anglicans, many denominations	Bible: Old Testament, New Testament	Priest, vicar, pastor, elder	Church, hall (Sabbath: Sunday)	Christmas, (birth of Christ Jesus), Easter (resurrection of Christ Jesus)	Baptism, confirmation, Holy communion, anointing of the sick, confession	Some denominations do not take intoxicants	Present new baby to church, baptism, paternal line of descent	In church by priest/vicar, sometimes civil ceremony followed by church blessing	Body washed and placed in a coffin, service followed by burial or cremation
Islam	One God, Allah, life after death	Muhammad	Muslims, Shiah, Sunni	Qur'an (Koran)	Imam	Mosque	Day of Arafat celebrates end of revelations made to Muhammad; Ramadan, month of fasting, Eid Ul-Fitr, end of fast	Ramadan a month of fasting, must not eat, smoke or have conjugal relations from dawn to sunset, Aqiqah, shaving of baby's head at seven days after birth; circumcision any time from eight days old to the age of ten years	Halal meat slaughtered in a certain way while God's name is pronounced, pig is forbidden, as is alcohol	Soon after birth the father whispers the call to prayer in both ears of the baby	Arranged marriage may occur but girl must give her consent	Body ritually washed and wrapped in white shroud, burial takes place because of belief in the resurrection
Hinduism	One ultimate being present in all things, manifests as many gods (e.g. Shiva, Brahman and Vishnu), atman karma, reincarnation	Nil	Hindus	Vedas, Upanishads, Bhagavada-Gita	Swamis, gurus, priests	Temple, home	Divali (festival of light)	Tenth to twelfth day after birth naming ceremony, first, third or fifth year head is shaved leaving a small tuft, idea to remove negative karma brought from previous birth	Strict Hindus are vegetarian, cow is sacred and must not be killed	Eighth month of pregnancy may offer cooked rice to Vishnu, tenth to twelfth day after birth naming ceremony	Strict Hindu parents continue to arrange marriages for their children	Cremation, if possible ashes are scattered on the Ganges
Buddhism	Nirvana	Buddha	Buddhists	Tripitaka	Monks, nuns	Temple	Wesak (Vesakha)	No universal ceremony but others have grown out of the adopted country's ceremonies		Child blessed at local temple	Blessed at the temple by monk following civil ceremony	Funeral very important led by monks, cremation

individual may live according to the spiritual values that underpin all religions and are found in religious and spiritual texts.

Multicultural, multi-ethnic society and multi-faith communities

The UK is a multicultural, multi-ethnic society and has multi-faith communities whose members practice a wide variety of religions. Religious values and beliefs continue to be influential in moulding the way society has developed and is developing. Religious and political persecutions have been one of the reasons why individuals from some countries have sought asylum in the UK. The nursing profession also includes a diverse range of ethnic, racial and cultural backgrounds. This cultural integration makes it very difficult for a nurse, no matter what their background, to know all the different beliefs and practices of all of the religions of the world. Many of the religions are made up of many sects; it would therefore be difficult for any of us to understand all of the different practices and beliefs of all the different religions that we come across. Yet if we are to deepen our understanding of our clients, it is important to increase our understanding of the main religions that may shape their world view.

As nurses, we cannot assume that someone from a particular cultural or ethnic background practices a particular religion. Many people from the Far East and Africa practice Islam or Christianity and many people from the West can be found in the Islamic mosque, the Hindu or Buddhist temple. Many people are turning away from traditional religions but are drawing on Eastern and Western religions, mysticism, Native American religions, early religions and Shamanism. Some call this movement the new age movement. This has enormous implications for psychiatry as we grapple with these issues. Fernando (2002) warns of practising 'psychiatric imperialism', which means trying to impose a Western reductionism viewpoint on an Eastern belief system that has been influenced by a particular religion such as Islam, Hinduism or Buddhism, which are holistic and not open to reductionism. Africa, Native America and Asia do not have a dichotomy between mind and body. Religion, medicine and ethics are integrated. The West views health as a matter of overcoming illness; Asia, Africa and Native America view health, and acceptance of emotions, nature and others, as striving for harmony within and between people, their surroundings, nature, spirits and the cosmos (Fernando, 2002).

Healing: therapeutic relationship

The use of psychoactive substances may offer a fleeting moment of euphoria and relaxation filling the spiritual vacuum, and strong enough to keep the client physically or psychologically dependent, despite the downward spiral of poor physical and psychological health, and deteriorating social circumstances. It is acknowledged that individuals with dual diagnosis may feel ambivalent about change; for the mental health team it means a long-term commitment; change will not happen overnight. The Department of Health (2002a) suggests that a harm reduction approach may be a more realistic goal than expecting total abstinence. Those of us without such problems will to varying degrees take care of our own needs. According to Maslow, it is difficult to appreciate the higher aspects of our nature, such as creativity, whilst we are focused on attending to our basic needs, such as finding food and a roof over our heads (Hurding, 1986). Building a therapeutic relationship is therefore fundamental to helping such clients address all these issues. There are several stages that a client may pass through on their road to leading a drug free life or achieving a goal of total abstinence. These include engagement, motivation (persuasion), active treatment and relapse prevention.

Engaging with the client is fundamental to helping the client change. It is therefore important to develop a relationship with the client. It is this relationship rather than any therapeutic model that could be the key to change (Clarkson, 1996). Writers cited by Hammond (2003) demonstrate the qualities thought to be fundamental to developing a therapeutic relationship: trust, compassion, agape (love of your neighbour, as opposed to romantic love), sensitivity, support, being friendly, accepting and caring, valuing clients, connecting and interconnecting with others and the environment, altruism, sharing with the client, being aware of the client's difficulties and circumstances (Elkins *et al.*, 1988; Anderson & Smereck, 1989; Burkhardt, 1989; Clark *et al.*, 1991; Bradshaw, 1994; Beech & Norman, 1995; Pejlert *et al.*, 2000; Wrigth & Sayre-Adams, 2000; Greasley *et al.*, 2001; Miller, 2002). Rogers (1995) identified four core conditions he believes help develop a counselling relationship: empathy, genuineness, respect and unconditional positive regard. Miller & Thoresen (2003) also suggest being non-judgemental, accepting, empathic; having an openness to listen and understand the client; familiarity with the values, beliefs and practices common to the client's culture and feeling comfortable talking to the client about spirituality.

Assessment

During the process of engagement and as the relationship develops the nurse will be in a better position to explore the client's religious and spiritual beliefs and needs. A spiritual religious assessment can be separated into a brief assessment and a longer, more in-depth assessment. The brief assessment may explore such issues as the client's religious practices, beliefs, special celebrations and religious leader. Bradshaw (1994) suggests that this is a structural functionist approach to spirituality/religion, the nurse being interested in supporting the client by putting them in touch with their religious network and supporting the client in their religious practice. This is about being actively involved rather than just asking after the client's religion. Perhaps no more is needed, as the client, their family and religious leaders will then be in a position to look after the client's spiritual needs. If it is apparent, following this brief assessment, that the client has either lost touch with their religious network or does not practice a religion, a more in-depth assessment can be made that explores the client's religious/spiritual beliefs from the point of view of the client. Bradshaw (1994) calls this the existentialist or sub-division transcendent approach. The former believes the spiritual dwells within the individual and the latter believes in a universal spirit. McSherry (2000) has drawn on work by a number of writers outlining the spiritual needs of a client (Table 21.3). Exploration of these aspects should be conducted by asking open-ended questions without imposing any personal beliefs on the client (Koenig *et al.*, 2001).

Table 21.3 Spiritual needs.

- Meaning and purpose
  Finding a purpose leading to fulfilment.
- Love and harmonious relationships
  Finding comfort, warmth and affection with humans, animals and creation generally.
- Need for forgiveness
  Unresolved anger and guilt may trigger psychological, physical and social problems. To maintain equilibrium there may be a need to resolve conflict and seek forgiveness and forgive.
- Need for source of hope and strength
  Beliefs and values, convictions and commitments that give hope and strength.
- Creativity
  To have the freedom to enjoy and find meaning, expression and value in literature, art, music and other activities, that allow the person to be in contact with their own emotions, communicate and find beauty in creation.
- Trust
  Important part of friendship and therapeutic relationships. Fundamental to existence and communication. Leads to self-worth, feeling valued and accepted.
- Maintain spiritual practices
  To have the freedom to take part in religious spiritual practices such as prayer or meditation, or church attendance, or non-religious spiritual practices, such as a walk that allows for spiritual well-being.
- Express one's own belief in God or a deity
  This may be in the religious sense of a belief in God or a deity or a it may be non-religious, the person finding spiritual motivation within their personal values.
- Ability to express one's own personal beliefs and values
  If this is restricted and suppressed it may lead to frustration and hostility.

Source: adapted from McSherry (2000).

Addressing ambivalence

Clients with a dual diagnosis may be ambivalent about change, they may feel demotivated because of a feeling of spiritual distress. Labun (1988) identified seven experiences that may trigger this: spiritual pain, alienation, anxiety, guilt, anger, loss and despair. McSherry (2000) also adds that when a client's values, belief system, and meaning and purpose they place on life has been challenged then the client may feel uncertain about their life, alone and afraid. A nurse who allows a client to talk about these issues, who values and cares for their client, and in so doing goes some way to increasing the client's self-esteem and self-efficacy, may increase the client's motivation to change (Miller & Rollnick, 1991). Hammond (2003) suggests that one way the nurse can address ambivalence is by helping the client reflect on such issues as what their illness means for them, what drug use means for them, what are their hopes and dreams, and what is blocking them from achieving them. Developing discrepancy may nudge the client into changing and help the client discover the meaning and purpose of their life. Yahne & Miller (2003) suggest that having hope and faith are important aspects of change. As the client makes positive changes, their self-efficacy will increase and they are more likely to continue making positive changes (Bandura, 1977; 1982).

Spiritual and religious problems

On a religious and spiritual esoteric level there are more similarities than differences between the schools of thought. Visions, hallucinations and other symptoms that may be thought of as psychotic phenomena, such as hearing voices, have been reported in religious texts and by eminent writers. The Bible describes the vision St Paul had on the road to Damascus and writers such as William James, Carl Jung (Fontana, 2003) and Bill Wilson, one of the founding fathers of Alcoholics Anonymous (Miller, 2002), have reported mystical, spiritual experiences. Some people might find these experiences rewarding and comforting; some may find them frightening. From time immemorial drugs have been used to trigger mystical experience. Unfortunately, drug use can also trigger a psychotic episode.

It may be difficult, sometimes, to separate what might be a normal religious, spiritual or mystical experience from an abnormal one. Family friends and health care workers may make a wrong diagnosis of a mental illness (Turner *et al.*, 1995). There are also other spiritual religious problems that the nurse or heath care worker might come across, such as a religious conversion, issues that may challenge the person's religious belief system, and bereavement and losses of other kinds. In the past the interpretation of what was normal and abnormal might have been determined by the subjective opinion of the doctor or nurse who might be from a different religious or cultural background and might misinterpret the symptoms. To help reduce making a wrong diagnosis, spiritual and religious problems have been incorporated into the DSM-1V (Turner *et al.*, 1995). Greenberg & Witzum (1991) suggest that psychotic experiences are more intense than religious experiences; are more terrifying and preoccupying; lead to a deterioration in the client caring for him or herself; and the client may believe that they are receiving special messages from religious figures. Lukoff (1985) suggested that the following issues should be taken into consideration during the assessment: good pre-episode functioning; acute onset of symptoms of three months or less; a stressful precipitant and a positive exploratory attitude towards symptoms. Austin (1998) has also differentiated between a mystical and psychotic episode (see Table 21.4).

Healing interventions

Research reviewed by Koenig *et al.* (2001), Fontana (2003) and Miller & Thoresen (2003) indicates that practicing religion or having a particular spiritual belief can have a positive benefit on physical and mental health, and substance misuse outcomes. The reasons for the positive relationship are not clearly understood. Despite this, Koenig *et al.* (2001) and Miller & Thoresen (2003) offer some reasons why this may be so: it provides a powerful source of comfort and hope for those with a chronic mental illness by enabling the individual to improve their functioning, reducing isolation and facilitating healing; individuals are less likely to have substance misusing friends; it offers a set of moral values; it increases coping skills and reduces the likelihood of turning to substances during stressful times. Prayer, meditation, reading religious and inspirational material and attending religious meetings has also been reported by Charters (1999) and Germer (1996), in studies exploring religious/spirituality in those with a mental illness. Germer (1996) also reported attending self-help groups, interacting with children and listening to inspirational music. Many people today use complementary medicine in conjunction with orthodox treatment; this is also true for those experiencing mental health problems. Russinova *et al.* (2002) surveyed clients with a history of mental health problems: those with bipolar affective disorder,

Table 21.4 Mystical path and psychotic episosdes.

	Mystical path	Psychosis in schizophrenia
General nature and duration	An ongoing, more orderly development	May be compressed, disorderly and disorganised
Hallucinatory phenomena	In general, more visual; not threatening	In general, more auditory; can be threatening
Ideas of self-reference	Enlightenment cuts off the personal connotations of stimuli	Stimuli generate ideas of self-reference, especially in paranoid schizophrenia
A gap is experienced that splits outer social reality from inner personal reality	1	3
Inhabiting only the inner world and being fearful of it	0–1	3
Degree of tolerance for inner experiences	Trained for and well tolerated	May be overwhelmed by them
Simplification of lifestyle and renunciation of worldliness	More under conscious control	More under unconscious control
Dissolution of social attachments	1	3
Re-entry into society, improved by the experience	The usual goal	Less common
Subsequent ongoing, fruitful, well-integrated contacts with society	2	1 or 0
Sense of unity with the environment	2 (partially cultivated)	Less commonly perceived
Cravings and aversions	Reduced	May be enhanced
Continued conscious control	Usual	Less effective

0 = none; 5 = maximal.

Source: adapted from Austin (1998).

schizophrenia and depression. The majority of respondents were female, white and employed. The findings indicated that 86% reported multiple practices of complementary/alternative therapies. The most frequently reported were that 50% practised religious/spiritual practices such as prayer, worship, spiritual reading, 43% practised meditation, 31% practised massage, 20% practised yoga, 18% used guided imagery, 16% used herbs, 13% used chiropractic and 13% used nutritional supplements. Other reported practices were aromatherapy, breath work, reiki, t'ai chi, past-life/regression therapy, homeopathy, ayurvedic medicine, acupuncture, acupressure and reflexology. Subjects with schizophrenia were less likely to use meditation and guided imagery, yet Marlatt & Kristeller (2003) have reported a positive experience by a client with a diagnosis of paranoid schizophrenia.

Complementary therapies, such as acupuncture, herbal teas and meditation are often available in substance misuse services. This has implications for those working with those who have a dual diagnosis who may request such treatments. Ryman (1996) also suggests that deep relaxation and visualisation is contraindicated in those with a history of psychosis. Hammond (2003) suggests that if the client requests such therapy the multidisciplinary team should be made aware, information needs to be gathered regarding the contraindication of such therapy and the client should be given this information so that they can make an informed choice. Such information can be gathered from complementary therapy registered bodies (see Rankin-Box, 1996). It is also worth noting that the code of professional conduct warns nurses about practising outside their professional competencies (NMC, 2002).

Art, music, dance and poetry have been an important part of religious practice, worship and healing from the earliest of times (Fontana, 2003). Although pharmacotherapy and cognitive therapy have revolutionised the treatment of mental illness and substance misuse, those with a dual diagnosis may not always respond to such treatments. Less invasive therapy that increases self-esteem is a distraction from problems, improves socialisation, reduces boredom and perhaps gives the client a way of self-expression that will improve self-esteem, confidence and self-efficacy, which may therefore reduce the rate of relapse. Research by Carter *et al.* (1996) reported that playing games or musical instruments, focusing on something other than the voices and listening to songs were methods rated most highly as being partially successful in helping cope with hallucinations. Alcoholics Anonymous is a spiritual based fellowship self-help group. Some fellowship members experiencing a dual diagnosis did not feel the fellowship met their specific needs and therefore set up Double Trouble (Vogel *et al.*, 1998). Groups similar to these that offer spiritual fellowship and support may be worth developing in the UK.

Conclusion

Religion has offered the world spiritual values that have also been adopted by those who do not practice their spirituality through religion and by those who do not believe in a god or a transcendent dimension. Religion may be described as the outward expression of the subjective spiritual experience. Spirituality is a subjective experience that has prompted many definitions, the common elements being a belief in a god, transcendent dimension or higher consciousness; having a meaning and purpose to life; feeling connected to and interconnected with and responsible for others, the environment and the universe. Some of the spiritual dimensions may be classified as psychological, but a step back in time shows that there is a bond in that both the theologian and psychologist have always been interested in the psychological well-being of the individual, one drawing on the divine, the other on the self. As we move into the world of quantum physics, we have discovered that both science and spirituality are compatible, both are working with the unseen and just because it is unseen it does not mean phenomena do not exist, which is what those with a belief in God or the universal spirit have always known. Psychologists and nurses are also realising that the removal of man-made boundaries allows us to work holistically, accepting the transpersonal and the mystical experiences of our clients.

The coexistence of substance misuse and mental health problems is not a new phenomenon and the dangers of psychosis caused by drug use have long been recognised. There have always been those that have turned towards the spiritual for help and those that have turned towards medicine for help, and others who have turned to both. In some ways medicine has replaced the role religion played in earlier times. The utilisation of a biopsychosocial approach to the understanding and treatment of those with a dual diagnosis should include the spiritual dimension. It is the spiritual that is the thread that unites the three fabrics of the biopsychosocial approach.

Spirituality can be integrated into the models of care recommended by the National Treatment Agency (Department of Health, 2002b; 2005). Building a therapeutic relationship based within the spiritual values of being non-judgemental, accepting and offering agape is fundamental to engaging with a client and generating change. It is also important to realise the religious and spiritual values of clients. This chapter suggests a brief assessment to explore the outward behaviours and practices, and liaising with the client's religious and spiritual leaders if appropriate. A more in-depth assessment exploring the client's subjective experience of the spiritual can be undertaken as the relationship builds. The in-depth assessment may include helping the client explore such issues as what meaning and purpose do they think life holds for them. In motivating the client to change, the chapter has offered Miller & Rollnick's (1991) motivational interviewing model and suggests that helping a client explore what their hopes and dreams are and what is blocking them from achieving them may also help motivate change.

Many practitioners, and clients, particularly in substance misuse, realise the limitations of orthodox medicine and are turning to complementary therapies as adjuncts to the orthodox. We cannot ignore this if our work is to be client centred and holistic. There are a variety of treatments on offer, such as cognitive behaviour therapy, family therapy and addressing the client's social and physical needs. We should realise that healing can also take place within less invasive therapies, such as art, dance, music and writing. Healing takes place as the nurse helps the client draw on their own inner resources to find and recognise their full potential. It is within this atmosphere of change that we can reduce relapse and help clients maintain any changes made.

But above all, it must 'entail renewed evaluation and understanding of our own spirituality, and our particular fears and prejudices in relation to spirituality of others, so that the spiritual care we offer is as unbiased and as informed as it can be' (Hollins, 2005). This is a challenge for nurses.

References

Anderson, M.D. & Smereck, G.A.D. (1989) Personalised nursing LIGHT model. *Nursing Science Quarterly*, 2 (3), 120–30.

Association of Hospice and Palliative Care Chaplains (2003) *Standards for Hospice and Palliative Care Chaplains*. AHPCC, London.

Austin, J.H. (1998) *Zen and the Brain*. The MIT Press, Cambridge, Mass., & London.

Bandura, A. (1977) Self-efficacy: towards a unifying theory of behavioural change. *Psychological Review*, 84, 191–215.

Bandura, A. (1982) Self-efficacy mechanism in human agency. *American Psychologist*, 37, 122–47.

Beech, P. & Norman, I. (1995) Patients' perceptions of the quality of psychiatric nursing care: findings from a small-scale descriptive study. *Journal of Clinical Nursing*, 4 (2), 117–23.

Beesley, R.P. (1980) *The Duty of Freedom*. Galilee Series 6. White Lodge Publications, Speldhust, Kent.

Boutell, K.A. & Bozett, F.W. (1987) Nurses' assessment of patients' spirituality: continuing education implications. *Journal of Continuing Education in Nursing*, 21, 172–6.

Bradshaw, A. (1994) *Lighting the Lamp. The Spiritual Dimensions of Nursing Care*. Royal College of Nursing Research Series, Scutari Press, London.

Burkhardt, M.A. (1989) Spirituality: an analysis of the concept. *Holistic Nursing Practice*, 3 (3), 69–77.

Capra, F. (1982) *The Tao of Physics*, 3rd edn. Flamingo, London.

Carson, V.B. (1989) *Spiritual Dimensions of Nursing Practice*. Saunders, Philadelphia.

Carter, D., Mackinnon, A., Copolov, D. (1996) Patients' strategies for coping with auditory hallucinations. *The Journal of Nervous and Mental Disease*, 183 (3), 159–64.

Charters, P. (1999) The religious and spiritual needs of mental health clients. *Nursing Standard*, 13 (26), 34–6.

Checinski, K. (2002) Treatment strategies and interventions. In: *Dual Diagnosis. Substance Misuse and Psychiatric Disorders* (Rassool, G.H., ed.). Blackwell Sciences, Oxford.

Clark, C.C., Cross, J.R., Deane, D.M. &. Lowry, L.W. (1991) Spirituality integral to quality care. *Holistic Nursing Practice*, 5 (3), 67–76.

Clarkson, P. (1996) The eclectic and integrative paradigm: between the Scylla of confluence and the charybdis of confusion. In: *Handbook of Counselling Psychology* (Wolfe, R. & Dryden, W., eds). Thousand Oaks, London & Sage Publications, New Delhi.

Coyle, J. (2002) Spirituality and health. *Journal of Advanced Nursing*, 37 (6), 589–97.

Department of Health (1999) *National Service Framework for Mental Health: Modern Standards and Service Models*. Department of Health, London.

Department of Health (2000) *The NHS Plan*. Department of Health, London.

Department of Health (2001) *Your Guide to the NHS*. Department of Health, London.

Department of Health (2002a) *Mental Health Policy Implementation Guide. Dual Diagnosis Good Practice Guide*. The Stationery Office, London.

Department of Health (2002b) *Models of Care*. Department of Health, London.

Department of Health (2003) *NHS Chaplaincy Meeting the Religious and Spiritual Needs of Patients*. Department of Health, London.

Department of Health (2005) *Models of Care for the Treatment of Adult Drug Misusers. Update*. Department of Health, London.

Dyson, J., Cobb, M. & Forman, D. (1997) The meaning of spirituality: a literature review. *Journal of Advanced Nursing*, 26, 1183–8.

Elkins, D.N., Hedstrom, L.J., Hughes, L.L., Leaf, J.A. & Saunders, C. (1988) Towards a humanistic phenomenological spirituality. Definition, description and measurement. *Journal of Humanistic Psychology*, 28 (4), 5–18.

Escohotado, A. (1999) *A Brief History of Drugs. From the Stone Age to the Stoned Age*, 2nd edn. Park Street Press, Rochester, Vt.

Fernando, S. (2002) *Mental Health, Race and Culture*, 2nd edn. Palgrave, Oxford.

Fontana, D. (2003) *Psychology, Religion, and Spirituality*. Blackwell, Oxford.

Germer, V. (1996) Psychiatric patients of spirituality in a group setting. IMAGE. *Journal of Nursing Scholarship*, 28 (3), 3.

Goldberg, B. (1998) Connection: an exploration of spirituality in nursing care. *Journal of Advanced Nursing*, 27, 836–42.

Granstrom, S. (1995) Spiritual care for oncology patients. *Topics in Clinical Nursing*, 7 (1), 39–45.

Greasley, P., Chiu, L.F. & Gartland, Rev. M. (2001) The concept of spiritual care in mental health nursing. *Journal of Advanced Nursing*, 33 (5), 629–37.

Greenberg, B. & Witzum, E. (1991) Problems in the treatment of religious patients. *American Journal of Psychotherapy*, 45 (4), 554–65.

Hammond, A.E. (2003) Substance misuse and serious mental illness: spiritual care. *Nursing Standard*, 18 (2), 33–8.

Harrison, J. (1993) Spirituality and nursing practice. *Journal of Clinical Nursing*, 2, 211–17.

Hollins, S. (2005) Spirituality and religion: exploring the relationship. *Nursing Management*, 12 (6), 22–6.

Hurding, R.F. (1986) *Roots and Shoots. A Guide to Counselling and Psychotherapy*. Hodder & Stougton, London.

International Council of Nurses (1973) *Code for Nurses, Ethical Concepts Applied to Nursing*. ICN, Geneva.

JCAHCO (Joint Commission on Accreditation of Health Care Organisations) (2003) *Comprehensive Accreditation Manual for Hospitals: The Official Handbook*. Joint Commission on Accreditation of Health Care Organisations, Oakbrook Terrace, Ill.

Koenig, H.G., McCullough, M.E. & Larson, D.B. (2001) *Handbook of Religion and Health*. Oxford University Press, New York.

Kurtz, E. (2003) The historical context. In: *Integrating Spirituality into Treatment* (Miller, W.R., ed.), 4th edn., pp. 19–46. American Psychological Association, Washington, DC.

Labun, E. (1988) Spiritual care: an element in nursing care planning. *Journal of Advanced Nursing*, 13, 314–20.

Lukoff, D. (1985) Diagnosis of mystical experiences with psychotic features. *Journal of Transpersonal Psychology*, 17 (2), 155–81.

McDonald, J. & Rassool, G.H. (1997) Complementary therapies. In: *Addiction Nursing: Perspectives in Professional and Clinical Practice* (Rassool, G.H. & Gafoor, M., eds). Stanley Thornes, Cheltenham.

McDowell, D., Galanter, M., Goldfarb, L. & Lifshutz, H. (1996) Spirituality and the treatment of dual diagnosis: an investigation of patient and staff attitudes. *Journal of Addictive Diseases*, 15 (2), 55–68.

McSherry, W. (2000) *Making Sense of Spirituality in Nursing Practice: an Interactive Approach*. Churchill Livingstone, London.

Marlatt, G.A. & Kristeller, J.L. (2003) Mindfulness and meditation. In: *Integrating Spirituality into Treatment*. (Miller, W.R., ed.), 4th edn. American Psychological Association, Washington, DC.

Miller, W.R. (1998) Researching the spiritual dimension of alcohol and other drug problems. *Addiction*, 93 (7), 979–90.

Miller, W.R. (2002) Spirituality and the treatment of addictions. In: *New Directions in the Study of Alcohol* (Aquarius, E.T.C., ed.), No. 26. New Directions in the Study of Alcohol group, Birmingham.

Miller, W.R. & Rollnick, M. (1991) *Motivational Interviewing. Preparing People to Change Addictive Behaviour*. Guilford Press, New York.

Miller, W.R. & Thoresen, C.E. (2003) Spirituality and health. In: *Integrating Spirituality into Treatment* (Miller, W.R., ed.), 4th edn. American Psychological Association, Washington, DC.

Nursing and Midwifery Council (2002) *NMC Code of Professional Conduct: Standards for Conduct, Performance and Ethics*. NMC, London.

Oldnall, A. (1996) A critical analysis of nursing: meeting the spiritual needs of patients. *Journal of Advanced Nursing*, 23, 138–44.

Pejlert, A., Norberg, A. & Asplund, K. (2000) From a psychiatric ward to a home-like setting: the meaning of caring as narrated by nurses. *Journal of Clinical Nursing*, 9 (5), 689–700.

Porter, R. (2002) *Madness: a Brief History*. Oxford University Press, Oxford.

Pullen, L., Tuck, I. & Mix, K. (1996) Mental health nurses' spiritual perspectives. *Journal of Holistic Nursing*, 14 (2), 85–97.

Rankin-Box, D. (1996) *The Nurses' Handbook of Complementary Therapies*, 2nd edn. Churchill Livingstone, London.

Rassool, G.H. (2000) The crescent and Islam: healing, nursing and the spiritual dimension. Some considerations towards an understanding of the Islamic perspectives on caring. *Journal of Advanced Nursing*, 32 (6), 1476–84.

Rogers, C. (1995) *On Becoming a Person. A Therapeutic View of Psychotherapy*. Houghton Mifflin Company, New York.

Russinova, Z., Wewiorski, N.J. & Cash, D. (2002) Use of alternative health care practices by persons with serious mental illness: perceived benefits. *American Journal of Public Health*, 92 (10), 1600–3.

Ryman, L. (1996) Relaxation and visualisation. In: *The Nurses' Handbook of Complementary Therapies* (Rankin-Box, D., ed.), 2nd edn. Churchill Livingstone, London.

Sayer-Adams, J. (1996) Therapeutic touch. In: *The Nurses' Handbook of Complementary Therapies* (Rankin-Box, D., ed.), 2nd edn. Churchill Livingstone, London.

Smith, H. (1991) *The World's Religions*. Harper, San Francisco and New York.

Stoll, R. & Stoll, I. (1989) The essence of spirituality. In: *Spiritual Dimensions of Nursing Practice* (Carson, V.B., ed.). W.B. Saunders, Philadelphia.

Swinton, J. (2000) *Resurrecting the Person: Friendship and the Care of People with Mental Health Problems*. Abingdon Press, Nashville, Tenn.

Swinton, J. (2001) *Spirituality and Mental Health Care, Rediscovering A 'Forgotten' Dimension*. Jessica Kingsley Publishers, London.

Swinton, J. (2002) Spiritual interventions and future directions for care. In: *Therapeutic Interventions for Forensic Mental Health Nurses* (Kettles A., ed. 2002). Jessica Kingsley Publishers, London.

Taylor, E.J., Amenta, M. & Highfield, M. (1995) Spiritual care practices of oncology nurses. *Oncology Nursing Forum*, 22 (1), 31–9.

Turner, R.P., Lukoff, D., Barnhouse, R.T. & Lu, F.G. (1995) Religious or spiritual problem. A culturally sensitive diagnostic category in the DSM-IV. *The Journal of Nervous and Mental Disease*, 183 (7), 435–44.

UKCC (United Kingdom Central Council) for Nursing, Midwifery and Health Visiting (1992) *Code of Professional Conduct*. UKCC, London.

Vogel, H.S., Knight, E., Laudet, A.B. & Magura, S. (1998) Double trouble in recovery: self-help for people with a dual diagnosis. *Rehabilitation Journal*, 21 (4), 356–64.

Warrier, S. & Walshe, J.G. (2001) Dates and meanings of religious and other multi-ethnic festivals 2002–2005. Foulsham Educational, London.

Whittemore, R. (1999) Natural science and nursing science: where do the horizons fuse? *Journal of Advanced Nursing*, 30 (5), 1027–33.

Wright, S. & Sayre-Adams, J. (2000) *Sacred Space. Right Relationship and Spirituality in Health Care*. Churchill Livingstone, London.

Yahne, C.E. & Miller, W.R. (2003) Evoking hope. In: *Integrating Spirituality into Treatment*. (Miller, W.R., ed.), 4th edn. American Psychological Association, Washington, DC.

22 Dual Diagnosis: Interventions with Carers

D. Manley & L.M. Rayner

Introduction

Falloon *et al.* (1996) define a carer as:

> 'the non-professional person in the community who is most involved with the everyday care of the person, and would be very likely to respond to any request for special assistance at any time, if such a request were made by that person.'

In their study Cresswell *et al.* (1992) stated that 'patients with severe psychotic disorders typically have small social networks containing disproportionately high numbers of relatives'. Other studies have shown that families have an important role to play in preventing readmission to hospital (Becker *et al.*, 1997). Offering supportive social networks to their relative with psychosis and substance misuse problems is an important part of the carer's role. However, supporting someone who experiences mental health difficulties and who takes substances in a problematic way can be a traumatic process. The social networks that carers provide are often in marked contrast to other social, often substance misuse related, networks the dual diagnosis client experiences. Families may be the only non-substance misusing people, other than professionals, that a service user has a relationship with.

In order to contribute this chapter the authors interviewed two separate families who cared for dual diagnosis clients and asked them for their opinions on the difficulties they had experienced and insights into what they felt had helped them to cope. Direct quotes from these interviews have been used throughout this chapter to illustrate the carers' experiences and to reinforce the suggested interventions. The aims of this chapter are to examine the burdens of the family facing dual diagnosis and describe the specific interventions and informal brief interventions with families.

Burden and the Family

> 'His aggression and his attitude were the most difficult things to deal with. He had no concerns about anything.' (E. & R.K., December 2004)

> 'He gets very distressed (when he takes drugs); he starts running around, eyes bulging, and I find dealing with it very difficult at times'. (A.P., December 2004)

Living with and caring for someone with substance misuse and mental health problems can have a profound effect on relatives. There is a comprehensive body of literature concerning the burden faced by families living with a relative who has a serious mental health problem (Creer *et al.*, 1982; Thompson & Doll, 1982; Fadden *et al.*, 1987; Lefley,

1989; Marsh, 1992) and though there is a lack of research with families where a person has both substance misuse and mental health problems, this literature is relevant. There is also the emotional effect. Carers will often feel anxious, fearful of the future, guilty and generally stressed. In addition, there will be an impact on family life in general. There may be constraints on social activities; friends and other relatives may not visit or be invited, due to the difficult behaviour of the service user. Routine household activities may be disrupted and there may be effects on relatives' employment, which may result in financial hardship. Relationships in the family may become strained and there may be an adverse effects on relatives' mental health. Relatives may have to deal with intolerable situations when the service user treats them with anger and disdain, completely disrupts daily life, denies that there is anything wrong and does things that are incomprehensible, distressing, illegal and dangerous.

Friends and families of dual diagnosis clients can find it difficult to cope with the complexity of providing care for such individuals (Graham, 2004). The interplay of mental health and problematic drug or alcohol use can cause an individual to be chaotic and unpredictable in their behaviour. A lack of knowledge and 'urban mythology' about substances of abuse may add to the confusion that carers feel about the effects that substances have upon their relative or friend. Under these circumstances carers may wish to take control of their relative/friend's substance misuse in a desire to be supportive. Recognising that the responsibility for change lies with an individual can be difficult for carers. Allowing the service user to develop their own motivation to change their drug-taking may be viewed by carers as tantamount to condoning substance misuse. The practitioner can have a central role in supporting and educating the family in supporting their relative to develop and maintain the motivation to change.

Confidentiality

The issue of confidentiality is often used by practitioners as a reason for not involving families as much as relatives would like. Clearly all professionals working in mental health services are bound by law and professional codes of conduct to a duty of confidentiality to their service users. The sensitive nature of mental health problems and substance misuse means that there can be particular difficulties in relation to confidentiality and the sharing of information. However, as current policy emphasises the importance of close collaboration between practitioners and families, confidentiality should not be used as a reason not to listen to the views of relatives and other informal carers. Also, it cannot be used as an excuse not to discuss with service users the need for their family to receive information so they can continue to support them.

Furlong & Leggatt (1996) suggest that dealing with the question of confidentiality presents the opportunity for practitioners to build quality relationships with both service users and their families. They report that services and practitioners who have a positive attitude to families do not generally experience problems with confidentiality. The Royal College of Psychiatrists, as part of their Partners in Care campaign, have produced a leaflet, *Carers and Confidentiality in Mental Health* (Royal College of Psychiatrist, 2004), which describes some specific examples of confidentiality issues and provides examples of good practice that may help to address them.

Background to family intervention

Over the past 30 years considerable research has been undertaken into interventions that can help families dealing with the difficult and stressful situations that can occur as a result of someone in the family having a serious mental illness. Initial studies in the late 1960s and early 1970s focused on the effect of family atmosphere on the course of schizophrenia. The term 'high expressed emotion' (high EE) was used to describe the responses of criticism and over involvement displayed by some family members to their relative. It was discovered that service users living with relatives that displayed these characteristics were more likely to relapse (Brown & Rutter, 1966; Brown *et al.*, 1972). Various studies have investigated whether a specific family intervention could reduce these levels of expressed emotion in family members that would then in turn prevent relapse in the service user. Studies undertaken by Falloon *et al.* (1982; 1985), Leff *et al.* (1982; 1985), Hogarty *et al.* (1986; 1991), Tarrier *et al.* (1988; 1989) showed that specific family interventions were effective in reducing relapse, compared to a control group.

However, family interventions of this sort have been criticised for a number of reasons. The concept of expressed emotion has been criticised for making families feel blamed. Though family work researchers have always been keen to emphasise that in their approach families are not seen as the cause of the illness, critics suggest that as high EE is seen as a factor that maintains mental illness, families may feel negatively labelled and alienated (Hatfield *et al.*, 1987). Johnstone (1993) criticises family intervention for its emphasis on compliance with medication. More recent family intervention studies have had less spectacular results in relapse prevention (Telles *et al.*, 1995; Szmuker *et al.*, 1996). A recent Cochrane review (Pharoah *et al.*, 2004) suggests that family intervention is less 'potent' in the hands of the second-generation researchers in comparison to their predecessors who developed the approach.

When we look specifically at dual diagnosis, with the exception of the study by Haddock *et al.* (2003), no research has examined families of individuals with both mental health and substance misuse problems. In fact, some studies identify substance misuse problems as exclusion criteria (Hogarty *et al.*, 1986; Glynn *et al.*, 1992; Linszen *et al.*, 1996; Hogarty *et al.*, 1997; Schooler, 1997). In Haddock *et al.* (2003) service users with dual diagnosis were randomised to either a treatment group of a motivational intervention, individual cognitive behavioural therapy (CBT) and family intervention, or a control group who received routine care. Results from the study demonstrated that there were significant improvements in service user functioning in the treatment group over the control at 18 months. However, there were no significant differences in the carer groups, though there was a trend towards a statistically significant difference on the carer needs measure for the group who received family intervention. Family intervention consisted of between 10 and 16 sessions, with a median of 11. The authors suggest that as the intervention was relatively short, a more intensive intervention is required to show statistical significance.

Research into family intervention has been influential in policy formation, for example *The National Service Framework for Mental Health* (NSF) (Department of Health, 1999). This ensures that carers have an assessment of their needs on an annual basis and they have a written care plan. The National Institute for Clinical Excellence (NICE) guidelines for schizophrenia advocate that family interventions should be available to the relatives of people with schizophrenia who are living with or who have close contact with the service user (NICE, 2002). The length of the intervention should normally be six months and include more than ten sessions. Therefore, as many of the service users will have substance misuse problems, family intervention will be offered to this group.

Family intervention: what is it?

There are various models of family intervention: Falloon *et al.* (1982), Hogarty *et al.* (1986), Barrowclough & Tarrier (1992), McFarlane *et al.* (1995), Kuipers *et al.* (2002). However, all these models have a number of key elements in common (World Schizophrenia Fellowship, 1997; Fadden, 1998).

- Serious mental illness is conceptualised as a condition with a neurobiological aetiology. A stress-vulnerability model is used to explain how, in a vulnerable person, stresses can bring on a psychotic illness or a relapse.
- Comprehensive approaches to care and treatment are provided. Family intervention is provided as part of a care package.
- An alliance is developed between family members, the service user and practitioners. Relatives are not blamed but viewed as therapeutic agents.
- There is a focus on working collaboratively: families and service users are seen as experts in dealing with mental illness and information about the illness is shared.
- Families and service users are seen to have both strengths and needs: strengths are used to tackle problems that the family is facing. A behavioural or cognitive behavioural approach is used to develop goals.

Which families are suitable for structured therapeutic approaches?

Though the NICE guidelines (2002) advocate that family interventions should be offered to all families who are living, or who have close contact, with a relative who has schizophrenia, many services will have to prioritise the families with the greatest needs. Kuipers *et al.*, 2002 advocate the use of a 'rule of thumb':

(1) Relatives living with patients who relapse more often than once a year despite being compliant with maintenance neuroleptics
(2) Relatives who frequently contact staff for reassurance or help
(3) Families in which there are repeated arguments that lead to verbal or physical violence, and any family that calls in the police
(4) A single relative, usually the mother, looking after a person with schizophrenia on her own

By using these criteria, practitioners will identify families where the service user has mental health and substance misuse problems.

Getting started – engagement

Families, despite facing difficult stressful situations, are often reluctant to engage in structured family work. There are various reasons for this. Families may have had negative experiences of previous contact with mental health professionals. This may be real or perceived. They may feel they are to blame for the illness and the situation they find themselves in. By agreeing to family interventions, they may also feel that they are admitting to having failed in some way. Families may have incorrect perceptions about family interventions. They may have a fear of being 'analysed' and that the work will entail an analysis of family dynamics and relationships.

In order to overcome difficulties with engagement, practitioners should approach families, giving them clear information about what the process will entail. Meeting with the whole family can be useful at this point, or meeting individually with family members, including the service user, may be more helpful for some. Whichever approach is used, the information given should provide an overview of what regular 'family meetings' would entail. It can be helpful to use this more informal term rather than 'family work' or 'therapy', which may have more negative connotations. As well as giving a verbal explanation, a written summary of the sessions and what they can expect should be left with the family.

There may be instances where some members of the family agree to the intervention, whereas others opt out. In this case, practitioners should go ahead with the meetings with those who are willing and leave the invitation open to the others to join at any stage. In the instance where service users decline, but other family members are keen, the meetings can go ahead, but practitioners and the family should be aware that the service user's absence will have an effect on the effectiveness of the intervention. It can be useful if the care coordinator discusses the issues concerning family meetings with the service user. Again the invitation to join should be left open.

Working in pairs

Advocates of family interventions recommend that practitioners should work in pairs with families. Though this may have resource implications, the advantages outweigh the disadvantages (Gamble & Brennan, 2000; Kuipers *et al.*, 2002). By working in pairs practitioners will be able to share the work in the meetings. Families can be powerful and at times overwhelming. Working in pairs, practitioners provide two views of the work and they also model how two people can work together. During family meetings it is important for all family members to feel supported; this can be difficult for one worker to achieve. In pairs, each practitioner can form alliances with different family members, to ensure that their views are heard and taken seriously (Leff & Gamble, 1995). Sometimes family meetings can get heated and families can get sidetracked; in these situations two workers can ensure that the focus is maintained and emotions are contained.

Assessment of families

Assessment of individual service users is the vital cornerstone on which all care and interventions are based. Similarly, assessment is a vital step in family intervention. Though practitioners, particularly the care coordinator, will have some idea of the challenges that the family is facing, it is important that enough information is obtained to develop an overall picture or case formulation for the family. Information covering the following areas should be obtained:

- Understanding: the family's level of understanding about the illness and the links with substance misuse
- Coping: how each family member copes with the stress that they are facing
- Distress: the sources of distress for each family member
- Dissatisfaction: what areas of family life they would like to change
- Strengths: what have they got going for them as a family, what resources have they got now or have used in the past

Both structured and informal assessment strategies can be used to build up this formulation, which can then be used to structure the family meetings. There are various structured family assessment tools, two of the most used and well known are the 'Relative assessment interview' and the 'Knowledge about schizophrenia interview' (Barrowclough & Tarrier, 1992).

The 'Relative assessment interview' is a semi-structured interview completed with individual relatives. It covers the following seven areas:

- Background to the service user and the family
- Background information and contact time
- Current problems/symptoms
- Irritability or quarrels in the household
- Relatives' relationships with the service user
- Effect of the illness on relatives

'Knowledge about schizophrenia' is a structured interview that covers the following areas:

- Diagnosis
- Symptomatology
- Aetiology
- Medication
- Course and prognosis
- Management
- Drug and alcohol use

Routine assessment that is undertaken as part of the care programme approach may be sufficient to ensure that the formulation contains the service user perspective. However the 'Knowledge about schizophrenia interview' can be adapted to be used with the service user and practitioners may find it helpful to use a structured mental state assessment like the KGV assessment scale (Krawiecka *et al.*, 1977).

The meetings

Following the assessments and the development of the formulation, regular family meetings are commenced. Meetings are usually held once a fortnight and last for an hour. Generally, the meetings are held in the family home. If the service user is not living with their family, the practitioners will need to negotiate with the family the most suitable venue. Family intervention uses an outreach model, so practitioners go out to visit the family, rather than expecting them to attend a team base for meetings. Usually, the first few meetings start with providing a psycho-education component. This seems to help the engagement process and can be a less contentious area to start with, rather than immediately starting with complex issues.

The meetings, regardless of the stage of family intervention, have a set format, starting with a review of events since the last meeting, planning the meeting, reviewing any tasks that the family may have undertaken since the last meeting, working through the agenda, setting a task to do before the next meeting and summarising the session. In order to ensure that the meeting runs smoothly, maintains its focus and that all family members are heard and supported it can be useful to introduce some ground rules or guidelines. Kuipers *et al.* (2002) suggest the following ground rules will help improve communication in the family:

- Only one person speaks at a time
- Talk to the person, not about them
- Speaking time should be shared out

Practitioners can introduce these ground rules at the beginning of the work, or they can be introduced when the need arises, that is if the family tend to all talk at once, or if one person tends to dominate the meetings. Additional ground rules can be established that meet the specific needs of family members. An example of this is where a service user tended to dominate meetings by talking about their voices; it was agreed that five minutes at the beginning of the meeting would be allocated to talk about the voices, but after this he would not mention them again in the meeting.

Psycho-education

This element of family intervention must be delivered flexibly to ensure that the needs for information are met for all family members. There will often be different levels of understanding about the illness and in particular its relationship with substance misuse problems. It can be useful to go through some education material quite formally with the family, but allowing time for questions and for the service user to relate the information to their own experiences. This can be important, as it can be the first time that family members have heard about the service user's own experience of psychosis. It is vital that at this stage information is included about substance misuse. Basic information about current knowledge of the role of drug-taking in mental health problems, particularly cannabis use in the cause of schizophrenia, should be included. Many families believe that their relative's mental health problems have been directly caused by drug misuse.

Psycho-education also provides the opportunity to discuss treatment and support options not only for the mental health problems but also for the problems of substance misuse. The meetings should provide an opportunity for the service user to talk about the reasons why they misuse substances. Often families are unaware that their relative is self-medicating against the distressful effects of psychotic experiences or the side effects of medication. Practitioners must handle this sensitively, ensuring that the service user does not feel pressurised into talking about or defending their substance misuse, and that the family listen carefully and are supportive. Practitioners can also stress that the treatment approach to the substance misuse is not necessarily one of total abstinence. The role of the family in supporting their relative and the treatment package can also be introduced at this stage.

Problem solving

Following a number of sessions focusing on psycho-education, family interventions move on to tackle the specific issues that they have identified. Using a specific problem-solving framework, the family is helped to identify specific areas of their family life that they would like to change. Practitioners guide them through the problem solving steps (Kuipers *et al.*, 2002):

- Specify in detail what the problem is
- Get everyone's view on the problem, particularly the service user's
- Elicit possible solutions
- Look at the pros and cons of each possible solution
- Compromise and agree on a desirable solution
- Anticipate any obstacles
- Spell out exactly what is to be done, how, by whom, where and when
- Assign the solution as a task that is to be completed before the next meeting

When working with families, where the service user has substance misuse problems, it is often these issues that are implicated in the problems that the family wishes to look at. One family, including the service user, identified the service user's difficulty in budgeting their benefits as causing some hardship to the family and causing tension. On gaining the specific detail of the problem, it was found that the service user spent most of his benefit on buying drugs and this also had a negative effect on him, as he had no spare cash to buy other things he needed, or to go out. Working through the problem-solving framework, the service user identified one possible solution: that of giving his mother some of the money to save in a building society account for him. When looking at the pros and cons of this solution, both his mother and a brother pointed out that there could be an argument when he pressurised his mother into withdrawing the money, when he was desperate to go and buy drugs. This discussion, conducted in an atmosphere that fostered support as well as challenge, allowed the service user to become aware of the impact his behaviour was having on his family. Later in the meeting family members suggested that he should try to reduce his drug use, which he agreed to do. Between meetings, as part of an inter-sessional task, he spoke to his care coordinator about possible strategies to do this. Other family members also helped in his efforts to reduce his drug misuse, by going out with him, something that had not been done for a number of years.

Problem solving can be a difficult and lengthy process; families can become disheartened when change is slow and improvement is not obviously apparent. Practitioners must foster optimism and hope (Drake *et al.*, 1993), highlighting even small changes in the client's attempt to control their substance misuse. Family interventions should complement the service user's care package and the family should be encouraged to support the staged interventions model, particularly as part of the problem solving process.

Family/carer support

Families may decline the offer of formal therapeutic interventions for the reasons outlined above. Support should still be offered, however, which though it may be less structured and informal, can be provided by mental health practitioners. This informal support should follow the principles inherent in structured family work, and will comprise similar interventions such as psychoeducation and problem solving.

> 'I felt initially that everybody didn't want to know. It was, oh that's horrible – I don't want that to touch my life. Everybody, friends, it was just a horror situation. You would go to one agency. They would say, "No, I'm sorry this is a psychiatric problem"; you would go to another agency and they would say it was a drug problem and I'd just be shouting for help when he was clearly very ill! Suddenly the dual diagnosis team appeared and it was like . . . yes! Somebody understands what I am saying here.' (A.P., December 2004).

Johnson (1997) has stated that, traditionally, service development in the UK is not structured to meet the specific needs of the dual diagnosis client group. The same could be said of the service's ability to meet the needs of carers, judging by the above quotation. The isolation that a carer can feel is illustrated by A.P.'s quote above. The carer interviewed clearly states that she has a need for continued support which she eventually received from a practitioner who was operating within an integrated model. There are, however, a number of important factors dictating the type of support offered.

Maintaining regular contact

> 'I think having somebody that you can ring up occasionally really helps. I did try one of these drug helplines, but I found it absolutely hopeless. You would get another mother like myself on the other end who was manning the line and you would just have another person's problems and stories. I'd think to myself, this is not what I want to hear now. What I needed was for somebody to be positive. Somebody to say, "right this is what is happening". Perhaps have some idea of a plan that you can work to so that you feel that you are not just wading through a quagmire as well.' (A.P., December 2004)

Contact should be provided regularly and consistently and will often include brief interventions, such as information giving, boundary setting and informal feedback. Informal support is not necessarily restricted to one-to-one or face-to-face contact. Access to someone to speak to on the telephone can be beneficial, as can email, and may provide vital support in times of crises. However, as the quote above illustrates, the service provider needs to be aware of the particular complex and distressing problems that caring for an individual with a dual diagnosis can pose. Mainstream drug or mental health telephone support/helplines may be able to offer appropriate help at times to carers of dual diagnosis clients. However, it is the authors' experience that in many cases the support offered does not meet the specific needs of carers whose relative/friend experiences substance misuse and severe mental health problems. The person or clinician who provides support, therefore, needs to be knowledgeable and empathic of the particular problems dual diagnosis poses.

Mainstreaming

> 'N.'s mental health care coordinator was a "family man" and he would come and see us quite

regularly. He would talk to us and since he was an artist himself, he and N. had a connection. N. enjoyed talking to him about art and he took him out to art exhibitions and got him more interested in work. He also kept talking to him about the effects of cannabis . . . He was fantastic, really good.' (E. & R.K., December 2004)

This quote reflects a central tenet of the Department of Health MHPIG (2002). The Department of Health have stated that mental health services should have the responsibility of supporting clients with dual diagnosis. They also maintain that integrated care or 'mainstreaming' is important. This means that a single person or team adapts both mental health and substance misuse approaches to meet the client's needs. This approach demands that the practitioner has a multitude of skills in both mental health and substance misuse which they can adapt to meet the needs of their clients. These skills would also be invaluable when working informally with carers and families.

Boundary setting

Families may find it difficult to identify and maintain strict boundaries in relation to substance misusing behaviour. These may in turn have concomitant effects on any boundaries the family have set in relation to behaviours associated with mental health. The altruistic desire to prevent their relative from getting into trouble, particularly criminal justice problems, can lead carers into breaching their own personal boundaries in order to help their relative. This help, whilst well meant, can lead to the steady erosion of previous boundaries and lead to confusion in the caring role. The practitioner has a role to play in helping the family establish boundaries to behaviours.

For example, it is not uncommon in the authors' experience for a carer to help their relative to procure drugs, by giving them money or even taking them to buy substances. This is often justified as a way to prevent the client from coming into harm from dealers, the criminal justice system or because the carer feels that if the client were to withdraw from drugs they may be at harm. However this 'help' is likely to reinforce the client's lack of responsibility in taking drugs. If, alternatively, the carer refuses to accept any responsibility, or help with acquiring drugs, this reinforces the client's responsibility and may eventually lead to positive changes to their substance misuse. This process of setting boundaries can be difficult for carers to adhere to as it may result in the deterioration of the client's situation. However, it is important to recognise with the carer that change in substance misuse is often engendered by a need to change, often caused by unpleasant experiences (for example being arrested). An empathic, supportive approach in helping the carer to explore these issues is most likely to result in appropriate boundary setting.

Structure and flexibility

The importance of *structured* family interventions has already been outlined in this chapter. However, informal carers' support does not necessarily need to be isolated to one-to-one unplanned individual sessions. Informal groups may also provide welcome release and sharing of ideas between peers and families. By engaging carers in this way practitioners may still leave the option of structured family intervention open at a later date.

Conclusion

Families provide support to their relatives 24 hours a day, often without a break; they are rarely given guidance on how to deal with strange and or problematic behaviour. The complexities that substance misuse combined with mental health problems can present to carers often further reinforce their feelings of helplessness and isolation. Practitioners need to be proactive in offering support and information.

> 'You do feel actually very alone and you feel as though you are battling with all of these problems, health, mental health and drugs. I feel that it was extremely helpful to have somebody to talk to'. (A.P., December 2004)

Some families/carers may benefit from a formal structured intervention, whereas others require more informal support. Whatever approach is adopted, a collaborative, integrated approach, which is optimistic of positive change, needs to be maintained over a long period.

The authors would like to extend their thanks to the relatives who took part in the interviews, which helped to structure and inform the content of this chapter.

References

Barrowclough, C. & Tarrier, N. (1992) *Families of Schizophrenic Patients: Cognitive Behavioural Interventions.* Chapman & Hall, London.

Becker, T., Thornicroft, G., Leese, M. *et al.* (1997) Social networks and service use among representative cases of psychosis in south London. *British Journal of Psychiatry*, 171, 15–19.

Brown, G.W. & Rutter, M. (1966) The measurement of family activities and relationships: a methodological study. *Human Relations*, 19, 241–63.

Brown, G.W., Birley, J.L.T. & Wing, J.K. (1972) Influence of the family on the course of schizophrenic disorders: a replication. *British Journal of Psychiatry*, 121, 241–58.

Creer, C., Sturt, E. & Wykes, T. (1982) The role of relatives. In: Long-term community care: experience in a London borough. *Psychological Medicine* (Wing, J.K., ed.) Monograph Supplement, 2, 29–39.

Cresswell, C.M., Kuipers, L. & Power, M.J. (1992) Social networks and support in long-term psychiatric patients. *Psychological Medicine*, 22, 1019–26.

Department of Health (1999) *National Service Framework for Mental Health.* HMSO, London.

Department of Health (2002) *Mental Health Policy Implementation Guidance; Dual Diagnosis Good Practice Guide.* Department of Health, London.

Drake, R.E., Bartels, S.J., Teague, G.B., Noordsy, D. & Clark, R.E. (1993) Treatment of substance abuse in severely mentally ill patients. *The Journal of Nervous and Mental Disease*, 181, 10.

Fadden, G. (1998) Family intervention. Chapter 8. In: *Serious Mental Health Problems in the Community: Policy, Practice and Research.* (Brooker, C. & Repper, J., eds) Baillière Tindall, London.

Fadden, G., Bebbington, P. & Kuipers, L. (1987) The burden of care: the impact of functional psychiatric illness on the patient's family. *British Journal of Psychiatry*, 150, 285–92.

Falloon, I.R.H., Boyd, J.L., McGill, C.W., Razani, J., Moss, M.B. & Gilderman, A.M. (1982) Family management in the prevention of exacerbations of schizophrenia: a controlled study. *New England Journal of Medicine*, 306, 1437–40.

Falloon, I.R.H., Jeffery, L.B., McGill, C.W. *et al.* (1985) Family management in the prevention of the morbidity of schizophrenia: clinical outcome of a two-year longitudunal study. *Archives of General Psychiatry*, 42, 887–96.

Falloon, I.R.H., Magliano, L., Graham-Hole, V. & Woodroffe, R. (1996) The stress of caring for disabling mental disorders in a home-based rehabilitation service. *Journal of Nervous and Mental Disease*, 184 (6), 381–4.

Furlong, M. & Leggatt, M. (1996) Reconciling the patient's right to confidentiality and the family's need to know. *Australian and New Zealand Journal of Psychiatry*, 30, 614–22.

Gamble, C. & Brennan, G. (2000) Working with families and informal carers. Chapter 11. In: *Working with Serious Mental Illness* (Gamble, C. & Brennan, G., eds). Baillière Tindall, London.

Glynn, S.M., Randolph, E.T., Eth, S. *et al.* (1992) Schizophrenic symptoms, work adjustment and behavioural family therapy. *Rehabilitation Psychology*, 37, 323–38.

Graham, H. (2004) *Cognitive-Behavioural Integrated Treatment (C-BIT). A Treatment Manual for Substance Misuse in People with Severe Mental Health Problems.* John Wiley and Sons, Chichester.

Haddock, G., Barrowclough, C., Tarrier, N. *et al.* (2003) Cognitive behavioural therapy and motivational intervention for schizophrenia and substance misuse. *British Journal of Psychiatry*, 183, 418–26.

Hatfield, A.B., Spariol, L. & Zipple, A.M.C. (1987) Expressed emotion: a family perspective. *Schizophrenia Bulletin*, 13, 221–6.

Hogarty, G.E., Anderson, C.M., Reiss, D.J. *et al.* (1986) Environmental/personal indicators in the course of schizophrenia research group. Family psychoeducation, social skills training and maintenance chemotherapy in the aftercare treatment of schizophrenia. *Archives of General Psychiatry*, 43, 633–42.

Hogarty, G.E., Anderson, C.M., Reiss, D.J. *et al.* and the Environmental-personal Indicators in the Course of Schizophrenia Research Group (1991) Family psychoeducation, social skills training and maintenance chemotherapy in the aftercare of schizophrenia. II. Two-year effects of a controlled study on relapse and adjustment. *Archives of General Psychiatry*, 48, 340–7.

Hogarty, G.E., Kornblith, S.J., Greenwald, D. *et al.* (1997) Three-year trial of personal therapy among schizophrenic patients living with or independent of family. I. Description of study and effects of relapse rates. *American Journal of Psychiatry*, 154 (11), 1504–15.

Johnson, S. (1997) Dual diagnosis of severe mental illness and substance misuse: a case for specialist services? *British Journal of Psychiatry*, 171, 205–8.

Johnstone, L. (1993) Family management in schizophrenia. Its assumptions and contradictions. *Journal of Mental Health*, 2, 255–69.

Krawiecka, M., Goldberg, D. & Vaughan, M. (1977) A standardised psychiatric assessment for rating chronic psychotic patients. *Acta Psychiatrica Scandinavica*, 55, 299–308.

Kuipers, L., Leff, J. & Lam, D. (2002) Family work for schizophrenia, 2nd edn. Gaskell, London.

Leff, J., Kuipers, L., Berkowitz, R., Eberlein-Fries, R. & Sturgeon, D. (1982) A controlled trial of social interventions in the families of schizophrenic patients. *British Journal of Psychiatry*, 141, 121–34.

Leff, J., Kuipers, L., Berkowitz, R. & Sturgeon, D. (1985) A controlled trial of social intervention in the families of schizophrenic patients: two-year follow-up. *British Journal of Psychiatry*, 146, 594–600.

Leff, J. & Gamble, C. (1995) Training of community psychiatric nurses in family work for schizophrenia. *International Journal of Mental Health*, 24 (3), 76–88.

Lefley, H.P. (1989) Family burden and family stigma in major mental illness. *American Psychologist*, 44, 556–60.

Linszen, D., Dingemans, P., Van der Does, J.W. *et al.* (1996) Treatment, expressed emotion and relapse in recent onset schizophrenic disorders. *Psychological Medicine*, 26 (2), 333–42.

McFarlane, W.R., Lukens, E., Link, B. *et al.* (1995) Multiple-family groups and psycho-education in the treatment of schizophrenia. *Archives of General Psychiatry*, 52, 679–87.

Marsh, D.T. (1992) *Families and Mental Illness: New Directions in Professional Practice*. Praeger, New York.

National Institute for Clinical Excellence (NICE) (2002) *Schizophrenia. Core Interventions in the Treatment and Management of Schizophrenia in Primary and Secondary Care*. National Institute for Clinical Excellence, London.

Pharoah, F.M., Rathbone, J., Mari, J.J. & Streiner, D. (2004) Family interventions for schizophrenia (Cochrane Review). In: *The Cochrane Library*, Issue 1. John Wiley & Sons Ltd, Chichester.

Royal College of Psychiatrists (2004) *Carers and Confidentiality in Mental Health*. Royal College of Psychiatrists and The Princess Royal Trust for Carers' Partners in Care campaign. RCP, London. www.partnersincare.co.uk

Schooler, N.J., Keith, S.J., Severe, J.B. *et al.* (1997) The effects of dose reduction and family treatment. *Archives of General Psychiatry*, 54, 453–63.

Szmuker, G.I., Herrma, H., Coulsa, S., Benson, A. & Bloch, S. (1996) A controlled trial of a counselling intervention for caregivers of relatives with schizophrenia. *Social Psychiatry Psychiatric Epidemiology*, 31, 149–55.

Tarrier, N., Barrowclough, C., Vaughan, C. *et al.* (1988) The community management of schizophrenia: a controlled trial of behavioural interventions with families to reduce relapse. *British Journal of Psychiatry*, 153, 532–42.

Tarrier, N., Barrowclough, C., Vaughan, C. *et al.* (1989) Community management of schizophrenia: a two-year follow-up study of a behavioural intervention with families. *British Journal of Psychiatry*, 154, 625–8.

Telles, C., Karno, M., Mintz, J. *et al.* (1995) Immigrant families coping with schizophrenia. Behavioural family intervention vs. case management with a low-income Spanish-speaking population. *British Journal of Psychiatry*, 167, 473–9.

Thompson, E.H. & Doll, W. (1982) The burden of families coping with the mentally ill: an invisible crisis. *Family Relations*, 31, 379–88.

World Schizophrenia Fellowship (1997) *Strategy Development. Family Interventions Work: Putting the Research Findings into Practice*. A report of the World Schizophrenia Fellowship. World Schizophrenia Fellowship, Christchurch, New Zealand.

23 Psychological Approaches in the Treatment of Dual Diagnosis

K. Barry

Introduction

It has now been stated that the number of people who suffer with enduring psychotic illness and who misuse substances is increasing yearly and much faster than the increases in the general population (Williams & Farrell, 2004). It has also been reported that as many as six out of ten people who misuse psychoactive substances suffer from a mental illness; also, research suggests between 25 and 60% of people with mental illnesses also have substance use disorders. The problem of substance misuse is now in a central position in mental health services and cannot continue to be the domain of a distant specialty (Appleby, 2000). It has been observed that doctors and other health professionals are rather poor at taking substance misuse histories in primary care, general hospital and mental health settings (Barnaby *et al.*, 2003).

This chapter aims to give the reader an overview of current thinking in relation to the treatment of the dually diagnosed client from a social learning, cognitive behavioural perspective. In this chapter dual diagnosis is used to describe people who have a mental disorder and who also have a problematic substance use. This use does not need to be at a dependence level and includes alcohol.

Integrated model

People with dual diagnosis have complex inter-related needs at varying levels; therefore, assessment and treatment should be integrated to address mental disorder, substance use and in some cases offending behaviour. People with dual diagnosis also often have complex social needs, such as unemployment, homelessness, violence and childhood trauma (Scottish Advisory Committees on Drug Misuse and Alcohol Misuse, 2003). Integrated treatment designed for those with dual diagnosis must support an approach based on assertive community treatment, and specific services must provide treatment for both disorders without cross referral to other agencies (Abdulrahim, 2001).

We also need to be sensitive to client experiences and streamline assessment procedures to avoid patients repeatedly having to tell their story, and give the same information to many different people. Therefore, services should encourage joint assessment and review information sharing procedures. A holistic approach to care is needed for the complexity of the dually diagnosed patient. Pharmacology and psychotherapeutic interventions need to be delivered hand in hand. Recent research has shown that clozapine was effective in reducing alcohol and drug misuse in patients with schizophrenia (Drake *et al.*, 2000). The introduction of the care programme approach (CPA) in mental health services in the UK should allow for an improvement in integrated care for the dually diagnosed client.

Social learning theory

Although originally formulated by Rotter (1954), social learning theory is generally associated with the American psychologist Albert Bandura (Hollin, 1990). This may be considered an interactionist theory. That is, the person, environment and behaviour all interact with each other to exert influences in all directions. The theory includes concepts derived from classical and operant conditioning, but it moves beyond these to assign importance to 'person factors', particularly cognitions (McMurran, 1997).

Operant conditioning

This refers to behaviour that is controlled by its consequences. Those that increase the frequency of the behaviour are termed reinforcers, and the behaviour that was instrumental in producing these consequences is said to be reinforced (Orford, 1985). For example, a person injecting cocaine (behaviour) gets an initial rush (reinforcer), because the rush is pleasant (positive reinforcer) the person may inject cocaine again (behaviour reinforced).

Intermittent reinforcement (non-receipt of reinforcer with each performance, but intermittently) results in stronger associative conditioning, and is therefore harder to extinguish. For example, someone who uses amphetamines (behaviour) receives reinforcement for this behaviour (getting a rush), and is likely to buy amphetamines in future. On subsequent uses, they may not get the same rush; however, at some point it is probable that use will receive reinforcement and the behaviour is therefore intermittently reinforced; this is similar to playing a one-armed bandit. The gradient of reinforcement is a phenomenon that helps to explain the paradox between the repeated use of substances that appear to produce harm or punishment in the long run. Behaviour may have both rewarding and punishing consequences, but it is the immediate consequences that are important in shaping habitual behaviour (Orford, 1985). For example, a cigarette smoker enjoys the proximal consequences of relaxation that outweigh the distal consequences of potentially developing certain types of cancers.

Secondary reinforcers help us to explain why certain people may take substances they do not enjoy or that act as punishers. For example, a young man on a stag night may drink whisky, which he detests, but he does so for the secondary reinforcing consequences of being part of the party where the rest of his peers are drinking whisky. The action of a drug as a primary positive reinforcer or a negative reinforcer to escape or avoid unpleasant situations could be responsible for the maintenance of drug-using behaviour (Orford, 1985).

Classical conditioning

The principles of classical conditioning are based on the work by Ivan Pavlov (1849–1936) and refer to learning by association. Pavlov noted in his experiments with dogs that they had learned to associate the sound of food bowls with the presentation of food, and would respond by salivating. The importance of the conditioned response in the addiction field is that specific stimuli, through being so often paired with substance use, may eventually elicit a desire to indulge in substance use (McMurran, 1997). For example, a cannabis smoker who regularly smokes whilst playing Mozart, walks down the high street and passes a shop playing the 'Magic Flute'. This serves as a cue, or discriminative stimulus, for cannabis smoking behaviour. Cue exposure used in relapse prevention is a technique where the therapist exposes the client to the discriminative stimuli that trigger the desire to indulge, but prevents the occurrence of the behaviour by breaking the association between the two (Table 23.1). These so-called cues can be known as discriminative stimuli.

The traditional operant and classical theories are reinforced by the environment; however, social learning theory uses the concept of motivation. Motivation can take three forms:

- External reinforcement
- Vicarious reinforcement
- Self reinforcement

Table 23.1 Coping strategies used in cue-exposure therapy.

- **Passive delay:** the client waits out the craving; cravings naturally dissipate over time.
- **Imagining negative consequences of substance use:** personally relevant negative outcomes are used as a focus to extinguish the cues (for example taking amphetamines has resulted in admission to hospital).
- **Imagining positive consequences of not taking substances:** personally relevant positive outcomes of not taking drugs/alcohol are used as a focus to extinguish the cues (for example 'I would have a better relationship with my family if I stopped drinking so much').
- **The craving is imagined to be an object**, such as a piece of paper, which can be screwed up and thrown away.
- **Imagining engaging in incompatible activities:** instead of responding to craving by taking the drugs the client imagines engaging in an incompatible activity, for example going swimming.
- **Mastery:** the client employs mastery statements that they can initially use verbally in practice but that they graduate on to using as a thought, for example 'I can beat this' or 'Jim stopped, so can I'.

Source: after Monti & O'Leary (1999).

External reinforcement is outlined in the section on operant and classical conditioning. Vicarious reinforcement is outlined in social learning theory and holds that behaviour can also be learned through observing the behaviour of other people, and particularly the consequences of such behaviour. Consequences that receive social reinforcement rather than punishment are more likely to lead to imitation by the observer. For example, a child may observe the effect that alcohol has on its parent's consumption of wine in the evenings at home for several years. The observed consequence of this behaviour may be that the parents become giggly. As a result of these observations, very few people come to their first drug experience completely inexperienced. This vicarious reinforcement may be one of initiation into substance use, as the person has developed certain expectations about a substance before actually using it.

Moral reasoning/self regulation

Bandura (1997a) also discusses moral reasoning, which refers to changes in moral judgements by changes in criteria for intentions. Moral judgements involve a complex process of considering and weighing various criteria in a given social situation. Thus, moral judgements are expected to be much more variable from time to time and from situation to situation (Miller, 1989). Moral judgements may be influenced by many factors: peers, long-range consequences, expected punishment or reward, past learned behaviour, or the environment as a whole. For example, a teenager may use amphetamines in the company of friends on a Friday night but does not use them when sitting down to eat Sunday dinner with grandparents.

Moral reasoning is one factor in a person's self-regulation, where people will commit themselves to a particular goal and evaluate their performance in relation to the goal. They will reward themselves with self-satisfaction if they attain their standard, but be dissatisfied and even punish themselves if they fail to attain it (Bower & Hilgard, 1981). For example, a heavy drinker may set a goal of abstinence, but a stressful event leads them to take a drink one day. They have failed at the goal of abstinence, and therefore punish themselves by continued drinking. The result is dissatisfaction with the self and leads to the development of a belief that they are useless for failing to maintain the goal. This phenomenon relates to the work of Marlatt & Gordon (1985) on the abstinence-violation effect.

Self-reinforcement

Self-reinforcement refers to a sense of pride, achievement or meeting one's own behavioural standards, and motivates the individual to behave similarly in the future (Hollin, 1990). For example, a person may have experienced a hard day at work and reward themselves with a large brandy. This experience may be rewarded in the future with the same behaviour.

Another important aspect of observational learning within social learning theory is that of modelling. Modelling is of particular importance in the initiation of drinking, and to a lesser extent, drug-taking (Velleman, 1996).

Self-efficacy

Self-efficacy is the strength of a person's belief in their effectiveness and ability to control actions in ways that create desired outcomes (Bandura, 1997b). A person's self-efficacy beliefs can be dependent on the following three factors:

- Magnitude: the perceived difficulty of the task
- Strength: the confidence of the performer in their ability to perform the task
- Generality: whether or not success in a given task is likely to generalise to success in other tasks

Expectations

Modern adaptations of learning theory place a larger emphasis on cognitive factors, such as expectations, than was the case with earlier, more behavioural learning theories (cited in Orford, 1985). Bandura (1997a) states that three factors determine a person's behaviour:

- The expectations the individual holds about the outcomes of the behaviour
- The value that the individual places on those outcomes
- The nature of the situation in which the person is behaving

These three factors underpin the cognitive behavioural view that man is an active and basically self-controlling organism, and that individuals process information and make decisions about their lives and their behaviour on the basis of that information (Velleman, 1996). For example, patients have often said to the author that they use cannabis to manage auditory hallucinations (expectancy), that they cannot function when suffering from voices, that cannabis is the only thing that helps (importance of outcome) and this usually happens when they are alone (situation).

As can be seen, these expectancies can lead to the maintenance of use and, perhaps in the case of the dually diagnosed, problematic use. Social learning theory is based on experimental evidence (Rassool, 1998). In this day of evidence based practices, utilising cognitive behavioural therapy from a social learning perspective may help the clinician provide proven methods of treatment.

Assessment

Assessment has been defined as a process designed to reach a thorough understanding of a person's problems in the overall context of their life, with the object of developing a treatment plan that stands the best chance of being helpful (WHO, 2002). Assessment is an integral part of treatment; right from the outset the assessor can use motivational techniques when assessing the dually diagnosed. Before we progress any further, the point must be made that whatever model of assessment or treatment the clinician uses, it will fail if they do not build a therapeutic relationship with the client. Clinicians must modify their assessments according to the client's mental stability. Assessment should be viewed as an opportunity to engage the patient, thus enabling a therapeutic relationship to be developed and to assess and harness motivation to change.

Once an assessment has been completed, a formulation of a hypothesis about the development and maintenance of substance use and its relationship with the patient's mental illness disorder can be completed; this can be termed as a case conceptualisation.

Cognitive behavioural therapy

Social learning theory gave rise to the cognitive revolution and in the clinical field has led to the development of many cognitive behavioural therapies. Cognitive behavioural therapy (CBT) aims to modify maladaptive thoughts that contribute to inappropriate behaviour or emotional states. Cognitive behavioural therapy for psychosis has developed rapidly in the past 25 years. CBT is now one of the best evidenced psychological treatments for schizophrenia (NICE, 2002). CBT for psychosis suggests that although psychosis may have an underlying biological origin, the symptoms are determined by environmental, cognitive, somatic and behavioural factors, which can be modified.

In CBT the clinician and the patient work together to reach an understanding of:

- The patient's beliefs and underlying assumptions about themselves, others and the world
- How these affect the patient's current behaviours, feelings and daily functioning
- Goals to be identified
- Agreeing on a shared treatment plan

It is possible to integrate motivational and cognitive behavioural treatment programmes for people

Table 23.2 Five general principles of motivational interviewing.

	Roadblocks
Express empathy: • Acceptance • Reflective listening • Ambivalence is normal Develop discrepancy: • Amplification of any discrepancies, create cognitive dissonance between present behaviour and set goals of the individual • Individual should present arguments for change • Awareness of consequences is important Avoid argumentation: • Arguments can lead to reluctance to change • Resistance is a signal to change strategies • Labelling is unnecessary Roll with resistance: • Respect for the individual • Perceptions can be shifted • New perspectives are welcomed but not imposed Support self-efficacy: • Belief in the ability to change • The individual is responsible for choosing and carrying out change • A range of alternative approaches	Ordering Directing Commanding Giving advice Lecturing Labelling Arguing Probing Judging Shaming Aggressiveness

with a dual diagnosis (Table 23.2) Treatment programmes should match the individual's needs, to help the client achieve their optimum level of functioning. This can be on an individual level, or in groups, or both. Another factor when deciding upon treatment is whether treatment can be offered in the community or whether the individual's needs warrant treatment within a hospital unit.

The use of motivational strategies, such as weighing up the pros and cons of using substances and the pros and cons of not using substances, can be one method used by the clinician to help the client look at the cost-to-benefit ratio of their drug use. Once the client has recognised that there may be more cost than benefit to their drug use, they may become motivated to want to make some change in relation to their substance use (see

Table 23.3 The pros and cons listed below are from patients with dual diagnosis.

Pros of taking the substance	Cons of taking the substance
Euphoria, it feels good Feels like I fit in and belong Have fun with others Worries go away Makes me feel better Gives me confidence	Lose family and friends Become ill No money Voices and paranoia Hospital No job No home More fights Lose respect of others
Pros of stopping substance	**Cons of stopping substance**
Healthier both physically and mentally More money Earn trust and respect of family and friends No need for crime to get money for substances Stay out of prison Stay out of hospital Find a partner who cares Get a place to live More prospects for employment	Fun element gone Have to find different friends Need to find different places to go Have to face up to dealing with situations and feelings without taking substances Finding something to replace the substances

Table 23.3). The use of diaries can be useful, not only as a means of self-reporting how much of a substance or substances an individual is using within a specified time, but they can also be used to identify substance related beliefs. In fact both of the above methods can be used in identifying substance related beliefs.

Discussing a person's substance use expectations may help in challenging beliefs associated with the relationship between their mental illness, symptomatology and substance use, thus opening the door for exploration of alternatives to using substances. Learning problem solving skills may be one way in which the individual can increase their self-efficacy. Problem solving will allow the person to think through situations and plan steps to take in advance of a situation that has caused them difficulties in the past. Table 23.4 is an example of problem solving where the clinician has helped a dually diagnosed client to:

Table 23.4 An example of some guidelines for problem solving.

(1) Identify the problem
- Be specific about the problem to address.
- What kind of problem is it?
- Who is involved?
- At what times is it a problem?
- Make sure that the problem you are addressing is not made up of lots of different problems; if it is then follow the process for each.

(2) Brainstorm all possible solutions to the problem
- Generate a list of solutions to the problem.
- Do not discard anything the patient may say even if it is an outrageous solution to the problem.

(3) Evaluate the possibility of using each solution
- Evaluate all possible solutions, weighing up the pros and cons for each.
- Reject those not suitable.
- Look at the ones that are left.
- Rank the solutions from least helpful to most helpful.

(4) Decide on which solution to use
- Take your first choice solution.

(5) Implement the chosen solution
- In very specific terms decide to implement the chosen solution.
- Decide upon who is going to do what, where, when and how?

(6) Review the success of the solution
- If successful, great.
- If not successful, go back to stage 4 and try again.
- In real life situations always have a back-up solution in case your first choice does not work.

- Identify the problem
- Brainstorm all possible solutions to the problem
- Evaluate the possibility of using each solution
- Decide on which solution to use
- Implement the chosen solution
- Review the success of the solution

Relapse prevention

Relapse prevention for the dually diagnosed client utilises a cognitive behavioural framework to help the individual maintain the goal they may have achieved in relation to changing their substance use. The interventions used should allow the client to explore high-risk situations that may lead to relapse into problematic substance use. Identifying triggers of mental illness relapse are also explored. Including partners, carers or others who care for and who are close to the dually diagnosed client in the relapse prevention programme can strengthen a relapse prevention plan. Family engagement in targeted treatment plays an important part in helping people with dual disorders decrease substance use (Clark, 2001). Kavanagh (1992) stated that stressful family relationships are connected with high levels of relapse.

Within the framework the following subjects are discussed and plans developed on how to manage them:

- Education about substances and their effects (especially on mental illness).
- The identification of high risk situations that may lead to substance use or/and destabilisation of mental state.
- Becoming aware of the difference between a lapse and a relapse and ways of learning from a slip.
- How to recognise urges and cravings; understand the difference between the two and develop coping strategies to deal with them (cue exposure).
- Look at and discuss what lifestyle changes may help in the individual maintaining their desired goal.
- Learning alternative coping strategies to substance use, for example distraction techniques, relaxation techniques, anger management, anxiety management, problem solving, managing auditory hallucinations and other psychotic symptomatology relevant to the individual.
- Identification of dysfunctional beliefs about prescribed medication, illness and substance use.
- Develop a lifestyle balance.
- Identification of people who can help and where to go for help.

For more in-depth reading on relapse prevention see Marlatt & Gordon (1985).

Conclusion

Nurses are at the coalface of patient care, and spend more direct time with the patient than any other clinical profession. This puts the nurse in a very powerful position in being able to help patients who have a mental illness and substance use problems, by utilising evidence based practices. It is hoped that this chapter has allowed the reader to gain an interest in integrated holistic approaches to care, using both motivational and CBT. The chapter does not set out to be a comprehensive piece of work on CBT. Instead, the author hopes that by giving examples of techniques used, the nurse will become motivated to explore integrated programmes of care and CBT in more depth.

Social learning theory is one way that helps us to understand how people may develop problematic substance use. Whereas motivational interviewing can help facilitate change in a person's substance use, CBT techniques can help to explore underlying assumptions that a person might have about themselves, their mental illness and their substance use, and substance use in relation to mental illness.

Relapse prevention incorporates cognitive behavioural strategies, such as problem solving and cue exposure to help the individual maintain their goal in relation to their substance use. Relapse prevention is also used to help the dually diagnosed to remain mentally stable. By using an integrated approach to care for the dually diagnosed patient, the nurse can help the patient understand all aspects of the complex interrelated factors that contribute to their presenting problems. Finally, in this day of evidence based practices, the nurse can now access cognitive behavioural programmes or techniques that have been proven to help those patients that fall under the umbrella of dual diagnosis.

References

Abdulrahim, D. (2001) *Substance Misuse and Mental Health Co-morbidity (Dual Diagnosis): Standards for Mental Health Services*. The Health Advisory Service, London.

Appleby, L. (2000) Safer services: conclusions from the report of the National Confidential Inquiry. *Advances in Psychiatric Treatment*, 6, 5–15.

Bandura, A. (1997a) *Social Learning Theory*. Prentice-Hall, Englewood Cliffs, N.J.

Bandura, A. (1997b) Self-efficacy: toward a unifying theory of behavioural change. *Psychological Review*, 84, 191–215.

Barnaby, B., Drummond, C., McCloud, A., Burns, T. & Omu, N. (2003) Substance misuse in psychiatric in patients: comparison of a screening questionnaire survey with case notes. *British Medical Journal*, 327, 783–4.

Bower, H.G. & Hilgard, E.R. (1981) *Theories of Learning*. Prentice Hall, London.

Clark, R.E. (2001) Family support and substance use outcomes for persons with mental illness and substance use disorders. *Schizophrenia Bulletin*, 27 (1), 93–101.

Drake, R.E., Xie, H., McHugo, G.J. & Green, A.L. (2000) The effects of clozapine on alcohol and drug use disorders among patients with schizophrenia. *Schizophrenia Bulletin*, 26, 441–9.

Department of Health (2002) *Mental Health Policy Implementation Guide: Dual Diagnosis Good Practice Guide*. Department of Health, London.

Graham, H., Copello, A., Birchwood, M. *et al.* (2004) *Cognitive Behavioural Integrated Treatment*. Wiley, Chichester.

Hollin, C.R. (1990) *Cognitive Behavioural Interventions with Young Offenders*. Pergamon Press, Oxford.

Kavanagh, D.J. (1992) Recent developments in expressed emotion and schizophrenia. *British Journal of Psychiatry*, 160, 601–20.

McMurran, M. (1997) *The Psychology of Addiction*. Taylor and Francis, London.

Marlatt, G.A. & Gordon, J.R. (eds) (1985) *Relapse Prevention: Maintenance Strategies in the Treatment of Addictive Behaviours*. Guilford Press, New York.

Martino, S., Carroll, K.M., O'Malley, S.S. & Rounsaville, M.D. (2000) Motivational interviewing with psychiatrically ill substance abusing patients. *American Journal on Addictions*, 9, 88–91.

Menezes, P., Johnson, S., Thornicroft, G. *et al.* (1996) Drug and alcohol problems among individuals with severe mental illnesses in south London. *British Journal of Psychiatry*, 168, 612–9.

Miller, P.H. (1989) *Theories of Developmental Psychology*, 2nd edn. Freeman, New York.

Miller, W.R. & Rollnick, S. (2002) *Motivational Interviewing: Preparing People for Change*, 2nd edn. The Guilford Press, London.

Monti, P.M. & O'Leary, T.A. (1999) Coping and social skills training for alcohol and cocaine dependence. *The Psychiatric Clinics of North America*, 22, 2, 447–70.

Mueser, K.T., Goodman, L.B., Trumbetta, S.L. *et al.* (1998) Trauma and post-traumatic stress disorder in severe mental illness. *Journal of Consulting and Clinical Psychology*, 66, 493–9.

National Institute for Clinical Excellence (NICE) (2002) *Schizophrenia: Core Interventions in the Treatment and Management of Schizophrenia in Primary and Secondary Care*. National Collaborating Centre for Mental Health, London.

Orford, J. (1985) *Excessive Appetites: A Psychological View of Addictions*. Wiley, Chichester.

Rassool, G.H. (1998) *Substance Use and Misuse: Nature, Context and Clinical Interventions*. Blackwell Science, London.

Rotter, J.B. (1954) *Social Learning and Clinical Psychology*. Prentice-Hall, Englewood Cliffs, N.J.

Scottish Advisory Committee on Drug Misuse (SACDM) and the Scottish Advisory Committee on Alcohol Misuse (SACAM) (2003) *Mind the Gaps: Meeting the Needs of People with Co-occurring Substance Misuse and Mental Health Problems*. Scottish Executive, Edinburgh.

Steadman, H.J., Mulvey, E.P., Monahan, J. *et al.* (1998) Violence by people discharged from acute psychiatric in-patient facilities and by others in the same neighbourhoods. *Archives of General Psychiatry*, 55, 393–404.

Velleman, R. (1996) *Counselling for Alcohol Problems*. Sage, London.

Ward, M. & Applin, C. (1998) *The Unlearned Lesson*. Wynne Howard Books, London.

Williams, A. & Farrell, M. (2004) Substance Use and Psychosis. *Psychiatry*, 3 (1).

World Health Organization (2002) Viewed at: //www.who.int/substanceabuse/topic assessment. htm psy

24 A Person Centred Approach to Understanding and Helping People with a Dual Diagnosis

R. Bryant-Jefferies

Introduction

This chapter will set out an overview of a person centred (sometimes referred to as client centred within therapeutic settings) perspective on dual diagnosis and how persons with such experiences and behaviours might be responded to from this theoretical perspective. The language of counselling and psychotherapy is used as this is the author's professional background; however, the attitudinal values of the person centred approach have application within all helping relationships.

The stance is taken that mental health problems may have biological causation, a life experience causation or a mixture of both. Human beings are complex and diverse products of nature and nurture, having natural and unique potential. However, mental disturbance can arise from a disturbance in nature or nurture, or both, equating with what are considered biological causes (organic, genetic, physical trauma) or life experience causes (psychological, relational). The natural and unique potential of the person may become encouraged, thwarted or distorted by the quality or lack of positive relational experience that is available, or the experience of problems within the brain chemistry and functioning that may significantly impact on the person's development and experience of self. Either way, damaging factors (biological or relational) can leave the person with a set of intimate experiences and behaviours that may be difficult to manage, and also difficult for other people to genuinely understand and empathise with. Such experience and behaviour can become diagnosed as mental illness. For the purpose of this chapter, substance misuse refers to the problematic use of drugs (prescribed or illicit) alcohol and/or volatile substances.

What is dual diagnosis?

The term 'dual diagnosis', which is also known as 'co-morbidity', is used with regard to people who are experiencing mental health and substance misuse problems concurrently. (For more elaborate explanations of the concept of dual diagnosis see Chapter 1.) It is important to highlight that dual diagnosis is not in itself a diagnosis, rather it is a recognition that an individual has a diagnosed mental health condition and substance misusing behaviours. It has to be recognised that each person with a 'dual diagnosis' will need to be treated as an individual, the causes and the resulting effects of their condition being unique to them, with treatment needing to be matched to their unique needs.

Whilst it is recognised that there will be certain conditions of mind that will require chemical interventions because the condition is the result of chemical imbalance or other biological abnormality, we should not allow this to blind us to the possibility that there are underlying environmental and experiential factors that have had a major contribution to a person's state of mind and emotion. I describe it thus because whilst emphasis is on mental health it is important to keep visible the fact that for many people their difficulties and psychological discomforts are strongly linked to problematic emotional experiences. It is also important to acknowledge that symptomatology might be better seen as a kind of experiential flashing neon sign, drawing attention to the fact that something is wrong. If our treatment responses are simply concerned with turning off the flashing light because it is a problem to us, rather than seeking the underlying reason for which it is flashing, then we have a system that goes no further than symptom management. Whilst this may well have a part to play in bringing a client symptom relief, it should not be confused with actual treatment of the underlying cause (Bryant-Jefferies, 2005).

The UK Department of Health's *Good Practice Guide* (2002) to dual diagnosis illustrates the scope of co-existent psychiatric and substance misuse disorders by describing four main groups of individuals, based on the severity of problematic drug misuse and the mental illness (Figure 24.1) taken from Minkoff (2002).

However, whilst this provides a framework for defining degrees of 'dual diagnosis' (although it does not make specific reference to eating disorders), what it does not do is provide a differentiation between the biological and life experience causation that can inform treatment choices. Each quadrant might be usefully modified to include this by adding a definition within each quadrant to differentiate those whose dual diagnosis condition is purely biologically/chemically caused, and those for whom it has developed in response to life experiences, as well as those for whom both are present as causative factors. In the context of an increasing emphasis on what are being termed 'psychosocial interventions' in substance misuse treatment in the UK (perhaps we should extend this to 'psychosocial therapeutic interventions) such differentiation would be both timely and appropriate.

Figure 24.2 provides an example of such a mapping. However, it should be recognised that biological and life experiences as causal routes for dual diagnosis conditions are by no means mutually exclusive; there may be an overlap with both present and both providing contributing factors. Widening the diagnostic lens to embrace both organic and life experience causal factors offers opportunity for treatment to be as focused on addressing the emotional-psychological relational components as it is on removing or managing symptoms. The patient with a dual diagnosis wants help to feel better as would the person with the broken leg. But with the person with the broken leg

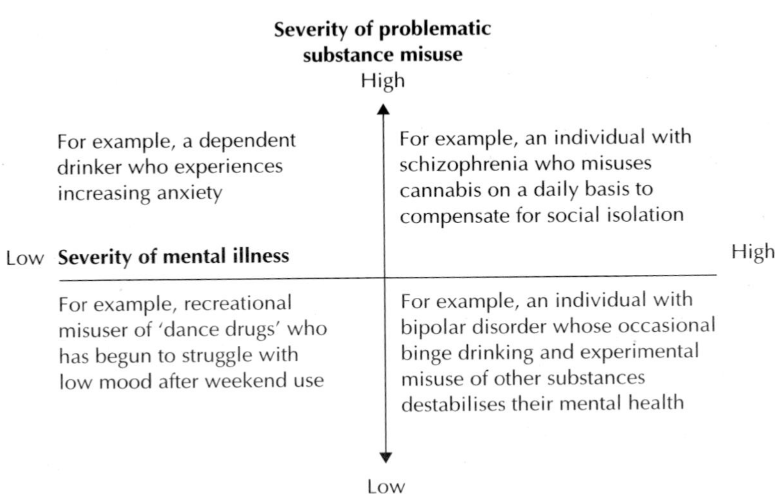

Figure 24.1 Severity of dual diagnosis.
Source: Department of Health (2002).

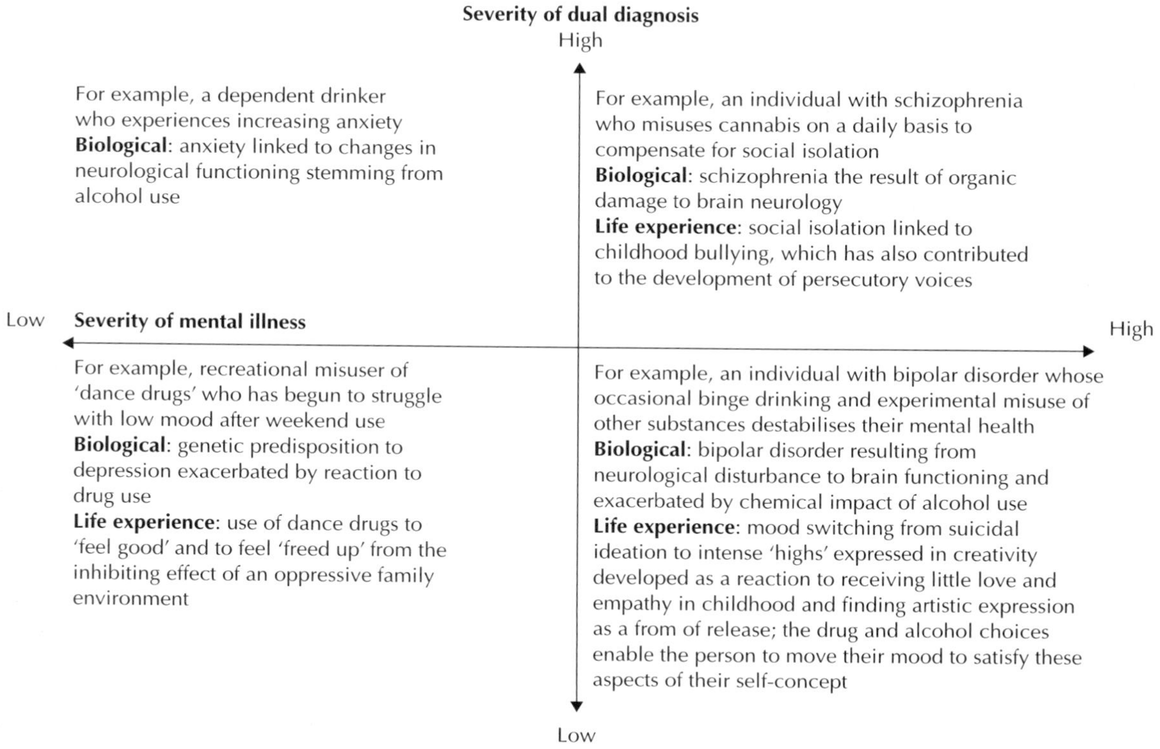

Figure 24.2 Biological and life-experience causation on the dual-diagnosis continuum.

we wouldn't simply medicate to remove the discomfort but offer treatment to heal the break. We can medicate to remove the discomfort of the dual diagnosis client, medicate to redress chemical imbalance and/or reduce the impact of organic damage, but we must also offer relational therapy to encourage the healing of the psychological breaks that may be present behind the dual diagnosis symptomatology.

Person centred approach to personality development

The person centred approach (PCA) is both a theory of personality development and a well established theory of psychological/therapeutic intervention. It was formulated by the psychologist Carl Rogers during the middle part of the twentieth century, and whilst his publications would be too numerous to reference in full, key elements of his developing theory can be found in Rogers (1951; 1957; 1959; 1961). Recently, Kirschenbaum (Carl Rogers' biographer) researched the number of books, papers and journals being produced on the person centred approach and it is clear that the trend is towards more publications of the approach. He concluded that the approach is experiencing 'something of a revival, both in professional activity and academic respectability' (Kirschenbaum, 2005). Perhaps this is indicative of greater recognition of a more relational approach to therapeutic practice. Joseph & Worsley (2005) have recently brought together a number of internationally renowned person centred writers and practitioners to demonstrate how the PCA can be applied to psychopathology, normally considered to be the remit of psychiatric services, conveying the depth, relevance and wide-ranging application of person centred theory and practice.

PCA differs from other approaches and theories in that fundamentally it is neither diagnostic nor an approach that seeks to treat and cure a specific disease, condition or dysfunctionality. Also, it is founded on the therapeutic stance of the client as expert and that if the right relational experience can be created for the client through therapy, then their potential for self-healing, for seeking more fulfilling and satisfying ways of being that match their increasing authenticity within their own psychological processes, will be released.

Rogers (1951)formulated the following propositional statements:

- Behaviour is caused, and the psychological cause of behaviour is a certain perception or a way of perceiving.
- The client is the only one who has the potentiality of knowing fully the dynamics of their perceptions and their behaviour.
- In order for behaviour to change, a change in perception must be *experienced*. Intellectual knowledge cannot substitute for this.
- The constructive forces that bring about altered perception, reorganisation of self and relearning, reside primarily in the client and probably cannot come from outside.
- Therapy is basically the experiencing of the inadequacies in old ways of perceiving, the experiencing of new and more accurate and adequate perceptions, and the recognition of significant relationships between perceptions.
- In a very meaningful and accurate sense, therapy *is* diagnosis, and this diagnosis is a process that goes on in the experience of the client, rather than in the intellect of the clinician.

He suggested that individuals develop their emotional and psychological structure of self and what they create is influenced by the conditioning effect of significant others. The person learns to think of themselves in a certain way, or to formulate behaviours to match the needs of others and to seek approval. This is obviously a significant feature of childhood, but patterns established early in life then become a feature of adulthood as well. For some people, these 'conditions of worth' can be first established in adulthood when the person is subjected to particularly intense, traumatising and undermining experiences. These 'conditions of worth' lead the person to symbolise in awareness a particular belief about themselves, for instance 'because no one shows me love, perhaps I am unlovable', and they may then instigate a lifestyle to maintain and reinforce this self-belief. It could be that they have been subjected to abuse and, for some of them, this is normalised and sought after, or, if occurring in early years, the person may develop dissociative states (Warner, 2000) that then encourage behaviours to enable that distinct sense of self within the structure of self to be maintained. Or they may have experienced a lack of empathy or 'empathic failure' in childhood, leaving them with the propensity for what has been termed 'fragile process' (Warner, 2000) where the person finds it difficult to contain emotions and is in extreme need to be empathically heard and understood.

These states or ways of processing experience, with the resulting behaviours that may follow, can be particularly significant for our understanding of people with what is often referred to as 'personality disorder'. In reality, the personality is not so much disordered, rather it is ordered but around a particularly intense and damaging set of relational experiences. Yes, there may be a chemical or biological explanation for a particular mental state, but it is not necessarily the whole picture; other experiential factors may need recognition, some of which if focused in dissociative states may be barely, if at all, present in the awareness of the client.

At the core of person centred theory is the notion that there exists what Rogers termed 'the actualising tendency'. This is a tendency within the person towards achieving a way of being that is optimally satisfying to them, in line with the structure of self that has been created, which is itself a complex result of genetic inheritance and reaction to life experience. The 'therapist trusts the actualising tendency of the client and truly believes that the client who experiences the freedom of a fostering psychological climate will resolve his or her own problems' (Bozarth, 1998). This is fundamental to the application of the person centred approach. Rogers (1986) wrote:

> 'The person-centred approach is built on a basic trust in the person . . . [It] depends on the actualising tendency present in every living organism – the tendency to grow, to develop, to realize its full potential. This way of being trusts the constructive directional flow of the human being towards a more complex and complete

development. It is this directional flow that we aim to release.'

Where there are distortions within the person's developing self-concept then the actualising tendency will still operate to seek to achieve what is most satisfying; however, the direction taken will then be strongly conditioned by the person's image of self. So, a person who has felt abandoned and bereft of emotional warmth, and who has an introjected belief that this is what they can expect, and is a key aspect of who they are, may not only seek an isolated lifestyle, but may also have developed little capacity to both feel warmth when it is shown, and also difficulty in expressing it. Having established a structure of self and a way of being that is rooted in a negative set of relational experiences, the person centred approach argues that it can take a relational therapeutic encounter to unravel the damage and help the person to free themselves from views that they have about themselves and relationships and the associated behaviours that have developed.

Where the developed concept of self or self-concept contains extremely painful elements the person can find themselves presenting to the outside world with behaviours and attitudes that, when assessed through the lens of mental illness, become assigned mental health diagnoses and treatments.

Setting aside those whose dual diagnosis is driven purely by organic factors requiring chemical/organic intervention (and research is needed to be clear just how many people this refers to) we then have a group who have been exposed to significantly problematic relational/emotional experiences in their lives, and often in childhood. For many within this group, mental discomfort will have preceded substance use, with their early use of substances bringing a sense of relief, of normality, of good feeling and perhaps even of well-being for some. These are profound and powerful experiences and, we might say, an effect of the person seeking that most satisfying experience of themselves that they can achieve. From this perspective, substance use can be seen as an attempt by the person to create a positive and satisfying experience of self. With many adult psychological difficulties and substance misusing behaviours developing out of problematic, conditional or abusive relational experiences (centred in childhood or later in life) the individual can remain driven to perpetually maintain a distorted perception of themselves and of their potential as a person. They will need to maintain and indeed protect their sense of identity as it has developed, whether it is a feeling of worthlessness, a normalising of anxiety states or depressive moods, coping with dissociated awareness, or coming to terms with a sense of self that is fundamentally fragmented by intensely damaging and painful experiences. The individual is emotionally and psychologically driven into thinking, feeling and acting in ways that enable them to maintain their self-beliefs and meanings, the condition of their structure of self. This is then lived out, possibly throughout life, with the person seeking to satisfy what they have come to believe about themselves.

A child exposed to difficult relational experiences in, for instance, school settings in the form of bullying and racial harassment, or at home where there is direct or indirect exposure to abuse, is likely to experience a profound sense of feeling flooded by intense feelings that undermine their sense of self, or force them to create one based on however they symbolise in their awareness what is occurring and what it means for and to them. Where their experience is that there is no one to turn to in order to stop it, then the negative internalising and symbolising process is deepened, with the effects taking deeper root in the child's developing structure of self. The impact of this can be lasting and can generate effects that can arguably be a basis for developing the kind of symptomatologies that are commonly associated with mental health diagnoses. This can occur to the point that in adulthood much work is required in order to recover it.

Some use substances, as mentioned before, to alleviate distressing mental symptoms. Others find that their early use seems to trigger symptoms of mental illness. Taking young people as an example, substance use and misuse is a growing phenomenon in many parts of the world. For some there can be a sense of alleviation from mental distress or disturbance; for others it can initially bring relief, but with this may then come added complications and more intense or wider-ranging problems and complex sets of symptoms. Then there are others whose first episode of psychosis, for instance, may be linked to skunk cannabis use, which, when stopped, enables the person's full mental health to be restored. Prolonged use, however, may leave the person more vulnerable to serious and enduring neurological damage. This is an area that demands more research.

For some people, their choice to use substances may be linked to other life experience factors, which, without the drugs, and whether or not there is organic impairment to brain function, will also need to be resolved therapeutically. Where the cause is linked to poor or abusive relational experiences then a relationship based therapy, such as the person centred approach, would be highly beneficial to help the person restore or recreate a fresh sense of self. This fresh sense of self would then develop through the new relational experience of themselves as they feel warmly accepted and empathically understood by a therapist who is authentically present with them, key elements in person centred therapy as we shall now see.

Person centred approach to therapy

Rogers proposed that certain conditions, when present within a therapeutic relationship, would enable the client to develop towards what he termed 'fuller functionality'. Over a number of years he refined these ideas, which he defined as 'the necessary and sufficient conditions for constructive personality change'. These Rogers (1957) described as:

(1) Two persons are in psychological contact.
(2) The first, who we shall term the client, is in a state of incongruence, being vulnerable or anxious.
(3) The second person, who we shall term the therapist, is congruent or integrated in the relationship.
(4) The therapist experiences unconditional positive regard for the client.
(5) The therapist experiences an empathic understanding of the client's internal frame of reference and endeavours to communicate this experience to the client.
(6) The communication to the client of the therapist's empathic understanding and unconditional positive regard is to a minimal degree achieved.

There is much to reflect on when considering a definition of 'contact' or 'psychological contact'. Rogers defined contact in the following terms: 'Two persons are in psychological contact, or have the minimum essential relationship when each makes a perceived or subceived difference in the experiential field of the other' (Rogers, 1959). This is important when we consider dual diagnosis, for there will be clients with whom the therapist may feel they have little or no contact. But is it for the therapist to judge this? Clients may be being positively affected even though they are unable to indicate that this is occurring. Also, within the discipline of the person centred approach, the use of 'pre-therapy' has developed, which will be discussed later in this chapter, but which is concerned with establishing psychological contact where it seems there is minimal, if any, impact being made on the awareness of the client by the presence of, and communication from, the therapist.

Rogers (1980) defined empathy as meaning:

> 'Entering the private perceptual world of the other . . . being sensitive, moment by moment, to the changing felt meanings which flow in this other person . . . It means sensing meanings of which he or she is scarcely aware, but not trying to uncover totally unconscious feelings'.

It is a very delicate process, providing a foundation block to effective working. The person centred practitioner's role is primarily to establish empathic rapport and communicate empathic understanding to the client. And this may be particularly important and highly relevant for clients with a dual diagnosis.

Within this relationship the counsellor seeks to maintain an attitude of unconditional positive regard towards the client and all that they disclose. This is not 'agreeing with', it is a warm acceptance of the client's way of being and perceiving. Rogers wrote that, 'when the therapist is experiencing a positive, acceptant attitude towards whatever the client *is* at that moment, therapeutic movement or change is more likely to occur' (1980).

Concerning congruence Rogers wrote 'genuineness, realness or congruence . . . this means that the therapist is openly being the feelings and attitudes that are flowing within at the moment . . . the term transparent catches the flavour of this condition' (Rogers, 1980). Elsewhere, Mearns & Thorne write that 'congruence is the state of being of the counsellor when her outward responses to her client consistently match the inner feelings and sensations which she has in relation to her client' (Mearns & Thorne, 1999). Any congruent expression by the counsellor of their feelings, thoughts or reactions:

> 'Has to emerge through the process of being in therapeutic relationship with the client. It is a disciplined response and not an open door to endless self-disclosure. Congruent expression is perhaps most appropriate and therapeutically valuable where it is informed by the existence of an empathic understanding of the client's inner world, and is offered in a climate of a genuine warm acceptance towards the client'.
>
> (Bryant-Jefferies, 2005)

It is interesting to note that in their recent paper, *The Effectiveness of Psychological Therapies on Drug Misusing Clients*, Wanigaratne *et al.* (2005) identify the 'following therapist factors which appear to contribute to good outcomes for clients. An effective therapist will:

- Be empathic and authoritative (Truax & Carkhoff, 1967).
- Be willing to participate in supervision (Luborsky *et al.*, 1985).
- Take a non-blaming, non-judgemental stance (Stanton & Shadish, 1997).
- Use motivational dialogue (Raistrick & Tober, 2004).
- Be a good listener.
- Be in good psychological health.
- Develop a helping alliance: a collaborative relationship between client and therapist.'

Apart from the reference to being authoritative (the PCA requires the practitioner to be authentically rather than authoritatively present) and the use of motivational dialogue (the person centred practitioner trusts the constructive flow and prompting of the actualising tendency to give the client direction), the other factors are key features of the PCA. However, it must be stressed that one of the core features of person centred therapy is that of the practitioner's non-directiveness and trust in the constructive influence of the therapeutic conditions; that when they are provided by the counsellor, and are experienced by the client, then constructive personality change is the likely outcome.

Case example

Mike is 36.

> 'I was taken into care when I was five, having been subjected to neglect and abuse from my parents. Got bullied at school and abused again whilst in care. Finally, got away when I was 14. Hated it, hated them, and hated myself. Tried to forget. Lived on the streets, drank, used drugs, anything, try to feel better, different, you know? The drugs made me forget sometimes, but made me feel bad too, worthless, hopeless, total failure. And I could hear their voices.'

Mike is unable to keep regular appointments and reacts badly to structure or to anyone who tries to control him or who he doesn't perceive as understanding him. His mood swings violently under the influence of substances. He has been diagnosed as having a personality disorder. He hates this, and part of him feels that it sums up who he is, a failed human being.

Person centred response

By offering empathy over the long term, and consistent warm acceptance whilst being utterly honest, and through flexibility in contact, which the client decided on, the person centred practitioner would offer an opportunity for Mike to experience himself as a valued human being. His self-concept contains powerful negative self-beliefs about himself and his expectation of how others will relate to him. At some deep level there may well be a human being craving for love, but it could be very childlike and this quiet but desperate voice may not emerge into awareness. The person centred practitioner will need to be very sensitive to this.

Mike is likely to push boundaries. There will be a need for flexibility to get alongside him. The person centred practitioner has to get alongside the client; they cannot expect the client to get alongside them.

Medication may suppress feelings, may manage symptoms and behaviours, but the disturbed and damaged personality will remain. For genuine healing to occur, Mike has to experience, at a very human level, the humanity of another human being. He will feel challenged by being offered unconditional positive regard. It will go against his concept of self as a worthless failure; it will threaten his accepted sense of self. There can be no quick fix to long-term damage from problematic relational experiences. Time will be required, and patience. Mike will need not simply to think differently about himself and the world around him, but to *feel* differently too. He will need a genuine, contrasting relational experience for this to develop and to have a chance of becoming a sustainable feature of a changing self-concept.

Pre-therapy

The development of what is termed 'pre-therapy' (Prouty, 2002; Prouty *et al.*, 2002) has provided a major theoretical development to the practice of working with clients for whom the nature, depth or even existence of psychological contact is under question. Within Rogers' system, psychological contact is the first necessary and sufficient condition for constructive personality change (Rogers, 1957). Prouty defines pre-therapy as:

> 'The development or restoration of the functions necessary for a therapeutic relationship and experiencing. Pre-Therapy, described in general terms, develops *the necessary psychological capacities for psychotherapy*. It assists those clients who are impaired in the psychological functions for treatment to occur'.
>
> (Prouty, 2002)

Prouty describes a series of contact functions, which he indicates as representing an expansion of Perls' concept of 'contact and ego function', these contact functions being 'conceived as awareness functions and described as reality, affective and communicative contact' and it is 'the development or restoration of the contact functions' that is 'the necessary pre-condition for psychotherapy'. It is the development or restoration of the contact functions that is the theoretical goal of pre-therapy (Prouty, 2002), and at the core of this process lies the notion of 'contact reflections'. These have 'the theoretical function of developing psychological contact between therapist and client when the client is incapable of reality, affective or communicative contact. They are applied when there is not sufficient contact to implement psychotherapy' (Prouty, 2002). There are five 'contact reflections' (Karon & Vanderbos, 1981): 'situational reflections, facial reflections, word-for-word reflections, body reflections and reiterative reflections.'

In the pre-therapy model, a distinction is drawn between 'empathy' and 'empathic contact'. In a situation in which 'the therapist does not know the client's inner frame of reference', then 'the empathy is for the client's effort at developing coherent experience and expression, perhaps a form of consolidating the self-formative tendency during these primitive phases of therapy'. Prouty goes on to suggest a second level of empathy, which he defines as being for 'the concrete particularity of behavioural expression', in other words, 'not focussed on the generalized "essence" of meaning, but on the literal expressive behaviour'. The third level of empathy concerns, he suggests, 'the increase in psychotic expression as a function of pre-therapy'. It is worth quoting verbatim what he has to say regarding this as it is clearly a view that many mental health professionals would find challenging:

> 'The client needs to get worse before she can get better. The therapist needs to be empathic to an increase in delusional and hallucinatory expression, as well as to an increase in bizarre communication (strange body language, postures, language disturbance, etc.). This means being empathic to the lived experience of the psychosis itself. This is, of course, the opposite of behavioural and chemical management.'
>
> (Prouty, 2002)

A Person centred view of mental illness, diagnosis and substance use

The person centred perspective may be deemed quite radical in its attitude towards the validity and helpfulness of diagnosis as it is an approach that seeks to help the person rather than treat a specific condition. Bozarth (2002) refers to his own studies of particular diagnostic concepts, which he contends do not evidence the clustering of symptoms in a meaningful way (Bozarth, 1998) and to those of others in relation to schizophrenia (Slade &

Cooper, 1979; Bentall, 1990), depression (Wiener, 1989; Hallett, 1990), agoraphobia (Hallam, 1983), borderline personality disorder (Kutchins & Kirk, 1997) and panic disorder (Hallam, 1989).

The PCA also recognises the negative impact of stigma inducing labels, of how they can dehumanise a person and reduce them to a diagnosis, with the attendant fear that once 'diagnosed', they will carry that diagnosis for life. In this respect, the genuine experiencing and offering of unconditional positive regard to the client, and the experience of its presence for them by the client, is an important feature of the PCA and a major contributing factor to the client developing 'unconditional positive self-regard'. Rogers argued that psychological diagnosis could place the client's locus of value firmly outside themselves and definitely within the diagnosing 'expert', leaving the client at risk of developing tendencies of dependence and expectation that the 'expert' will have the responsibility of improving the client's situation (Roger, 1951). Vincent argues that '*therapist* diagnosis, evaluation and prognosis clearly do not respect the inner resources of *clients* and their potential and capacity for self-direction, as there is an obvious implication that actually the therapist, not the client, knows best' (2005). Returning to Rogers (1946):

> 'If we can provide understanding of the way the client seems to himself at this moment, he can do the rest. The therapist must lay aside his preoccupation with diagnosis and his diagnostic shrewdness, must discard his tendency to make professional evaluations, must cease his endeavours to formulate an accurate prognosis, must give up the temptation subtly to guide the individual, and must concentrate on one purpose only; that of providing deep understanding and acceptance of his attitudes consciously held at this moment by the client as he explores step by step into the dangerous areas which he has been denying to consciousness.'

Also to be recognised as radical is the non-directive nature of the person centred approach. A person centred assessment process is a direct challenge to the usual medical assessment where specific questions are asked to elicit specific information in order for a diagnosis to be made. The person centred counsellor will learn about their client as the client chooses to disclose, encouraging the client's autonomy within the relationship. The client will be assessing their situation and what they experience their needs as being. Assessment is an internal process for the client as they assess themselves, the therapist, their experience, what they feel they need and what they feel is unhelpful. We often read or hear of people talking of being 'patient centred' or 'client centred', but what this can refer to is a directive process in which the practitioner listens to the client, but forms their own diagnosis and then works with the client to get them to agree to a treatment plan essentially formulated by the diagnostician.

Sommerbeck (2003) contends that whilst 'psychiatric diagnosis is of no issue in client centred theory and therapy', the client centred therapist working in a psychiatric setting should not be ignorant about the diagnoses that are employed by others within that particular health care setting, or regard such diagnoses as unnecessary. 'In the medical model setting of a psychiatric hospital, for example, it is necessary for the client centred therapist to acknowledge the necessity of psychiatric diagnostics for other professionals and to know about the main psychiatric diagnoses.' She continues by stressing that 'the conditions necessary and sufficient for facilitation of the client's most constructive potentials are trusted to be the same for everybody, irrespective of diagnosis'. There are going to be diagnoses that are specific and measurable conditions: biological, genetic, physical trauma damage. Within a medical model setting the diagnostic language facilitates communication, though it might not necessarily facilitate understanding. It is important for the therapist to be able to be part of and to understand discussions with colleagues as part of the multidisciplinary process. For the person centred therapist, their language will be more in terms of the causal life experiences, and how these relate to symptomatic effects.

Stevens, in Rogers & Stevens (1973), quotes from a letter by Gendlin who brings the human and the relational elements alive to our interpretation of the way of being that may be diagnosed as schizophrenic:

> 'I believe that schizophrenia is *the absence of* (or greater narrowing of) that felt experiential interaction process which we are as people and which

we feel as our concrete selves. When an individual is stuck in a hurtful relationship situation so that he can neither leave it nor feel and relate himself sufficiently to it, then he becomes deadened and empty inside, reports that he is "not himself." The ongoing feeling process on which we all rely inside becomes muddy, swampy, unreliable, or stopped, and feeling contents become stuck, frozen, unowned, seemingly alien, static places, rather than fluidly functioning feeling . . .

This definition of schizophrenia as an *absence* of a certain type of felt interaction (an absence rather than an illness or a content) has important consequences. It seems that we think of ourselves not so much as working with something ill in the person, but rather as providing the necessary personal relationship in the context of which someone can again come alive as a person.'

This is a challenging and yet optimistic perspective, and fully in line with the person centred view of the person as a process of being tending towards fullness, wholeness and complexity, a tendency that can lean towards fullest functionality within the context of the relational experience that contains the core conditions of empathy, congruence and unconditional positive regard. The healing process that occurs through the constructive relational experience enables the 'damaged' individual to self-heal, to fill the gaps, the emptiness, the loneliness that can lie at the heart of some forms of mental disturbance. It is, then, not so much a case of there being a specific 'illness' to treat, but rather the need for a relational experience to encourage greater wholeness.

Interestingly, Mearns & Thorne express the opinion that 'congruence as a therapeutic condition becomes more critical with psychotic clients', a view that they emphasise as being supported by the study of person centred therapy with schizophrenic clients. They draw from Rogers (Rogers *et al.*, 1967) in pointing out that:

'Those patients who perceived a high degree of congruence in their therapist were independently rated as showing the greatest degree of change. Furthermore, those patients who were in relationships where the therapist exhibited low congruence showed no change or even *regressive* change'.

(Mearns & Thorne, 1999)

Elsewhere, I have argued that the therapeutic condition that is most effective for a given client will be that which is the opposite to the deficiency that caused the damage to the client (Bryant-Jefferies, 2005). The implications of this are, in my view, far reaching and highly significant for therapeutic responses to people with a dual diagnosis. It would mean that:

'The psychotic client who has developed high levels of incongruence will be most positively affected by the congruent therapist; the client who was adversely affected by a lack of warmth and prizing will require a therapist able to offer high levels of unconditional positive regard; the client who was not listened to or heard during their early development will need high levels of accurate empathic understanding within their therapeutic experience; and the client who withdraws into their own reality and away from external contact will need a therapist who can work effectively within a relational experience of minimal psychological contact by staying close to the client without threatening to invade their psychological world.'

(Bryant-Jefferies, 2005)

When working with clients who are evidencing 'psychotic' symptoms (withdrawal into a reality that seems alien to the socially accepted 'norm'), or who have a 'personality disorder' (where the personality characteristics, we might say the structure of self, has developed in such a way due to, for instance, often traumatic and undermining experiences, that the person's ability to function without constant distress or as a social being is greatly impaired), the counsellor can be greatly challenged. It can be an intensely demanding, frustrating and disorientating experience. With regard to working with the psychotic client, Lambers (1994a) writes of the challenge to the 'counsellor's ability to create the therapeutic conditions' and of the 'fundamental challenge to the therapist's understanding and expression of the conditions' (1994b). She writes of how, 'at the core of the self-concept of the client with personality disorder', there is 'a profound sense of worthlessness. A central issue in the counselling relationship is acceptance. The counsellor is likely to experience challenge of her ability to offer acceptance; the client will be challenged in his ability to experience being accepted'.

Schlien's (1961) paper *A Client Centered Approach to Schizophrenia: First Approximation*[1] captures something extremely valuable when thinking about 'psychosis' and 'paranoia':

> 'That which we call "psychosis" is not a disease. It is a learned behaviour, exaggerated to a point of no return, i.e., where control is lost and the exaggerated behaviour "takes on a life of its own" temporarily. Because this exaggeration is so overwhelming, so much beyond our ordinary capacity to assimilate, it appears to us that we are no longer dealing with, for instance, ordinary suspicion, but something *quite* different – "paranoia". Then it appears that psychosis is not of the same order, not on the same continuum, as "normal" or "neurotic" behaviour. But as psychotic behaviour becomes more common it is seen as a form of maladjustment similar in kind to lesser degrees of maladjustment, though so much greater in quantity that it seems different in *quality* too.'

He then continues to describe metaphorically how 'in one sense . . . it *is* different':

> 'A boulder balanced on the edge of a precipice can be pressed ounce by measured ounce towards rolling off. Each ounce is just like the last, but when the quantity of pressure totals to the "breaking point", the quality of the *consequences* changes radically. No longer will the relief or counter-pressure of one ounce recover the balance. Even if the boulder is not smashed in the fall, an enormous effort is required to restore it to its original position. It is because of this effort (which so few can make, and so many need) that it is necessary to prevent the "psychotic situation" in life. The "psychotic situation" is a precondition to the psychotic state, which may or may not follow.'

Of course, the mental and emotional state of the client combined with substance use adds to the complexity of the condition and the nature of treatment responses. The client will need to be helped to understand their condition, what is happening for them and feel part of the collaborative decision making process insofar as what treatment responses will be most helpful. For many dual diagnosis clients, their substance use has been their solution and they may be reluctant to give it up. The symptoms that it alleviates may sometimes be memories of past experiences that invade their awareness. For others, the substance misuse may trigger a release into awareness of memories and feelings that had previously been denied to awareness. Experiences that are not consistent with a person's self-concept may be denied in this way, particularly painful and distressing ones. Their release back into awareness can be not only psychologically distressing but also, in extreme cases, increase the risk of a psychotic breakdown.

Rogers wrote of the process of psychological breakdown and disorganisation. He expressed four stages to this process, the first two stages of which 'may be illustrated by anxiety producing experiences in therapy, or by acute psychotic breakdowns'.

> (1) If the individual has a large or significant degree of *incongruence between self and experience* and if a significant experience demonstrating this *incongruence* occurs suddenly, or with a high degree of obviousness, then the organism's process of *defense* is unable to operate successfully.
> (2) As a result *anxiety is experienced*, as the *incongruence* is subceived. The degree of anxiety is dependent upon the extent of the *self-structure* which is *threatened*.
>
> (Rogers, 1959)

As a result of this process, Rogers then went on to describe the effect this has on the individual's self-structure and subsequent behaviour. He writes:

> (3) The process of defence being unsuccessful, the *experience* is *accurately symbolised* in *awareness*, and the gestalt of the *self-structure* is broken by this *experience* of the *incongruence* in *awareness*. A state of disorganisation results.
> (4) In such a state of disorganisation the organism behaves at times in ways which are openly consistent with experiences which have hitherto been distorted or denied to awareness. At other times the self may temporarily regain regnancy, and the organism may behave in ways consistent with it. Thus, in such a state of disorganisation, the tension between the

[1] This passage is taken from the abridged version that appears in Rogers, C.R. & Stevens, B. (1973) *Person to Person: The Problem of Being Human*. Souvenir Press, London; the full paper having appeared in *Psychotherapy of the Psychoses*, edited by A. Burton, Basic Books Inc., 1961.

concept of self (with its included distorted perceptions) and the experiences which are not accurately symbolised or included in the concept of self, is expressed in a confused regnancy, first one and then the other supplying the "feedback" by which the organism regulates behaviour.

(Rogers, 1959)

It then becomes an interesting question to consider the impact a mood altering substance might have on this process and which substances (illicit or prescribed) will have the tendency to open up an individual's awareness to the incongruence within their self-structure, rooted in those experiences that have been denied to awareness, and which substances will in some way enhance the internal defences. Could it be that, for some people, the use of cannabis, particularly skunk cannabis, weakens the defences and causes incongruence to break into awareness, thereby precipitating a psychotic event? Does the disinhibiting effect of alcohol have a similar effect, or could its depressive effect drop the person into depths of despair already present within their inner world though outside their normal awareness?

Interestingly, Rogers cited sodium pentathol therapy, under the influence of which the client could reveal experiences that he had previously denied to himself, but which were clearly linked to 'incomprehensible elements in his behavior'. Faced with this material in his normal state of mind, the individual could no longer deny the authenticity of what had come into awareness and his 'defensive processes could not deny or distort the experience, and hence the self-structure was broken, and a psychotic break occurred' (Rogers, 1959). Given the amount of drug use in society today, and the numbers of young people presenting with forms of mental disturbance, there is scope here for serious research. Perhaps those whose structure of self is riddled with incongruence rooted in early life experience and who use substances may be more at risk of experiencing symptoms associated with mental illness. Certainly, the fact that some people use cannabis without experiencing a problematic mental health reaction, whilst others do experience psychotic effects (and similarly with other substances) demands further investigation in terms of the formative relational experiencing of the individuals concerned.

Conclusion

The person centred approach offers a relational theory for the development of mental disturbance and symptomatology, together with a therapeutic system for responding to the whole person so affected. The use of substances to alleviate mental distress by clients can bring relief, but it can also complicate the condition and, in some instances, rather than suppress experiences it may actually disinhibit the person in such a way that awareness can become flooded by material that has been denied to awareness and that can actually threaten the person's structure of self. The approach emphasises the need for a therapeutic relational response so that the person can be offered the opportunity to feel understood and understandable, to feel that as a person they can be and are warmly accepted and may begin to feel warmly accepting of themselves, and that they can be treated respectfully and with genuine authenticity, with the likelihood that greater authenticity may become possible within the client. Results or outcomes may be very subjective, not necessarily outwardly measurable and yet highly significant for the client in terms of their internal relationship with themselves, and with their symptoms, should they persist.

None of this is to suggest that working with clients who have experiences, perceptions and behaviours that come within the medical definition of dual diagnosis is easy. The need for patience is vital. Often these are the most complex individuals, badly damaged by life experience and whose substance use or misuse has been their best attempt to cope, alleviate symptoms or make the best of their lives. They deserve and require society's compassion and the very best that therapy and other forms of treatment can offer.

References

Bentall, R.P. (1990) The syndromes and symptoms of psychosis. In: *Reconstructing Schizophrenia* (Bentall, R.R., ed.). Routledge, London.

Bozarth, J. (1998) *Person Centred Therapy: a Revolutionary Paradigm*. PCCS Books, Ross-on-Wye.

Bozarth, J. (2002) Empirically supported treatments: epitomy of the specificity myth. In: *Client Centred and Experiential Psychotherapy in the Twenty-first Century: Advances in Theory, Research and Practice*. (Watson, J.C.,

Goldman, R.N. & Warner, M.S., eds), pp. 168–81. PCCS Books, Ross-on-Wye.

Bryant-Jefferies, R. (2005) *Responding to a Serious Mental Health Problem: Person Centred Dialogues*. Radcliffe Publishing, Abingdon.

Department of Health (2002) *Dual Diagnosis Good Practice Guide*. Department of Health, London.

Hallam, R.S. (1983) Agoraphobia: deconstructing a clinical syndrome. *Bulletin of the British Psychological Society* 36, 337–40.

Hallam, R.S. (1989) *Classification and Research into Panic*. In: *Panic Disorder* (Baker, R. & McFadyen, M., eds). Wiley, Chichester.

Hallet, R. (1990) Melancholia and depression. A brief history and analysis of contemporary confusions. Unpublished Masters thesis, University of East London.

Joseph, S. & Worsley, R. (2005) *Person Centred Psychopathology: A Positive Psychology of Mental Health*. PCCS Books, Ross-on-Wye.

Karon, B. & Vanderbos, G. (1981) *Psychotherapy of Schizophrenia*. Aaronson, New York.

Kirschenbaum, H. (2005) The current status of Carl Rogers and the person centred approach. *Psychotherapy*, 42 (1), 37–51.

Kutchins, H. & Kirk, S. (1997) *Making us Crazy: DSM: the Psychiatric Bible and the Creation of Mental Disorders*. The Free Press/Simon Schuster, New York.

Lambers, E. (1994a) Personality Disorder. In: *Developing Person Centred Counselling* (Mearns, D., ed.). Sage, London.

Lambers, E. (1994b) Psychosis. In: *Developing Person Centred Counselling* (Mearns, D., ed.). Sage, London.

Luborsky, L., McLellan, A.T., Woody, G.E. *et al.* (1985) Therapist success and its determinants. *Archives of General Psychiatry*, 42 (6), 602–11.

Mearns, D. & Thorne, B. (1999) *Person Centred Counselling in Action*, 2nd edn. Sage, London.

Minkoff, K. (2002) *CCISC Model – Comprehensive, Continuous, Integrated System of Care Model*. www.kenminkoff.com/ccisc.html

Prouty, G. (2002) The Practice of Pre-therapy. In: *Rogers' Therapeutic Conditions: Evolution Theory and Practice* (Rogers, C.R., ed.), Vol. 4, *Contact and Perception* (Wyatt, G. & Sanders, P., eds). PCCS Books, Ross-on-Wye.

Prouty, G, Van Werde, D. & Pörtner, M. (2002) *Pre-therapy: Reaching Contact Impaired Clients*. PCCS Books, Ross-on-Wye.

Raistrick, D. & Tober, G. (2004) Psychosocial interventions. *Psychiatry*, 3, 36–9.

Rogers, C.R. (1946) Significant aspects of client-centred therapy. *American Journal of Psychology*, 1, 415–22.

Rogers, C.R. (1951) *Client Centred Therapy*. Constable, London.

Rogers, C.R. (1957) The necessary and sufficient conditions of therapeutic personality change. *Journal of Consulting Psychology*, 21, 95–103.

Rogers, C.R. (1959) A theory of therapy, personality and interpersonal relationships as developed in the client centred framework. In: *Psychology: A Study of a Science*, Vol. 3, *Formulations of the Person and the Social Context* (Koch, S., ed.), pp. 185–246. McGraw-Hill, New York.

Rogers, C.R. (1961) *On Becoming a Person: a Therapist's View of Psychotherapy*. Constable and Co. Ltd, London.

Rogers, C.R. (1980) *A Way of Being*. Houghton-Mifflin Company, Boston, Mass.

Rogers, C.R. (1986) A client-centered/person-centered approach to therapy. In: *Psychotherapists' Casebook* (Kutash, I. & Wolfe, A., eds), pp. 236–57. Jossey Bass, New York.

Rogers, C.R., Gendlin, E.T., Kiesler, D.J. & Truax, C.B. (eds) (1967) *The Therapeutic Relationship and its Impact. A Study of Psychotherapy with Schizophrenics*. University of Wisconsin Press, Madison, Wis.

Rogers, C.R. & Stevens, B. (1973) *Person to Person: the Problem of Being Human*. Souvenir Press, London. Originally published in 1967 by Real People Press, USA.

Schlien, J.M. (1961) A client-centred approach to schizophrenia: first approximation. In: *Person to Person: The Problem of Being Human* (Rogers, C.R. & Stevens, B., eds). pp. 151–65. Souvenir Press, London.

Slade, P.D. & Cooper, R. (1979) Some difficulties with the term 'schizophrenia': an alternative model. *British Journal of Social and Clinical Psychology*, 18, 309–17.

Sommerbeck, L. (2003) *The Client Centred Therapist in Psychiatric Contexts: a Therapists' Guide to the Psychiatric Landscape and its Inhabitants*. PCCS Books, Ross-on-Wye.

Stanton, M.D. & Shadish, W.R. (1997) Outcome, attrition, and family/couples treatment for drug abuse: a meta-analysis and review of the controlled, comparative studies. *Psychological Bulletin*, 122, 170–91.

Truax, D.B. & Carkhoff, R.R. (1967) *Toward Effective Counseling and Psychotherapy*. Aldine Publishing Company, Chicago, Ill.

Vincent, S. (2005) *Being Empathic*. Radcliffe Publishing, Abingdon.

Wanigaratne, S., Davis, P., Pryce, K. & Brotchie, J. (2005) *The Effectiveness of Psychological Therapies on Drug Misusing Clients*. National Treatment Agency for Substance Misuse, London.

Warner, M. (2000) Person centred therapy at the difficult edge: a developmentally based model of fragile and dissociated process. In: *Person Centred Therapy Today* (Mearns, D. & Thorne, B., eds). Sage Publications, London.

Wiener, M. (1989) Psychopathology reconsidered. Depression interpreted as psychosocial interactions. *Clinical Psychology Review*, 9, 295–321.

25 Motivational Interviewing

P.G. Mason

Introduction

As nurses we can do much to assist our clients who have coexisting mental health and substance use disorders. However, for us to help we usually need the clients to take some action on their own behalf or at least to cooperate with our efforts. One of the big frustrations is the client who will not do so; who repeatedly fails to keep appointments, does not attend support services, takes medication only sporadically or even refuses to acknowledge that there is a problem to be addressed in the first place. These people are sometimes considered to be 'unmotivated' or 'in denial' and nurses become discouraged in their attempts to help them.

Motivational interviewing (Miller & Rollnick, 2002) is a counselling approach that helps clients to explore what they really want and direct their energy into taking action that will help them to achieve it. It was originally developed in the specialist addictions field but has since been found to have wider application. It can be used to help clients who are considering a specific behaviour change such as:

- Committing themselves to a particular treatment programme
- Taking long-term medication
- Changing their alcohol or drug use

It is not possible to do justice to the complexity of motivational interviewing in a few hundred words. This chapter merely outlines the key principles of this approach and looks at how it can be used in the context of dual diagnosis. You can find further explanations of motivational interviewing in Miller & Rollnick (2002) or Rollnick *et al.* (1999). Specific ideas on integrating motivational interviewing into work with clients with a dual diagnosis can be found in Sciacca (1997), Martino *et al.* (2002) and Graham (2003).

The spirit of motivational interviewing

The spirit of this approach is very important. It is not a set of tricks to make clients take advice. It certainly carries no guarantees that everyone who receives such an intervention will come round to the health professional's point of view and become compliant. Motivational interviewing has its roots in person centred approaches to counselling and therapy, and enables people to make their own decisions. As a way of working it doesn't suit all health professionals. To see if you would be comfortable using this approach consider the following statements. If you mostly agree with them, or think they are interesting, challenging and worth considering, you might be comfortable with it. If you find them at odds with your own views, motivational interviewing is probably not for you.

- People have the right to live their lives in their own way (provided they do not infringe others' rights, in which case society imposes sanctions).
- It is rarely clear-cut what someone ought, or ought not to do.
- Responsibility for change lies with the client.
- Health (either physical or mental) is not everyone's top priority.
- Health professionals do not always know what is best for their patients.
- Patients often do know what would be best for them.
- Health professionals are not failures just because they cannot persuade people to change.
- Motivation is not an 'all or nothing' concept. It is a continuum and subject to change.
- Change is a process, not an event.
- Successful change occurs only when the person has made up their own mind that it is what they really want.

Motivational interviewing invites people to look at their lives differently and consider new options. It supports them through the inner conflicts and uncertainties of the change process. It does not seek to impose new perspectives.

Ambivalence – a key concept

It is important to our understanding of motivation that we recognise how often we are torn two ways about making changes. We can see advantages of change but also disadvantages. There are some good things about the current situation that we do not want to lose. Maintaining long-term changes can be a constant internal battle. Consider the client who is expected to attend a day centre twice a week to get support from peers and engage in some purposeful and rewarding activity. He wakes up and lies in bed thinking about going.

> 'I should get up and go. They are expecting me and I'll have to come up with a good excuse if I don't. I know it's helping me too. I've been feeling more confident since I've been going.
>
> It's raining. I hate waiting for the bus. I always feel really awkward, as if everyone is looking at me and knows where I'm going. The bus always seems more crowded when it's raining too. I hate that.
>
> I know I'll feel better when I get there though. It's good to have company and something to do.
>
> I don't like that new woman though. She's a bit too pushy for me. If she's there today it'll get on my nerves.
>
> It's lovely and warm in bed. I'd really like to stay here and not have to bother getting up and getting dressed. It's too much like hard work getting out and getting organised. I don't even know if I've got a clean shirt to wear.
>
> I'd get bored if I stayed here all day though. I want to get better and they do say this place will help me.
>
> But there are some people there who've been going for months and they don't seem to be getting very well. Maybe it won't work for me after all.'

And so it continues. This is not pathology. It is normal ambivalence. It is probably not much different to the internal dialogue all nurses have when they have to get up for an early shift. He wants to go to the day centre *and* he wants to stay in bed. He is motivated to get better but he doesn't, just now, want to engage in this particular activity that might help him do so. He also has some doubts about whether it really will help if he does go.

Sometimes the ambivalence goes deeper. The client described above wants to get better. Sometimes there is even ambivalence about this. There can be both good and bad things about recovering from long-term problems and rejoining life as a healthy, responsible adult. Motivational interviewing is an approach that accepts ambivalence and helps the client to explore and resolve it. Change is the responsibility of the client and is unlikely to take place unless he or she really wants it. One way of helping someone express this ambivalence is to complete a 'decisional balance' matrix, discussing with them what would go in each of the boxes and how important each item is to them (see Table 25.1).

Table 25.1 Pros/cons of current behaviour: pros/cons of change.

Pros of current behaviour	Cons of current behaviour
Pros of change	Cons of change

Seeing the ambivalence mapped out in black and white can help clients weigh up what is most important to them and begin to problem-solve to overcome the obstacles to change. It is important to remember that this exercise is a highly individual and subjective process and is only meaningful when counsellors seek to understand how clients see things in the context of their own lives and value systems. What the counsellor sees as a major advantage of change may be of little interest to the client.

The principles of motivational interviewing

The four principles of motivational interviewing are:

(1) Express empathy
(2) Develop discrepancy
(3) Roll with resistance
(4) Support self-efficacy

Various tools and strategies have been developed to help apply these principles. These include pencil and paper exercises, structured questions and focused reflections.

Principle 1: express empathy

This is a principle that motivational interviewing upholds in common with other counselling approaches. The counsellor tries to understand the client's position as well as possible and to convey this understanding to them. Core counselling skills such as open questions and reflection are essential, and nurses may have learned these skills from other approaches. In particular, the counsellor expresses empathy with the clients' ambivalence, being willing to listen to and understand why they are reluctant to change, as well as why they are keen to do so. When clients know they are being listened to they are encouraged to explore more deeply their readiness to change. One of the challenges this approach often poses for nurses is the need for the counsellor to listen attentively to the client's point of view, resisting the temptation to try to talk the client into accepting the health professionals' view. Advanced reflective listening skills are an important prerequisite for motivational interviewing.

Principle 2: develop discrepancy

This principle is related to the concept of cognitive dissonance. In motivational interviewing, counsellors seek to encourage clients to explore the conflicts between their beliefs and their behaviours. The importance of change increases as people become more aware of discrepancies between where they are and where they would like to be. The woman in the example above wants to be able to cope and to feel in charge of her life. She realises that she doesn't feel able to cope at present and although she drinks to try to help herself she can see that the drinking is making things worse, not better. The more people become unsettled by this awareness the more they will think seriously about change. The task of developing discrepancy is a delicate one as will be seen when we look at resistance below.

Principle 3: roll with resistance

Resistance refers to the common experience of people opposing others' efforts to impose change. When people are ambivalent about something they are, in effect, in conflict with themselves. *I want to do it and I don't want to do it.* If another person comes in and takes one side of this argument there is a tendency to take the opposite side. For example, someone is being encouraged to try a new medication and their decisional balance looks like Table 25.2.

If the health professional tries to talk the client into changing, the conversation might go like this.

> I don't know whether I want to take this new medication or not.
> **You should give it a try. It helps a lot of people with problems like yours and you only have to take it once a day, so you won't forget so often.**
> But I've got used to the old tablets and I don't want a whole lot of side effects. I don't forget them that often anyway.
> **You might not get any side effects. Not everyone does.**

Table 25.2 Pros and cons of staying on drug A/B.

Pros of staying on drug A	**Cons of drug A**
Familiarity Better the devil you know . . . The side effects are manageable	Needs to be taken several times a day Doesn't seem to be working as well as it might, perhaps because of poor compliance Some side effects
Pros of drug B	**Cons of drug B**
Only needs to be taken once a day; easier to remember It's a new drug and seems to be helping other people who were not doing well on drug A	Untried on this particular client Some people get troublesome side effects

But I did with the stuff you gave me a couple of years ago. They were horrible. I didn't feel like myself at all.
But you're really not all that well at the moment. Surely it's worth a try. They might make you feel better.
I'm OK really. Just because I had a bit of a bad spell the other week. Everyone has good days and bad days.

The internal argument has become externalised and the more the health professional promotes drug B the more the client resists change, supporting the pros of drug A and the cons of drug B. 'Denial' about the recent relapse is looming on the horizon.

Rolling with resistance is a metaphor taken from the 'soft' martial arts, where rolling out of the way of an attack is more effective than fighting back. An important aspect is listening to and actively reflecting the resistance, giving the client the opportunity to put both sides of the argument themselves. Here is how the conversation might go.

How do you feel about trying this new drug?
Well, I'm not sure really.
It sounds as if you think it might be worth a try but you've got some reservations.
I've got used to the tablets I'm on and I'm worried about a whole new set of side effects.
You feel its better the devil you know than the devil you don't!
I suppose so.
But in some ways you're tempted to give the new ones a try . . .
Well, they might work better than the ones I'm on now.
So, you're not totally happy with the ones you're on at the moment.
Well it's hard to remember to take them regularly and if I miss too many they don't work properly. The other week is an example. That was horrible.
So a tablet you only have to take once a day might be a better option for you as long as it doesn't have bad side effects.
Perhaps. What do you think I should do?
Well, I can't guarantee how they'll work for you. All I can tell you is we've got a few patients on them now and all except one have found them helpful. But it's your decision. If you gave them a go you'd need to give it a couple of weeks for them to start working and to know if they're going to agree with you. Is there anything else I can tell you to help you make your mind up?

The counsellor has listened to the client's ambivalence and reflected the reservations. This has facilitated the contemplation of change and the client has begun to express some positive views about the change in medication.

Principle 4: support self-efficacy

People are only motivated to attempt change if they have faith in the possibility of achieving it. There are two types of self-efficacy (Bandura, 1977): belief that they can achieve the behaviour change and belief that if they do so there will be a beneficial outcome. The client above needs to have sufficient confidence that:

- I *could* take this drug regularly.
- If I took it regularly it *would* help me.

The client described earlier, who is thinking about stopping drinking needs to have confidence that:

- She *can* do without a drink.
- Changing her drinking *would* have a beneficial effect on her mental health and her social circumstances.

Counsellors aim to support what self-efficacy

clients have, encouraging them to talk about past successes, their strengths and the support they can enlist. So, in the example of the woman who drinks, the counsellor might encourage her to talk about the possibility of success and to think about things that would help.

> What is the longest you have been without a drink recently? What sort of things have you found help you cope when you haven't got a drink?
>
> You say you used to cope better than you do at the moment. What were you like at that time? What sort of things did you do to help yourself then? Could you do any of them now if you were to give up the drinking?
>
> You say that some of your friends and family have been keeping their distance a bit since you've been drinking so much. I wonder if any of them would renew their support if you told them you were going to stop drinking? What would that be like?
>
> What would be the good things for you about drinking less?

Exploring importance and confidence

Motivation arises out of a combination of beliefs. I am motivated to change when I believe that:

- The way I am now is unsatisfactory to me. (*importance*)
- I will be better off if I change. (*importance*)
- If I decide to change I can do it. (*confidence*)

For example, the client who has been drinking in an attempt to cope with anxiety and depression might be ready to change when she believes that:

> The drinking doesn't really help me after the first hour or so. In fact it tends to make me worse. I feel dreadful in the mornings. It's causing me more problems because I run out of money, don't eat properly, forget to take my tablets and my family are losing patience with me because I'm always drunk.
>
> If I stopped drinking I would have to face up to my problems, which would be hard, but I would get more support from my family, would be able to look after myself more and get some of my self-esteem back. I'd feel more in control and if I took my pills regularly maybe they would work better.
>
> I know I can get by without a drink. Often I run out of money and have to go a couple of days without and I cope with that. I get by because I have to. That means I could get by all the time if I wanted to. Five years ago I hardly drank at all and with the help of the counsellors at the centre I do believe I could get back to being the person I was then.

People who are not motivated may lack one or more of these beliefs. It is very important to some people to change, but they really do not believe they can do it. They will only become motivated when their self-efficacy or confidence increases. A sense of hopelessness is common in clients with dual diagnosis (Kofoed, 1997). Others believe that they could make a particular change any time they choose but are not convinced that they would benefit from doing so. These will only be motivated when the disadvantages of their current behaviour become important to them or the advantages of change seem really attractive. Motivational interviewing helps people to clarify how motivated they are, using the dimensions of importance and confidence. It then enables them to explore what it will take to resolve the ambivalence and find the courage to move forward.

One way of helping people to understand their own position is to ask scaling questions similar to those used in solution focused therapy (De Shazer *et al.*, 1986). These use the concept of a continuum to assess importance and confidence and then ask questions that encourage people to talk positively about their interest in change. When enquiring about importance the counsellor might ask questions like this:

> Do you mind if I ask you a bit about how you feel about making this change? If I was to ask, on a scale of 1–10 where 1 is 'It's not at all important to me' and 10 is 'It's the most important thing in my life right now' what number would you give it? Why would you give it that number rather than a 0 or 1?
>
> What puts it as far up as that?
>
> What would it take to move it up a step?
>
> What number would it need to be before you'd have a go at making this change?

Then similar questions about confidence:

> If I was to ask a similar question about how confident you feel about being able to do it, on a scale of 1–10, where 1 is 'I really don't think it's possible' and 10 is 'I could definitely do it if I really wanted to' what number would you give it?
>
> Why would you give it that number rather than a 0 or 1?
>
> What puts it as far up as that?
>
> What would it take to move your confidence up a step?
>
> What number would you need to be on before you'd have a go at making this change?

People are ready to change when both importance and confidence are high. These questions can be brought together in summary by asking:

> 'So, where does this leave you now? How ready are you to do it?'

And if the client found the scaling idea useful they can be asked to put a number on this readiness too. Prochaska & DiClemente (1986) have developed a model that explains readiness to change in terms of stages through which people move. From *precontemplation*, when the person is not interested in change there is a move through *contemplation*, *determination* (or *preparation*), *action* and *maintenance*. Sometimes the change attempt leads to a long-term *termination* of the behaviour and sometimes it ends in *relapse* and recycling back through the earlier stages. Figure 25.1 shows a model of the process of change. Motivational interviewing can be seen as a counselling style that supports the client through these stages.

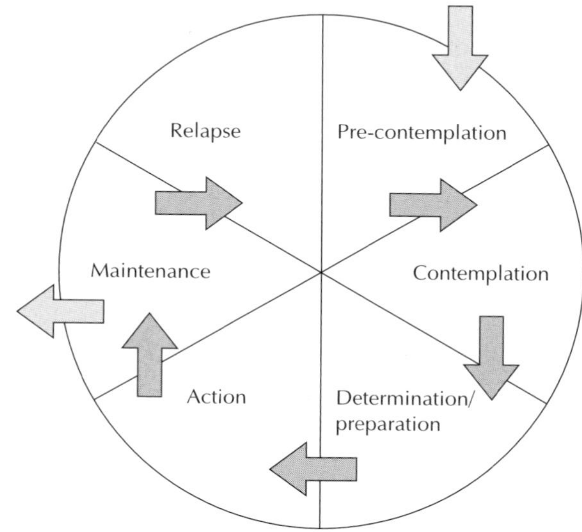

Figure 25.1 A model of the process of change.
Source: Prochaska & DiClemente (1986).

Some guidelines

Be clear about the agenda

It is important to set the agenda clearly at the beginning. There may need to be a negotiation about which of several possible behaviour changes to discuss. Some dual diagnosis clients will be most ready to discuss behaviour change around their substance use and others will want to talk about how they can help their mental health problem. The client will be in a different stage of change about each of the behaviour changes that are on the table and the ambivalence issues will vary, so both should be clear what the current topic of discussion is. All things being equal, it is most productive to follow the client's interest and energy and let them choose the agenda. Distressed and anxious clients can feel so overwhelmed by their problems that they find it hard to keep focused on one thing at a time. The nurse may then need to take responsibility for keeping to the chosen agenda.

Remain client centred

Skilled motivational interviewers do not follow a set routine for employing the strategies described above. The first principle is empathy and client centeredness, and techniques should support this principle, not impede it. For example, having a discussion with a client around joining a day programme focused on mental health issues, the counsellor might use scaling questions on importance and confidence. On discovering that the client is perfectly confident that he could enrol and take part but does not consider it important to do so the counsellor might move to looking at the pros and cons of being on the programme, being careful to roll with resistance.

In a discussion with another client around cannabis use the counsellor rapidly discovers that the client knows the cannabis is contributing to their mental health problems and wants to stop but has a circle of friends who use regularly and cannot imagine how she could get out of the pattern of using. The focus shifts to supporting self-efficacy and exploring options for avoiding or resisting peer pressure.

Avoid rushing into action

It is important not to push clients prematurely into action. It can be tempting to move rapidly into discussion about *how* to change before the person has decided whether or not they *want* to change. When this happens the ambivalence has not been resolved and the client either begins to resist, or complies half-heartedly only to relapse.

The evidence for using motivational interviewing with dual diagnosis clients

Motivational interviewing has been evaluated in a range of settings and a full description of the research findings can be found in Miller & Rollnick (2002). Three key areas of behaviour change have been examined in the context of work with dual diagnosed clients:

- Taking medication as prescribed
- Attending and participating in treatment programmes
- Engaging with outpatient services after an in-patient stay

So far, many of the studies in this area have been pilots with small numbers of clients involved. Handmaker *et al.* (2002) reviewed the evidence. Motivational interviewing, when integrated into treatment services, shows potential for increasing client involvement with treatment both as in-patients and outpatients. Interestingly, Steinberg *et al.* (2004) found motivational interviewing effective in motivating schizophrenic patients to seek help to give up smoking. The evidence for it improving medication adherence is less clear, although UK studies (Kemp *et al.*, 1996; 1998) have shown that an adaptation of motivational interviewing improved compliance rates. Research in this specialist area has not, then, been into the evaluation of motivational interviewing as a treatment per se, but as an adjunct, to enhance client engagement with the actual treatment process. In other contexts it has shown its worth as a treatment in its own right. One concern expressed about the use of decisional balance techniques with mentally disordered individuals is that there may be such severe deficits in their thinking processes that they cannot be realistic about the pros and cons of their behaviour. However Carey *et al.* (1999) found that schizophrenics with substance abuse problems were able to engage usefully with this process. Martino *et al.* (2002) found that their dually-diagnosed patients found the 2 × 2 matrix 'confusing and redundant' and responded better when the matrix was reduced to just the pros and cons of the anticipated change. Coming at this from a different angle, an Italian study (Solomon & Fioretti, 2002) applied the principles of the stages of change and motivational interviewing to facilitate change in a psychiatric system of health care delivery, with the aim of incorporating substance use treatment into existing mental health services.

Conclusion

Motivational interviewing has been found to be a useful approach to counselling clients with concurrent mental health and substance use problems. It provides a way of engaging with clients who do not share the health professional's view of what the problem is or who are reluctant to engage in treatment. It is not magic and does not guarantee compliance, but encourages the client to make an informed and considered decision, reducing the risk of eliciting resistance and denial.

References

Bandura, A. (1977) Self-efficacy: toward a unifying theory of behavioural change. *Psychological Review*, 84, 191–215.

Carey, K.B., Purnine, D.M., Maisto, S.A. & Carey, M.P. (1999) Decisional balance regarding substance use among persons with schizophrenia. *Community Mental Health Journal*, 35, 289–99.

De Shazer, S., Berg, I., Lipchick, E. *et al.* (1986) Brief therapy: a focused solution development. *Family Process*, 25, 207–22.

Graham, H. (2003) Cognitive-Behavioural Integrated Treatment (C-BIT). A Treatment Manual for Substance Misuse in People with Severe Mental Health Problems. Wiley, Chichester.

Handmaker, N., Packard, M. & Conforti, K. (2002) Motivational interviewing in the context of dual disorders. In: *Motivational Interviewing* (Miller, W. & Rollnick, S., eds), Guilford, New York.

Kemp, R., David, A. & Hayward, P. (1996) Compliance therapy: an intervention targeting insight and treatment adherence in psychotic patients. *Behavioural and Cognitive Psychotherapy*, 24, 331–50.

Kemp, R., Kirov, G., Everitt, B., Hayward, P. & David, A. (1998) Compliance therapy in psychotic patients: randomised controlled trial. *British Medical Journal*, 312, 345–9.

Kofoed, L. (1997) Engagement and persuasion. In: *The Principles and Practice of Addictions in Psychiatry* (Miller, N.S., ed.), 214–20. W.B. Saunders, Philadelphia.

Martino, S., Carroll, K., Kostas, K., Perkins, J. & Rounsaville, B. (2002) Dual diagnosis motivational interviewing. A modification of motivational interviewing for substance-abusing patients with psychotic disorders. *Journal of Substance Abuse Treatment*, 23, 297–308.

Miller, W. & Rollnick, S. (2002) Motivational Interviewing. Guilford, New York.

Prochaska, J.O. & DiClemente, C.C. (1986) Towards a comprehensive model of change. In: *Treating Addictive Behaviors: Processes of Change* (Miller, W.R. & Heather, N., eds). Plenum, New York.

Rollnick, S., Mason, P. & Butler, C. (1999) *Health Behaviour Change, a Guide for Practitioners*. Churchill Livingstone, Edinburgh.

Sciacca, K. (1997) Removing barriers; dual diagnosis and motivational interviewing. *Professional Counsellor*, 12 (1), 41–6.

Solomon, J. & Fioretti, A. (2002) Motivational interviewing as applied to systems change: the case of dual diagnosis. *Substance Use and Misuse*, 37 (14), 1833–51.

Steinberg, M.L., Ziedonis, D.M., Krejci, J.A. & Brandon, T. (2004) Motivational interviewing with personalized feedback: a brief intervention to smokers with schizophrenia to seek treatment for tobacco dependence. *Journal of Consulting and Clinical Psychology*, 72 (4), 723–8.

26 Relapse Prevention in Dual Diagnosis

D. Manley & J. McGregor

Introduction

Of all the possible outcomes of treatment for substance misuse problems, relapse is often the most common. If someone with mental health problems relapses into substance misuse it is often associated with deterioration in their mental health. Poor concordance with treatment and a reluctance to take prescribed medication can result from the chaos associated with substance misuse and severe mental health problems (Drake *et al.*, 1989). Conversely, poor concordance may also be at the root of mental health crises and may compel the client to take substances. The risk of relapse may be increased for individuals with substance misuse and psychosis if they choose to take substances in an attempt to self-medicate for their symptoms. This would suggest that control of their substance misuse is dependent upon the stability of their mental health. Furthermore, psychoactive substances can have a significant impact upon an individual's mental health and may be a destabilising factor for some people. Clearly, substance misuse and mental health problems have complex interdependencies for people who are regarded as having a dual diagnosis. Ongoing relapse prevention for these individuals should therefore address both their substance misuse and their mental health, holistically.

The consequences for relapse into substance misuse are highly significant for this client group, given that it may also lead to, or compound, mental health crises. These crises may in turn result in compulsory admission to hospital. Intoxication can have a significant effect on an individual's behaviour, which may also be interpreted as deteriorating mental health. Evidently the picture is complex.

Traditionally, there has been an onus on people with psychiatric problems to become completely abstinent from substances that may negatively affect their mental health. Abstinence, it is suggested, is the only safe, sensible and risk free course for psychiatric clients. However, whilst being abstinent may be good advice it is not always the most pragmatic. Clients who engage in drug and alcohol taking often become disillusioned with service providers when they try to impose abstinence as the only choice. Clients may regard professionals who pressure them to be abstinent as lacking in empathy and the client may subsequently disengage from services. It is perhaps better to see abstinence as part of the continuum of possibilities for individuals. Any attempt at control of substance intake can be viewed as a positive progression to a less problematic state, which requires the client to adopt new skills and motivation to maintain stable mental health. These new skills are the bread and butter of relapse prevention work. This chapter will examine the interventions that nurses can employ with their clients to help minimise the risk and impact of relapse into substance taking and the associated mental health issues.

As already noted in this book, psychiatric service users experience a number of factors that may affect their desire to engage with services. Continued support is an essential factor in addressing relapse of both the client's mental health and their substance misuse. The next part of this chapter will examine some of the potential barriers to continued engagement with services to prevent relapse.

Negative experiences of services/treatment

Dually diagnosed clients can have negative perceptions of services and treatment. Often this is a result of repetitive episodes of psychiatric treatment and a resulting loss of self-efficacy. Clients who are pessimistic about the outcome of treatment are likely to be resistant to change and unlikely to fully engage in the change process. It may therefore be helpful to gauge from the client their fears and concerns when engaging in dialogue about changing any behaviour that is significant to them.

Social isolation

Dually diagnosed clients have often had the invalidating experience of combined social stigma associated with their substance use and psychotic disorders (Evans & Sullivan, 1989). Service users are often confused by service arrangements and this results in a 'misfit' to treatment systems that do not have integrated dual diagnosis care (Ridgely *et al.*, 1990). Many clients sense acutely a social exclusion at some level, be it derived from the stigma of having a mental health diagnosis, from heightened vulnerability to abuse from others, or from environmental and social factors, such as unemployment or criminal offending as a result of drug-taking behaviour. Problematic drug use tends to create marginalisation for the user, but coupled with mental health problems the individual can often find themselves cut off from mainstream society.

Empathy

It is important in these circumstances to understand clients' difficulties within the context of their mental health problems. As previously noted, if a client feels that the practitioner is not empathic about both their mental health problems and their drug-taking then that may be a barrier to establishing a therapeutic alliance.

Dealing with cognitive impairment

Cognitive impairments among dually diagnosed clients may include problems with attention and concentration, short-term and working memory, organising and abstracting information, and mental flexibility (Seidman *et al.*, 1993; Bell *et al.*, 1994; Lysaker *et al.*, 1995; Green, 1996). Disordered thinking may include thought blocking or other psychotic symptoms, such as paranoia or grandiosity, that may impede the motivational enhancement process. Interviews that have insufficient structure or that excessively delve into emotionally laden material or psychotic belief systems may heighten the client's psychotic symptoms and reduce the effectiveness of the health practitioner to motivate the client for change. Trying to follow the client's conversational lead when the client continues to veer from a logical pathway may be very difficult for the health practitioner and client, and result in the health practitioner becoming confused about which part of the client's conversation to reflect.

Recognising fluctuations in motivation

Motivation is not a static phenomenon for any of us, and in dually diagnosed clients motivation may fluctuate, especially in relation to changes in their mental health. Interventions designed to enhance motivation, whilst aiming to strengthen confidence in the change process, should undoubtedly play a vital role in the therapeutic process. The process of motivational interviewing, which forms a central part of helping a client maintain control of their substance abuse, is examined later in this chapter.

Concepts of relapse prevention in dual diagnosis

Graham (2004) proposes a modified cognitive model of problem substance misuse after Beck *et al.* (1993). In this model (see Figure 26.1) triggers or stimuli are cues that become associated with drug

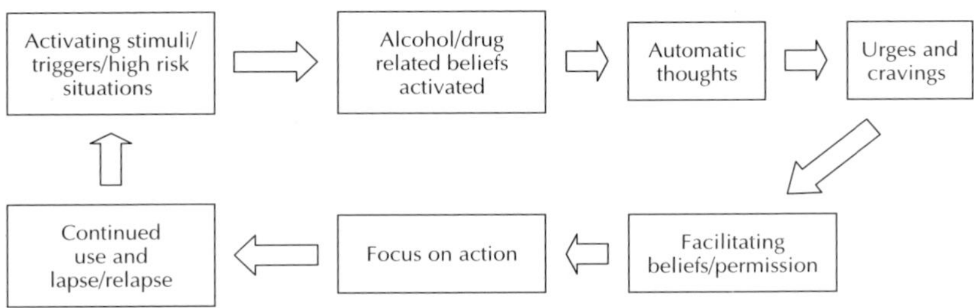

Figure 26. 1 Cognitive model of problem substance use.
Source: Graham (2004).

or alcohol taking (Coombs *et al.*, 2001). Through the process of classical conditioning these cues, associated with drug-taking and withdrawal, come to elicit a conditioned desire or craving in long-term drug users (Modesto-Lowe & Kranzler, 1999). Triggers activate alcohol or drug-related beliefs, usually positive, which in turn will induce involuntary thoughts and usually lead to cravings or urges to take their drug of choice. (Interventions to help the client deal with these cues are examined later in the chapter.)

In the above model these urges lead on to facilitating beliefs, where the client gives themselves the permission to take drugs/alcohol. At this stage the client is also likely to minimise the negative consequences of indulging their craving. Following this part of the process a likely lapse or relapse becomes inevitable as the individual becomes completely focused on obtaining their substance. The possibility of relapse avoidance is lost. Continued lapse or relapse is then only a step away as the client gives themselves the 'permission' to continue (see rule violation experience below). The great advantage of this model is that it allows the clinician and client an opportunity to evaluate the process that may lead to a lapse. Once these risk areas are established the possibility for intervention at all stages to prevent the 'inevitability' of relapse can be planned with the client. This chapter will explore interventions used to support relapse planning and prevention in greater depth.

The rule violation experience

Marlatt & Gordon (1985) put forward the idea that there is a strong cognitive link to behaviour in misuse of drugs and alcohol. They have suggested that when a client relapses in their endeavour to become abstinent or control their substance misuse there is a strong cognitive basis in their belief that they have failed. In other words they have violated the rule that they originally set for themselves, which is 'once stopped I must stay stopped'. In this case the client may go on to link the idea of failure with worthlessness, inability and meaninglessness. In the face of these feelings it is easy for an individual to convince themselves that their attempt at control or abstinence has completely failed and is always doomed to fail. At this juncture it is natural for the individual to extend this belief to reinforce continued use of substances, leading them into a full blown relapse.

Marlatt & Gordon (1985) argued that if the client is led to believe that rather than experiencing a full relapse they are merely lapsing then this may be less catastrophic to the client. This in turn offers the client the opportunity, facilitated by the practitioner, to learn from their experiences and employ their understanding of previous lapses to avoid future risks. A simple intervention with a client is to explain this process to them and to examine their beliefs and previous experiences of relapse. This process often helps to break down the 'catastrophisation' of lapse and begin the process of learning how to cope with the risk of relapse for the client.

Relapse prevention in practice

By the time you begin to address the potential for relapse with your client you should have already thoroughly examined their positive reasons for taking substances. Individuals with mental health problems often begin taking substances problematically for similar reasons to those drug/alcohol users who do not experience mental health problems. However, some individuals with mental health problems have a preference for specific substances that they believe help them cope with their individual circumstances, in particular their mental health problems. Clients may self-medicate in an attempt to cope with the negative symptoms of their illness. Alternatively, clients may choose to self-medicate in an attempt to deal with extrapyramidal side effects of drugs that they have been prescribed. An example of this is illustrated by the case vignette below.

Jason is a 22-year-old-man who has a diagnosis of schizophrenia. At the age of 18 he started injecting amphetamines ('speed') and occasionally smoking cannabis. With the help of his care coordinator, Ian, Jason identified numerous positive factors he associated with taking drugs. One factor he identified was that when he took 'speed' he felt less stressed by the voices that he hears. In addition to this, Jason also completed drug diaries and he noted, when evaluating these with the help of Ian, that he was injecting more amphetamines in the three or four days immediately prior to his depot injection. When he explored this further it came to light that at times he felt over sedated by his monthly depot and he resorted to the amphetamines to cope with the sedation. Jason decided to stop taking amphetamines for a week. However, after a while he began to feel that his prescribed medication made him feel so stupefied that he craved the lift that the stimulants gave him. In addition to this, Jason struggled to cope with the voices he heard and his desire for the confidence to deal with his hallucinations that amphetamines had previously given him, increased his craving. Within a few days Jason began injecting stimulants once more.

The next part of this chapter will examine specific skills and therapeutic approaches that can be employed to help your client maximise their ability to maintain control of their substance misuse and avoid relapse.

Relapse prevention planning

Relapse prevention is a term used to refer to a wide range of eclectic interventions, which include cognitive behavioural strategies. In the substance misuse field, much relapse prevention work is based on the theoretical model of the relapse process proposed by Marlatt & Gordon (1985). In dual diagnosis it can be helpful to view relapse not in terms of a recurrence of old behaviour after a period of changed behaviour, but in terms of a failure to reach targets/goals set by the individual over a given period of time. Cognitive behavioural approaches tend to assume that it is largely psychological factors, such as thinking processes and mood following a relapse, that determine whether the individual returns to previous behaviours.

One of the most important interventions with clients at this stage is to help them assess risks that may be associated with relapse. A useful tool that can be employed in this assessment is the *Inventory of Drug-Taking Situations* (IDTS) (Annis *et al.*, 1997). The IDTS is a 50-item self-assessment clinical tool that is used to identify situations that may pose risks to the client. The IDTS is primarily aimed at those individuals who experience substance misuse rather than a dual diagnosis, but as with other interventions in this book it can be adapted to meet the needs of this specific client group. Clients may need support to identify risks associated with their substance misuse and the clinician should ensure that mental health related risks are included in the evaluation. Once these risks are identified the client and clinician should negotiate an appropriate relapse prevention plan. The plan should be owned by the client as this will help to empower them and increase their self-efficacy. An important part of any plan should include social skills training, for example assertiveness work, and social inclusion, such as attending college and peer support. The plan can also include specific interventions to help motivate the client to deal with their substance misuse.

Motivational interviewing (MI)

MI is a brief psychotherapeutic intervention for helping clients change addictive behaviours. Conceptually, it is a blend of principles drawn from motivational psychology, Rogerian therapy (1951), and the stages of change model (Prochaska & DiClemente, 1986). MI aims to facilitate and enhance the client's intrinsic motivation to change problem behaviours by engaging the client in an empathically supportive, but strategically directed, conversation about the client's use of substances and related life events. MI is a skill that is used throughout interactions with the dually diagnosed client, but is particularly important in maintaining motivation in relapse prevention. Typically, the MI practitioner uses a variety of techniques to help increase intrinsic motivation for change. These techniques can be divided into two categories: micro-skills and strategies (Rollnick *et al.*, 1992).

Motivational interviewing micro-skills serve to facilitate an open discussion with the client about problems they may be experiencing. These skills include the use of open-ended questioning, reflective listening, using affirmations and summarising the patient's comments in a balanced manner. The MI practitioner uses these skills to accurately understand the client's perceptions about a problem, heighten the client's recognition of their problems and resolve their ambivalence about changing it. The MI practitioner's competent use of micro-skills is essential in the creation of MI's highly empathic and collaborative style. In a subsequent section of this chapter we highlight an adapted motivational approach (Martino *et al.*, 2002). This places more emphasis on the strategic nature of guiding the conversation with the client in a manner that promotes the client's logical organisation and reality testing, without sacrificing the collaborative and respectful nature of MI.

Towards a model of intervention

Motivational interviewing modifications

Martino *et al.* (2002) describe an adapted motivational approach, which they name dual diagnosis motivational interviewing (DDMI). The following section outlines suggested modifications to MI to meet the needs of people who experience mental health problems. Asking open-ended questions, listening reflectively (including summarising), and affirming the client care are MI micro-skills. These micro-skills are also fundamental to the DDMI approach, so the practitioner may consider first providing the client with a brief and simple introduction to DDMI before asking open-ended questions and beginning the reflective listening process. The collaborative MI style of interaction established by the MI practitioner's use of micro-skills often is unfamiliar to clients with dual disorders, who may have become accustomed to a more directive and authoritarian style of interviewing from mental health services.

Simplifying open-ended questions

After the opening remarks, the MI practitioner typically begins with an open-ended question (for example 'What brings you here today?'). Asking open-ended questions is a primary MI strategy, particularly at the early stages of the interview when a practitioner encourages the client to talk about their perception of specific problem areas (Miller & Rollnick, 2002). Open-ended questions are questions that result in more than a yes/no response and that encourage the patient to elaborate on a topic rather than to provide very specific information. These types of questions generally provide the client with opportunities to express their viewpoint, uninterrupted by the practitioner. Whilst fairly straightforward, open-ended questions are most effective when the practitioner asks them in very clear terms and avoids compound questions that may be difficult for psychotic patients to follow. For example, the question: 'What types of psychiatric symptoms do you experience and how does your use of cocaine affect your symptoms in the short and long term?' is overly complex and may overwhelm the client's organisational capacity to respond. DDMI practitioners try to avoid these types of open-ended questions and aim to simplify them where possible (Martino *et al.*, 2002).

Refining reflective listening skills

To listen reflectively means that the practitioner takes time to carefully understand what the client has said and confirms this understanding with them by repeating it back to them in similar (simple reflection) or somewhat transformed ways (restatement, paraphrasing, double-sided reflection). The practitioner uses this structure as a foundation from which to identify and resolve ambivalence towards change. In MI, competent reflective listening is a difficult task that requires keen practitioner attention and ability to organise and rephrase what the client has said. Clients with psychotic disorders may exhibit some degree of disordered thinking and poor reality testing that might unravel further in the absence of a sufficiently structured interview. To address this, DDMI incorporates strategies of repetition, use of simple and concrete verbal and visual materials, and breaks within sessions. To emphasise this point, the following recommendations are considered important:

(1) Use simple and concise language.
(2) Reflect often.
(3) Use metaphors where possible.
(4) Avoid excessive focus on despairing client statements and negative life events.
(5) Logically organise clients' statements with summaries.
(6) Give clients enough time to respond to reflections.

Heightening emphasis on affirmations

Another MI micro-skill is affirming the client. The health practitioner affirms the client by acknowledging their personal qualities and efforts. In DDMI heightened emphasis is placed upon affirming clients during the interview process (Martino *et al.*, 2002). For example, a practitioner might express appreciation to a client who has had a history of treatment non-compliance for attending a session or taking medications as prescribed. Reflecting such achievements reinforces progression and positive change.

Providing feedback that addresses dual diagnosis concerns

DDMI incorporates many of the commonly used MI strategies, including a variety of techniques for skilfully handling resistance. Dually diagnosed clients often express resistance in reaction to perceived coercion compelling them to make changes (from case managers, psychiatrists, probation officers, etc.). The practitioner, it is suggested, places great effort in developing discrepancy in the client's perceptions of his or her problems and provides personalised feedback as a means to alter the client's view that substance use or psychiatric issues are not problematic. Feedback typically involves a practitioner providing a structured review of objective assessment results in an empathetic and collaborative style (for example showing the client and talking through urine screen results). The health practitioner explores with clients their reaction to the feedback and the possible relationships between the client's use of substances, their problems or concerns, and their intention to change their behaviour. The feedback needs to be simple in presentation and capable of compelling clients to look at their long-standing problem areas in a renewed light (Martino *et al.*, 2002).

Other clinical considerations

The modifications described above help practitioners use MI more effectively in relapse prevention with dually diagnosed clients. However, clients must have sufficient psychiatric stability to benefit from MI's ample use of verbal persuasion and logical reasoning. When clients are too psychotically disorganised to remain based in reality, it is not appropriate to use DDMI and they may require other types of intervention (for example crisis intervention, pharmacotherapy) first. In addition to psychotic exacerbation, dually diagnosed clients have higher rates of suicide (Drake *et al.*, 1989; Lyons & McGovern, 1989; Turner & Tsuang, 1990) than substance abusing clients without co-occurring psychiatric conditions. Therefore, DDMI requires that practitioners are capable of performing risk assessments of clients' dangerousness to self and others, and are knowledgeable about the policies and procedures for handling clients who are at imminent risk.

Motivational interviewing is a promising treatment approach to use with dually diagnosed clients although it requires modifications to accommodate the special needs of substance using clients who have psychotic disorders. The complex and severe problems experienced by dually diagnosed clients may limit the ultimate capacity of a brief intervention like DDMI to render beneficial impact. Nonetheless, studies of brief motivational interventions have shown the intervention's effectiveness in reducing substance use outcomes with high average effect sizes comparable to more extensive treatments (Bien *et al.*, 1993), particularly when they are used to enhance engagement in intensive treatment as usual (Dunn *et al.*, 2001).

Cue exposure therapy (CET)

CET is a cognitive behavioural intervention that endeavours to equip the client with skills that they can employ to resist drug-related stimuli. Cue exposure treatment, based on a Pavlovian extinction paradigm, involves exposure of the patient to cues that induce drug craving whilst preventing actual drug use and, therefore, the experience of drug-related reinforcement (Niaura *et al.*, 1988). In contrast to counselling, which often encourages clients to avoid drug-related cues, CET involves the client in inducing triggers (or cues) under controlled, supported circumstances. The client is then encouraged to develop a variety of coping strategies that they can use to extinguish their craving. In essence the client is encouraged to engage and work through their cravings instead of avoiding and fearing such stimuli.

Some clinicians have concerns that CET, which is designed to elicit cravings, might provoke relapse before any therapeutic benefit is achieved (Coombs *et al.*, 2001). However, avoidance of all substance related cues is nearly impossible, as not only can ordinary everyday items be used as drug-taking paraphernalia but cues may also be negative emotional states. It is the author's experience that CET can be particularly useful in helping the client break the link between substance misuse and negative emotional states associated with their mental health problems. Cue exposure has been used as part of relapse prevention therapy with clients who use a variety of substances: stimulants, alcohol, opiates and nicotine (O'Brien *et al.*, 1990).

The process of CET is usually conducted over several (eight or ten) 45-minute individual sessions. Initially, the client is taught to measure their level of craving and their ability to cope with the cravings (self-efficacy). The client is introduced to a 10-point rating scale for craving (0 = no craving, 10 = the worst craving they have ever experienced) and a similar 10-point scale for measurement of self-efficacy (0 = I couldn't resist the desire at this time, 10 = I could easily resist the craving). A 'baseline' rating is taken at the start of every session. The client and clinician use this baseline as a point to which the client is returned at the end of every session. This essentially acts as a safety net, ensuring that the client's cravings and ability to cope with them is always at a level that they experience naturally on a day-to-day basis.

Initial sessions of CET involve an in depth assessment of paraphernalia that the client uses to take substances, and related emotions and situations that act as cues. The process of conducting this assessment may induce craving for the client so a baseline needs to be taken before commencing such an assessment. The assessment should be as detailed as possible as it is important that cues are meaningful to each individual. For example, the difference between one type of syringe and another is likely to be highly significant to the injecting drug-taker. The client is taught a variety of coping mechanisms (outlined in Table 26.1 below) before the actual exposure to cues begins. Once the client has a good understanding and can practice these coping strategies exposure sessions can commence. Sessions typically involve two or three cue exposure episodes, repeating the same cues or adding new ones. Clients are asked to monitor their craving

Table 26.1 Coping strategies used in CET.

- **Passive delay**: the client waits out the craving; cravings naturally dissipate over time.
- **Imagining negative consequences of substance use**: personally relevant negative outcomes are used as a focus to extinguish the cues (for example taking amphetamines has resulted in admission to hospital).
- **Imagining positive consequences of not taking substances**: personally relevant positive outcomes of not taking drugs/alcohol are used as a focus to extinguish the cues (for example 'I would have a better relationship with my family if I stopped drinking so much').
- **The craving is imagined to be an object**, such as a piece of paper, which can be screwed up and thrown away.
- **Imagining engaging in incompatible activities**: instead of responding to craving by taking the drugs the client imagines engaging in an incompatible activity for example going swimming.
- **Mastery**: the client employs mastery statements that they can initially use verbally in practice, but that they graduate on to using as a thought. For example 'I can beat this' or 'Jim stopped, so can I'.

Source: after Monti & O'Leary (1999).

and self-efficacy at regular points throughout sessions (every two or three minutes is preferable, every five minutes may be more practical). This self-assessment allows for evaluation of ongoing craving and it also gives the client and clinician insight into strategies that work best. The first one or two sessions usually comprise exposure to photos of substances being taken, photos of paraphernalia or drugs which act as stimuli. Once the client is comfortable that they have mastered photos they can move on to exposure to actual paraphernalia (for example injecting/smoking equipment or 'mocked up' drugs). The final stages of cue exposure involve the strongest stimuli, using imagined cues.

Important factors when conducting CET

- Cues must be as realistic and meaningful to the client as possible.
- Practising mastery of cues in a clinical setting can lead to the client being able to generalise their new skills to less supported settings. Trying to 'generalise' skills should be avoided in the initial stages until the client has gained greater self-efficacy. As the sessions progress the client may be asked to practice outside structured sessions in order to enhance their level of confidence.
- Throughout CET sessions the client should be asked *not* to expose themselves to strong cues.
- CET can be initiated on in-patient units to positive effect. The additional support that a client receives outside CET sessions may be very beneficial in the short term. However, clients will need to be 'psychiatrically stable' to engage in this therapy.
- Evaluation is an important part of CET. Clinicians should keep copious and specific notes on sessions so that progress can be reflected to the client as part of a supportive intervention.
- Clinicians may prefer to work in pairs when conducting sessions in order to aid observations and feedback to the client.

Conclusion

Clinicians can employ a number of effective interventions to help reduce the risk of relapse for their clients. Effective relapse prevention should be based upon thorough assessment of associated risks related to drug/alcohol taking *and* risks of relapse in mental illness. The interdependency of these factors should not be ignored as they affect each other significantly. Positive outcomes of relapse prevention are likely to be related to an integrated approach that encourages the client to take ownership of their drug/alcohol and mental health problems. A client centred approach is the best way to encourage self-efficacy for the client and is likely to raise self-esteem and the belief that being substance free is achievable and sustainable. Ultimately though, the success of relapse prevention in this client group is intrinsically linked to the stability of their mental health.

References

Annis, H.M., Turner, N.E. & Sklar, S.M. (1997) *IDTS Inventory of Drug-Taking Situations. A User's Guide.* Addiction Research Foundation, Ontario.

Beck, A.T., Wright, F.D., Newman, C.F. & Liese, B.S. (1993) *Cognitive Therapy of Substance Abuse.* Guilford, New York.

Bell, M.D., Lysaker, P.H., Milstein, R.M. & Beam-Goulet, J.L. (1994) Concurrent validity of the cognitive component of schizophrenia: relationship of PANSS scores to neuropsychological assessments. *Psychiatry Research*, 54, 51–8.

Bien, T.H., Miller, W.R. & Tonigan, J.S. (1993) Brief interventions for alcohol problems: a review. *Addiction*, 88, 305–25.

Coombs, N., Manley, D. & Rosenberg, H. (2001) Resisting reaction; acting on cue. *Drug Link*, 16 (2).

Drake, R.E. & Wallach, M.A. (1989) Substance abuse among the chronically mentally ill. *Hospital and Community Psychiatry*, 40, 1041–6.

Drake, R.E., Osher, F.C. & Wallach, M.A. (1989) Alcohol use and abuse in schizophrenia: a perspective community study. *Journal of Nervous and Mental Disease*, 177, 408–13.

Dunn, C., Deroo, L. & Rivara, F.P. (2001) The use of brief interventions adapted from motivational interviewing across behavioral domains: a systematic review. *Addiction*, 96, 1725–42.

Evans, K. & Sullivan, J.M. (1989) *Dual Diagnosis: Counselling the Mentally Ill Substance Abuser.* Guilford Press, New York.

Graham, H., Copello, A., Birchwood, M. *et al.* (2004) *Cognitive Behavioural Integrated Treatment.* Wiley, Chichester.

Green, M.F. (1996) What are the functional consequences of neurocognitive deficits in schizophrenia? *American Journal of Psychiatry*, 153, 321–30.

Lyons, J.S. & McGovern, M.P. (1989) Use of mental health services by dually diagnosed patients. *Hospital and Community Psychiatry*, 40, 1067–9.

Lysaker, P.H., Bell, M.D., Zito, W.S. & Bioty, S.M. (1995) Cognitive deficits in schizophrenia. Prediction of symptom change for participators in work rehabilitation. *Journal of Nervous and Mental Disease*, 183, 332–6.

Marlatt, G.A. & Gordon, J.R. (1985) *Relapse Prevention: Maintenance Strategies in the Treatment of Addictive Behaviors*. Guilford Press, New York.

Martino, S., Carroll, K., Kostas, D., Perkins, J. & Rounsaville, B. (2002) Dual diagnosis motivational interviewing: a modification of motivational interviewing for substance abusing patients with psychotic disorders. *Journal of Substance Abuse Treatment*, 23, 297–308.

Miller, W.R. & Rollnick, S. (2002) *Motivational Interviewing: Preparing People for Change*, 2nd edn. Guilford Press, New York.

Modesto-Lowe, V. & Kranzler, H.R. (1999) Using cue reactivity to evaluate medications for treatment of cocaine dependence; a critical review. *Addiction*, 94, 1639–52.

Monti, P.M. & O'Leary, T.A. (1999) Coping and social skills training for alcohol and cocaine dependence. *The Psychiatric Clinics of North America*, 22, 447–70.

Niaura, R.S., Rohsenow, D.J., Binkoff, J.A., Monti, P.M., Pedraza, M. & Abrams, D.B. (1988) Relevance of cue reactivity to understanding alcohol and smoking relapse. *Journal of Abnormal Psychology*, 97, 133–52.

O'Brien, C.P., Childress, A.R., McLellan, T. & Ehrman, R. (1990) Integrating systemic cue exposure with standard treatment in recovering drug dependent patients. *Addictive Behaviour*, 15, 355–65.

Prochaska, J.O. & DiClemente, C.C. (1986) Towards a comprehensive model of change. In: *Treating Addictive Behaviors: Processes of Change* (Miller, W.R. & Heather, N., eds). Plenum, New York.

Ridgely, M.S., Goldman, H.H. & Willenbring, M. (1990) Barriers to care of persons with dual diagnoses. *Schizophrenia Bulletin*, 16, 123–32.

Rogers, C.R. (1951) *Client Centred Counselling*. Houghton-Mifflin, Boston, Mass.

Rollnick, S., Heather, N. & Bell, A. (1992) Negotiating behaviour change in medical settings: the development of brief motivational interviewing. *Journal of Mental Health*, 1, 25–37.

Seidman, L.J., Pepple, J.R., Farone, S.V. *et al.* (1993) Neuropsychological performance in chronic schizophrenia in response to neuroleptic dose reduction. *Biological Psychiatry*, 33, 575–84.

Turner, W.M. & Tsuang, M.R. (1990) Impact of substance abuse on the course and outcome of schizophrenia. *Schizophrenia Bulletin*, 16, 87–95.

Part 5

Professional Development

Chapter 27 Educational Development and Clinical Supervision

Chapter 28 The Role and Competencies of Staff in the Treatment of Coexisting Problems of Mental Health and Substance Misuse

27 Educational Development and Clinical Supervision

G.H. Rassool

Introduction

The issue of dual diagnosis is one of the most pressing concerns facing the substance misuse and mental health fields at the current time. The care and management of individuals with dual diagnosis are being poorly addressed and there is reluctance and resistance from practitioners to become more involved. One of the aims of the equality framework for the NHS *The Vital Connection – An Equality Framework for the NHS* (Department of Health, 2000) is to recruit, develop and retain a workforce that is able to deliver high quality services that are fair, accessible, appropriate and responsive to the diverse needs of different groups and individuals. This has implications and relevance for workforce development on ethnicity, mental health and substance misuse. The challenge is therefore how to enable existing services to address dual diagnosis more effectively through capacity and competency building. Education and training are central to the long-term strategy to overcome the problems, but the organisational culture needs to be re-examined. Resistance by individuals needs to be addressed through training and clinical supervision. The central themes that guide the professional development of mental health and addiction nurses, as specialist practitioners, are based upon their educational preparation, continuing professional development and clinical supervision.

The aims of this chapter are to examine issues for professional development in relation to education and training and clinical supervision. In addition, the types of education and training and those who need training will be examined. Finally, a framework for dual diagnosis courses at foundation and advanced level will be presented.

Education and training

Since substance misuse is more likely to be the norm than exception amongst individuals with mental health problems, there is a pressing need for mental health practitioners to develop their knowledge and clinical expertise in substance misuse in order to respond effectively to the needs of this group of patients. It is also acknowledged that addiction nurses and other professionals need to update their knowledge on mental health aspects relevant to working with individuals with dual diagnosis.

Many reports have recommended that professional bodies in health and social work continue to design training in the early identification of drug and alcohol misuse and appropriate referral skills for professionals working in health, social care and the criminal justice system (Rassool, 2002). The Department of Health report *Working in Partnership* (Department of Health, 1994) emphasises that mental health nurses encounter substance use problems as part of their workload and recommends that all mental health nurses should be capable of prevention, recognition and early intervention. The report also states that there is an urgent need to prepare mental health nurses and others in the primary health care teams in dealing with substance misusers.

In the *National Alcohol Training Strategy* report (Alcohol Concern, 1994), it is stated:

> 'The basic training which is provided for professional staff such as doctors, nurses, social workers and probation officers ensures that they are competent in the performance of their professional role. It does not, however, always include the competencies required for the early identification of alcohol misuse, for offering appropriate response, and for making appropriate referrals where indicated. Professional staff also need opportunities for post-basic training to enable them to specialise in work with alcohol misusers.'

The report on *Alcohol Harm Reduction Strategy* (Prime Minister's Strategy Unit, 2004) stated that at present there is little training on alcohol issues for health professionals. Many health professionals acknowledge that they need more training, and studies indicate that some do not feel adequately trained to deal with alcohol-related problems.

The All Party Parliamentary Drugs Misuse Group report (2000) recommended that

> 'Better training in substance misuse and dual diagnosis for doctors, nurses, social workers, probation officers, police and prison officers and voluntary sector personnel would assist in the early recognition of the condition and better accessibility to appropriate treatment provision.'

The recent report of the working party of the Royal College of Psychiatrists and Royal College of Physicians (2000) suggested that both addiction and psychiatric services serve dual diagnosis poorly and consider that 'the management of problem drug and alcohol misuse must become more central to the training of all mental health professionals, particularly those working in community psychiatric services'. There is an urgent need to increase the availability of training courses on dual diagnosis at all levels and to ensure access for professionals working in both rural and urban settings.

There are recent recommendations from the Health Advisory Service (2001) and the Department of Health (2002) *Dual Diagnosis Good Practice Guide* for the training and ongoing professional development of staff to be prepared adequately to work with individuals with coexistence of mental health and substance misuse problems. Furthermore, it is recommended that each local area should develop a training strategy to identify the training needs of all staff and professional groups working in statutory and non-statutory organisations. It has been argued that a substance misuse component should be integrated far more extensively into the undergraduate and postgraduate training programmes of mental health professionals (Rassool, 1993; 1997a; 1999; Crome, 1999).

However, education and training in substance use and dual diagnosis have been largely patchy and limited, and have lagged behind the growth in service provision. There is evidence to suggest that mental health service workers lacked the knowledge and skills for assessment and treatment of substance misuse and were insufficiently aware of the available resources and how to access substance misuse services (Maslin *et al.*, 2001). Dual diagnosis is often not picked up by substance misuse or mental health services, indicating needs for improvement in staff training and routine assessment and recording (Weaver *et al.*, 2002).

Identifying and meeting training needs

Education and training in dual diagnosis, at a local level, should not be ad hoc but based upon systematic planning. Initially, purchasers should develop an educational strategy with local authorities, educationalists and providers of services to identify the target needs and the planning of an educational programme. It is acknowledged that although this process is complex and time consuming, it is invaluable in the delivery of high quality training and is service driven. A training needs analysis of each team or service is of paramount importance and should be part of a coherent strategy. This analysis should focus on the mapping of skills, experience and attitudes.

The targeted audience for training should be staff working in community mental health teams, in-patient services, assertive outreach teams, early intervention teams, crisis resolution teams, primary care, mental health services for older people, independent mental health projects, accommodation services, day care services, statutory drug and alcohol services and independent drug and alcohol service providers (Department of Health, 2002) and those working in hostel accommodation, housing, prisons, health care, probation and others in the criminal justice system. In effect, all those who come into contact with dual diagnosis patients, generic and specialist staff, in both hospital and community settings. The question here is not who needs training in dual diagnosis but what kind and levels of training are required?

Theoretical and skills based training

The needs analysis, including attitude analysis, would provide an adequate mapping of the theoretical content and skills development in each team in either substance misuse or mental health services. Issues raised by individuals, service users and carers can also form the basis of learning and teaching activities. Thus, training can be tailored to meet the individual needs of each part of the service, depending on the context and nature of the staffs' roles and responsibilities. If effective collaborative working is to take place it will also be important to learn about the roles of other agencies and the framework of their assessment and interventions. It is important to acknowledge and build upon the existing knowledge and competencies of each team. There is bound to be a mix of skills and experience in teams, as individual levels of knowledge of mental health or substance misuse may be variable within teams. It has been suggested that, where possible, whole teams should be trained together to ensure a cohesive approach is adopted and that team members share an understanding of the theoretical basis of the approach so that they can support each other in their daily work (Department of Health, 2002).

Core competencies

The goal of education and training in substance use and mental health problems (Rassool, 2002) would be to:

(1) Provide an increased awareness and recognition of the needs of the patients
(2) Enhance the shared care and collaborative approaches between the different disciplines
(3) Improve the evidenced based intervention strategies required in dealing with such complex problems
(4) Provide high quality care for those with dual diagnosis

Training will need to adopt a two-tiered approach as individuals working within mental health services will, by definition, need a higher emphasis on training around substance misuse and vice versa for individuals working in substance misuse services (Department of Health, 2002). Individuals working in mental health services will need a broad programme, based on needs analysis, that will include knowledge of dual diagnosis, drug and alcohol, assessment skills for substance misuse, risk assessment and management, management of substance misuse problems, detoxification procedures, motivational interviewing, relapse prevention, self-help groups, shared care approach and care coordination. Individuals working in substance misuse services will need training on knowledge of mental health, assessment skills for mental health problems, psychosocial interventions, pharmacological treatments, medication management, early warning sign monitoring and relapse prevention for mental health problems and mental health legislation.

The following core competencies that are relevant to all staff in all settings have been suggested by the Department of Health's *Dual Diagnosis Good Practice Guide* (2002). The core competencies for training in dual diagnosis are presented in Table 27.1.

The core competencies for staff would need to be modified, based on training needs, according to which part of the service they work in. For example, staff working in assertive outreach teams will require intensive training on the assessment, engagement and management of individuals with a dual diagnosis, whereas training for in-patient staff may focus on the detection and assessment of substance misuse, with less emphasis on longer-term treatment options.

Inter-agency training has also been suggested to provide the foundation of the training strategy (Department of Health, 2002). The aim is to foster

Table 27.1 Core competencies for training in dual diagnosis.

- Knowledge of dual diagnosis
- Drug and alcohol awareness
- Assessment skills for substance misuse
- Assessment skills for mental health problems
- Risk assessment and management
- Knowledge of the management of substance misuse problems
- Knowledge of the management of mental health problems
- Engagement skills
- Care coordination
- Motivational enhancement strategies including motivational interviewing
- Relapse prevention for substance misuse
- Early warning sign monitoring and relapse prevention for mental health problems
- Mental health legislation

Source: Department of Health (2002).

Table 27.2 Inter-agency training agenda to meet the following training needs.

- Raise awareness of mental health issues and therapeutic responses
- Raise awareness of drug-related issues and therapeutic responses
- Raise awareness of the relationship between substance misuse and mental health problems
- Challenge negative attitudes and prejudices around both mental health problems and substance misuse
- Increase staff confidence and reduce fear and anxiety in relation to working with people with complex needs
- Joint/shared training on assessment and referral
- Knowledge of other relevant services and referral criteria
- Cross-cultural and gender issues
- Accessing users' views
- Scope and limitations of compulsory powers under mental health legislation

Source: Department of Health (2002).

closer working alliances between teams, services, prisons and all agencies, whether statutory or independent sector, for mental health and substance misuse. Considerable effort may be required in some services to ensure all professional groups are involved with the training strategy and key representatives of each profession need to be involved with strategy development. This may be done through a journal club or forum to share information about capacity development and to discuss current working practice and professional boundaries. The inter-agency training agenda (Department of Health, 2002) is presented in Table 27.2.

Ongoing supervision, continuing professional development and peer support is vital if training is to be effective in developing a competent practitioner.

New problem, new danger

One of the training agenda of inter-agency training is to challenge negative attitudes and prejudices around both mental health problems and substance misuse. Despite the magnitude of the problem, and even when substance use problems are identified, health care professionals may be reluctant to respond appropriately due to the lack of adequate preparation and negative attitudes towards substance misusers. Social prejudice, negative attitudes and stereotyped perceptions of substance misusers (Hanna, 1991; Carroll, 1996; Rassool, 1998; Selleck & Redding, 1998) and dual diagnosis patients (Williams, 1999) are widely held amongst health care professionals and this may lead to minimal care being given to this population. Overtly self-abusive behaviour, particularly when it involves illicit drugs, is dealt with in a suppressive and moralistic way by many health care workers not least of all nurses, probably out of a sense of frustration or inadequacy about their ability to effect any change (Gafoor, 1985).

Studies support the development of a more positive and non-judgemental attitude, and confidence and skills in identifying and working with substance misuse and related problems may be partly related to the provision of education and training (Cartwright, 1980; Hagemaster *et al.*, 1993; Rassool, 1993). However, much professional education and training reinforces the view that dealing with substance misuse is the job of a specialist (Rassool, 1993; 2000). In the case of dual diagnosis patients, the responsibility for health and social care provision is being shifted from one discipline to another and the 'diffusion of responsibility' is all too apparent.

Practice development and clinical supervision

For the application of theory derived from training programmes to clinical practices, staff from mental health or substance misuse services need to be supported by ongoing clinical supervision. This is an essential element for new ideas to be embedded in clinical applications and in the development of professional competence in clinical practice. Addiction and mental health nurses, like any other nurse specialists, are envisaged to be autonomous practitioners with professional competence in the delivery of care and accountable to the clients and the profession. Generally, health and social care professionals (non-substance misuse specialists) feel overwhelmed and deskilled in working with substance misusers. It is through both the process of training and supervision that the barriers to practice can be eliminated and confidence in existing skills can be enhanced. This is part of the component in transforming the 'culture and context' of care for individuals with coexisting substance misuse and mental health problems.

Several reports have highlighted the importance of clinical supervision and recommended that nurses, midwives and health visitors should embrace the concept of clinical supervision and incorporate it as an integral part of their practice (Department of Health, 1993; UKCC, 1995). Faugier (1994) argues that, despite increasing recognition of the importance of clinical supervision, few mental health nurses have access to skilled, sensitive and formal supervision. Those who work in a developmental nursing specialty, such as addiction nursing, have derived a need for clinical supervision because of the nature of their work within a multidisciplinary framework and the multiple roles they operate (Rassool, 1997b). The reality of clinical supervision is that it is seldom clear-cut in the context of addiction nursing and substance misuse. Staff (1997) states that:

> 'The opportunity for independent autonomous working practices in a specialism where the patient or client group is frequently operating in an illegal underworld or subculture is a danger, and becoming over involved stretches the boundaries of professional conduct'.

Clinical supervision as a priority for nurses working with individuals with coexisting substance misuse and mental health problems can no longer be ignored.

What is clinical supervision?

The definitions of supervision are many, and are sometimes based on the nature of the professional discipline. These definitions are often conflicting and contradictory and this is augmented by the negative connotations attached to the concept. In its simplest form clinical supervision refers to a process of practising, experiencing and reflecting upon clinical practice (Rassool, 1997b; 1998). Clinical supervision can be seen as a formal process whereby a worker and an experienced practitioner meet to examine and reflect on the management of clients and the refinement of therapeutic skills.

In the context of clinical supervision in nursing, Butterworth & Faugier (1992) describe supervision as 'an exchange between practising professionals to enable the development of professional skills'. This seems to suggest that there must be a formal way and a logical approach to reviewing one's professional work with a more experienced colleague. It has also been described as a formal process of professional support and learning that enables practitioners to develop knowledge and competence, assume responsibility for their own practice and enhance consumer protection and safety of care in complex situations (Department of Health, 1993). Bond & Holland (1998) describe clinical supervision as regular, protected time for facilitated, in-depth reflection on clinical practice aimed to enable the supervisee to achieve, sustain and creatively develop a high quality of practice through the means of focused support and development. Although the above definitions adequately stress the importance of personal support, they omit the wider functions of educative, supportive and managerial relationships in clinical supervision as described by Kadushin (1976).

Purpose of supervision

An important and central focus of clinical supervision is to enhance the quality of services to clients or patients and it is generally acknowledged that introducing clinical supervision in clinical practice would provide benefits for both practitioners and the client.

Barker (1992) argued that clinical supervision is needed 'to protect patients from nurses and nurses from themselves'. Nurse practitioners, with the help of clinical supervision, would be able to develop professional competencies in specific areas of their work, and with adequate supervision and support, stress and burnout are reduced. It is argued that practitioners who are well supported, up-to-date and professionally aware, as a result of having access to effective clinical supervision, will benefit the organisation (UKCC, 1995). Moreover, it is stated that supervision has the potential to reduce litigation and complaint levels (Tingle, 1995) and supervision correlates with job satisfaction (Cherniss & Egnatios, 1978). The task of supervision is not only to develop the skills, understanding and reflective practices of the supervisee, but may have other functions depending on the settings. Kadushin (1976) describes three main roles of supervision: educative, supportive and managerial.

In the nursing profession it is common to have a combination of these three roles in dealing with a supervisee. This may be achieved through the system of personal tutorial (educative and supportive) and clinical supervision (educative, managerial and supportive). There is also the assertion that a good deal of supervision takes place in the areas where managerial (quality control function), supportive and educative considerations all intermingle (Hawkins & Shohet, 1989). In summary, the purpose of clinical supervision includes the maintenance of clinical standards, development of professional competence, reducing stress and burnout and provides support and job satisfaction.

Approaches to clinical supervision

There are many forms of clinical supervision: self-supervision, one-to-one, co-supervision, group supervision and peer supervision. The one-to-one supervision and group supervision are common in mental health nursing and addiction nursing. A summary of approaches to clinical supervision is presented in Table 27.3.

Table 27.3 Approaches to (models of) clinical supervision.

Individual	Meeting one to one with a more experienced clinician acting as supervisor
Peer	Meeting one to one with an equally experienced clinician
Group (led)	Meeting as a group with a more experienced clinician acting as supervisor
Group (peer)	Meeting as a group of similar level experience with no designated supervisor or group leader
Team	Meeting as multidisciplinary clinical team to address clinical issues, either with or without designated supervisor

Self-supervision

This is a form of 'self-reflecting in action' that is important in personal and professional development, and can occur in a variety of different contexts. This form of self-supervision is valid to the individual; and the ability to explore our own thoughts, feelings and actions with self-evaluation is seen as therapeutic. Self-supervision should always be accompanied by one or other forms of supervisory practices. What is essential for all forms of self-supervision is giving oneself enough time and also being willing to confront one's own ways of working with a healthy 'internal supervisor' (Kagan, 1980; Hawkins & Shohet, 1989).

One-to-one supervision

This is the most common form of supervision that is given and received on an informal basis by practitioners in the helping profession. It is acknowledged that one-to-one clinical supervision will become a model in most branches of nursing, but on a formal and regular basis. For example, a student receives clinical and academic supervision by one or more supervisors. A clinical nurse specialist provides clinical supervision to a drug and alcohol worker.

Co-supervision

As in co-counselling, co-supervision involves two practitioners. Both practitioners alternate the role of supervisor and supervisee in providing clinical supervision for each other. This form of supervision usually occurs on an informal basis amongst practitioners working in the community.

Group supervision

Group supervision is common in mental health nursing, whereby a supervisor or consultant external to the agency or with a different orientation is responsible for the facilitation of the group. The group facilitator negotiates the allotted time with the supervisee for the presentation of casework. The consultation group can arrive at formulations and strategies that provide the group members with new understanding and action plans.

Geller (1994) asserts that group supervision augments traditional supervision and is an effective tool for teaching students about group work; thus, students are sensitised to group processes as a medium for growth and change. The advantages of group supervision over one-to-one supervision include: cost effectiveness in terms of time and money; supportive environment; opportunity to test out or check emotional and intuitive responses with other members of the group; receiving feedback and input from group members and the facilitator; provision of a wider range of life experiences; and use of group and action techniques. However, group supervision is less likely to mirror the dynamics of the individual session, and the dynamics of the group could become a preoccupation to members, with less time for individual members to have supervision (Hawkins & Shohet, 1989).

Peer supervision

Peer supervision is common in substance misuse agencies in an informal context, where the multidisciplinary team shares the responsibility for providing clinical supervision within a group context. The potential problems of using only peer supervision are that current norms of practice may be perpetuated, and the exploration of innovative or alternative practices is less likely to occur (Devine & Baxter, 1995). It is argued that peer supervision is not recommended for the novice, the newly qualified practitioner or those who lack adequate skills and professional competence. In a study by Benshoff (1993) on peer supervision in counsellor training, it was found that 70 subjects out of a total sample of 81 students reported that peer supervision had been very helpful in developing their skills and the understanding of counselling concepts. However, it was also found that subjects who received peer supervision did not rate themselves higher on counselling effectiveness than those who received traditional supervision.

Models of clinical supervision: a review

The model of supervision and supervisory practices used by supervisors is largely dependent on their orientation to a particular school of counselling and psychotherapy. Some supervisors would use an integrated or eclectic model of clinical supervision based on the humanistic, psychoanalytical, transpersonal and behavioural schools of psychology. Others would base their supervisory practices upon the framework and philosophical underpinnings of one particular school of psychology.

A number of models of supervision can be identified in the literature: growth and support model (Faugier, 1992); interactive model (Proctor, 1991); triadic model (Milne, 1986); multicultural model (Ramirez, 1991); and integrative model (Hawkins & Shohet, 1989). Some of the nursing based literature includes descriptions of clinical supervision in the psychotherapy mode. Dombeck & Brody (1995) describe the principles and process of a model of clinical supervision for psychotherapy, drawing heavily on Peplau's (1952) theory of interpersonal relations and Bowen's (1978) family systems theory.

Rich (1993) describes an integrated model of supervision that identifies basic requirements. In the organisational context in which it is embedded, clinical supervision fulfils four functions:

- Facilitating a supportive learning and work environment
- Fostering staff development
- Providing a means for the professional socialisation of staff
- Ensuring the delivery of effective client services

The UKCC's statement on clinical supervision also argues that there is no single model that can be used in every clinical setting and that local practitioners will need to develop an approach that suits their particular needs. Powell & Brodsky (1993) argue that the substance misuse field requires a model of supervision that synthesises all the (developmental, psychodynamic, skills and family therapy) traditions into a coherent whole that reflects the principles and practices specific to alcohol and drug abuse counselling. They have designed a comprehensive, 'blended' model, and offer guidelines for its use with substance abuse workers and counsellors.

Choosing a supervisor

It is acknowledged that a novice practitioner should always be accommodated with an advanced practitioner, that is, the less experienced should be supervised by an experienced and competent practitioner. Supervisors in nursing and other health care professions should possess a first level registration with the recommended requisite of attending formal educational preparation in clinical supervision. The process of supervision depends very much on the supervisor and supervisee's levels of motivation, development and past experiences of supervision.

Watkins (1995) reviewed four models of supervisor development and found that all supervisors begin in a state of uncertainty, insecurity, anxiety and inexperience. They wrestle with various issues; progress by means of time, experience and struggle; and ultimately forge a supervisory identity and become competent. According to Devine & Baxter (1995) the nurse supervisor should meet the following criteria:

- Receive supervision
- Have some form of preparation
- Be trained or have identifiable skills/qualifications
- Demonstrate facilitation skills
- Be a reflective and proactive practitioner
- Be chosen by the supervisee
- Be willing to give supervision
- Understand the privilege of the position
- Be worthy of respect
- Respect confidentiality
- Utilise research findings

However, it is the supervisor's skills and the relevance of his/her experience and expertise to the supervisee that are of prime importance (Kohner, 1994). There are, however, organisational factors and inherent ambiguities in this managerial relationship and supervisory situation where conflicts may inhibit the learning process. The contemporary clinical supervision in nursing and allied professions has focused heavily on the management accountability and quality control, with other aspects in teaching and consultation. The UKCC (1995) has stated that clinical supervision should not be an exercise of managerial responsibility and managerial supervision, or a system of formal individual performance review procedures, or hierarchical. The choice of having a line manager as supervisor can lead to difficulties, since a conflict of interests may arise between the needs of the substance misuse agencies and the needs of the supervisee. The UKCC's position statement on clinical supervision states that practitioners should have a say in who acts as their clinical supervisor, and although the supervisor will normally be a registered nurse, they may be a clinician from another profession in exceptional cases. This is applicable for addiction nurses as in many community oriented substance misuse teams, where there may be only one nurse as a full member of the team.

Perception of addiction nurses

There is an assumption that nurses are generally inclined to embrace and to receive clinical supervision. Hawkins & Shohet (1989) identified interpersonal, organisational and professional factors that may cause reluctance to give and receive supervision. These barriers may be applicable to addiction nurses and include:

- Previous experience of supervision
- Personal inhibitions
- Difficulties in the supervisory relationship
- Organisational blocks
- Practical block
- Culture of the organisation
- The professions' being antithetical to supervision

Nurses' beliefs and attitudes are highly significant towards the positive acceptance of clinical supervision as an integral part of professional practice. There is a paucity of literature on the attitudes of nurses towards clinical supervision, and few studies on the nature of clinical supervision in mental health nursing. Pesut & Williams (1990) administered the Nursing Clinical Supervision Questionnaire to 61 clinical nurse specialists and found that supervision seemed to be highly valued, although many did not feel well prepared to assume the role of the clinical supervisor. There were disagreements on such items as structuring the supervisory session.

A study was undertaken to explore and examine the perception of addiction nurses towards clinical supervision (Rassool & Lind, 2000). An opportunistic sample of 40 addiction nurses completed a self-reported questionnaire: the Clinical Supervision Perception Questionnaire (CSPQ). A focus group was also used to elicit further content and themes regarding clinical supervision. The sample consisted of 22 females (55%) and 18 males (45%); 75% of the subjects had worked in the field of addictions for less than five years; 25% of the sample had six or more years' experience in addiction services.

The findings showed that 92.5% of the subjects had a clear understanding of the concept of supervision and perceived clinical supervision as distinct from other support systems. The subjects viewed supervision as something more than an informal chat and different from counselling in both its nature and its process. The type of clinical supervision preferred by addiction nurses in combined services (drug and alcohol agencies) and those more experienced in addictions, was found to be the non-managerial role as described by Kadushin (1976) and Proctor (1991). This finding is similar to that of Bishop (1994) who, in a study of clinical supervision with a sample of 534 nurses, also revealed a clear preference for the non-managerial type of supervision. However, as to the question of whether managerial supervision was more appropriate in addiction nursing the group as a whole was split evenly, indicating that there may be a place for 'managerial' supervision in both types of agencies. It would also appear that one-to-one clinical supervision was a popular choice with practitioners. This approach to supervision offers the potential to meet individual clinical practice developmental needs without the apprehension of formal assessment of work performance.

The findings also show that 44% of subjects working in a single substance agency were satisfied with the level of supervision they received, compared with only 37.5% of those working in combined services. This raises the question as to whether addiction nurses in combined agencies required additional supervision in order to address the more varied nature of their work. The complexities of working with those with a dual diagnosis of alcohol and drug misuse presented more challenges in meeting the needs of the client group. In addition, 56% of subjects working in a single substance service (drug or alcohol agencies) found managerial supervision appropriate to their type of work, compared with only 25% of those working in combined agencies. This may also indicate that addiction nurses working in combined agencies have different supervisory needs compared with those working in single drug or alcohol agencies. This study also confirms that the value of clinical supervision was highly regarded by addiction nurses working in combined agencies. Supervision was perceived as an integral part of their nursing practice by 71% of those working in combined agencies, compared with only 37% of subjects working in a single substance agency.

Addiction nurses with more experience in the field have less preference for their senior manager to be their supervisor; 70% of subjects compared with 30% with less than five years' experience. This may indicate that the nurses with more experience require a different style or form of supervision and also that those experienced nurses who are more autonomous in their delivery of care require a more educative and supportive role from their supervisor. The focus here is that more experienced addiction nurses require less monitoring in relation to balancing the workload, administrative procedures, audit activity and meetings, compared with less experienced addiction nurses.

In summary, this exploratory study does indicate that some addiction nurses are receiving clinical supervision on a regular basis; however, less than half the subjects were satisfied with the style and form of that supervision. The study also reveals different supervision requirements amongst the different subgroups, for example nurses working in combined drug and alcohol services, and nurses who have worked in the field for longer, having different needs and perceptions of supervision.

Conclusion

In this chapter the emphasis has been on the importance of professional development in relation to training and clinical supervision. If clinical supervision is to remain an integral part of the lifelong learning process, there is a need to develop standardised training and clinical standards in practice. There are few studies that directly examine the relationships of the supervisee performance to patient outcomes. There is a need for a shared understanding of the tasks and purposes of clinical supervision in nursing, especially for those undertaking undergraduate professional courses. Although some form of supervision is grounded in mental health nursing, it remains underdeveloped in addiction nursing. Existing models of supervision, either integrated or developmental models of clinical supervision, could be adapted to fill the gap in supervision framework and delivery. It is hoped that clinical supervision as a developmental activity, in the substance misuse field, will generate more research. The focus should be based not only on the effectiveness of educational programmes but also on whether improvement of professional competence, as a result of supervision, has a direct benefit for the client in the delivery of quality care.

Professional development will always be most effective when it is part of a strategic plan to create an organisational learning culture (Rassool, 1997a). The consequences of lack of adequate education and training in substance use and misuse, at all levels, are a self-perpetuating cycle. Where a low priority is accorded to both policy and educational development in this area, there is no opportunity for health and social care professionals to develop role adequacy. This results in reinforcing the negative attitudes and the reluctance of health care professionals to respond effectively to substance misusers (Rassool, 1993; 2000). It is argued that the dual development and integration of a substance misuse curriculum at pre-registration and post-registration levels should be part of a parallel process of change (Rassool, 1993). If education and training in addiction for all health care professionals is to become a reality, policy-makers, professional associations, educationalists and clinicians need to capitalise on the current political climate to focus on an effective strategy for enhancing substance misuse education on the professional agenda. Health and social care professionals have a dissonance between their personal belief (therapeutic pessimism), and their professional roles. That is, they think that there is nothing that can be done or should be done, and feel de-skilled and lacking in confidence (Rassool, 2000). This statement is highly significant in working with individuals with coexisting substance misuse and mental health problems.

Due to the nature and extent of dual diagnosis, a cultural shift is required in many of the paradigms that have traditionally guided the work of health and social care professionals. This cultural paradigm needs to focus on equality of access to services, diversity issues, social inclusion, 'beyond professional boundaries', cultural competence and above all to have therapeutic optimism in dealing with the complexities of dual diagnosis.

References

Alcohol Concern (1994) *A National Alcohol Training Strategy*. Alcohol Concern, London.

All Party Parliamentary Drugs Misuse Group (2000) *Report on Drug Misuse and Mental Health: Learning Lessons on Dual Diagnosis*, (April). All Party Parliamentary Drugs Misuse Group, London.

Barker, P. (1992) Psychiatric nursing. In: *Clinical Supervision and Mentorship in Nursing* (Butterworth, T. & Faugier, J., eds). Chapman & Hall, London.

Benshoff, J. (1993) Peer supervision in counsellor training. *Clinical Supervisor*, 11 (2), 89–102.

Bishop, V. (1994) Clinical supervision questionnaire results. *Nursing Times*, 90, 40–2.

Bond, M. & Holland, S. (1998) *Skills of Clinical Supervision for Nurses*. Open University Press, Milton Keynes.

Bowen, M. (1978) *Family Therapy in Clinical Practice*. Aronson, New York.

Butterworth, T. & Faugier, J. (eds) (1992) *Clinical Supervision and Mentorship in Nursing*. Chapman & Hall, London.

Carroll, J. (1996) Attitudes to drug users according to staff grade. *Professional Nurse*, 11, 718–20.

Cartwright, A. (1980) The attitude of helping agents towards the alcoholic client: the influence of experience, support, training and self-esteem. *British Journal of Addiction*, 75, 413–31.

Cherniss, C. & Egnatios, E. (1978) Clinical supervision in community mental health. *Social Work*, 23 (2), 219–23.

Crome, I.B. (1999) The trouble with training: substance misuse training in British medical schools revisited. What are the issues? *Drugs: Education, Prevention and Policy*, 6 (1), 111–23.

Department of Health (1993) *Working in Partnership: A Review of Mental Health Nursing*. HMSO, London.

Department of Health (1994) *Working in Partnership: a Collaborative Approach to Care: a Report of the Mental Health Review Team*. HMSO, London.

Department of Health (2000) *NHS The Vital Connection – An Equality Framework for the NHS*. Department of Health, London.

Department of Health (2002) *Mental Health Policy Implementation Guide: Dual Diagnosis Good Practice Guide*. Department of Health, London.

Devine, A. & Baxter, D. (1995) Introducing clinical supervision: a guide. *Nursing Standard*, 9 (40), 32–4.

Dombeck, M.T. & Brody, S.L. (1995) Clinical supervision: a three-way mirror. *Archives of Psychiatric Nursing*, 9 (1), 3–10.

Faugier, J. (1992) The supervisory relationship. In: *Clinical Supervision and Mentorship in Nursing* (Butterworth, C.A. & Faugier, J., eds). Chapman & Hall, London.

Faugier, J. (1994) Thin on the ground . . . clinical supervision in mental health nursing. *Nursing Times*, 90 (20), 64–5.

Fox, P. (1995) Nursing developments: trust nurses' views. *Nursing Standard*, 9 (18), 31–4.

Gafoor, M. (1985) Nurses' attitudes to the drug abuser. Letter to *Nursing Times*, 30 Oct.

Geller, C. (1994) Group supervision as a vehicle for teaching group work to students: field instruction in a senior centre. Special issue: field instruction in social work settings. *Clinical Supervisor*, 12 (1), 199–214.

Hagemaster, J., Handley, S., Plumlee, A., Sullivan, E. & Stanley, S. (1993) Developing educational programmes for nurses that meet today's addiction challenges. *Nurse Education Today*, 13, 421–5.

Hanna, Z.E. (1991) Attitudes towards problem drinkers revisited: patient-therapist factors contributing to the differential treatment of patients with alcohol problems. Alcoholism. *Clinical and Experimental Research*, 15 (6), 927–31.

Hawkins, P. & Shohet, R. (1989) *Supervising in the Helping Professions*. Open University Press, Milton Keynes.

Health Advisory Service (2001) *Substance Misuse and Mental Health Co-morbidity (Dual Diagnosis). Standards for Mental Health Services*. Health Advisory Service, London.

Kadushin, A. (1976) *Supervision in Social Work*. Columbia University Press, New York.

Kagan, N. (1980) Influencing human interaction – eighteen years with IPR. In: *Psychotherapy Supervision: Theory, Research and Practice* (Hess, A.K., ed.). Wiley, New York.

Kohner, N. (1994) *Clinical Supervision in Practice*. King's Fund Centre, London.

Maslin, J., Graham, H.L., Cawley, M.A.C. *et al.* (2001) Combined severe mental health and substance use problems: what are the training and support needs of staff working with this client group? *Journal of Mental Health*, 10 (2), 131–40.

Milne, D. (1986) *Training Behaviour Therapists: Methods, Evaluation and Implementation with Parents, Nurses and Teachers*. Brookline, Cambridge.

Peplau, H. (1952) *Interpersonal Relations in Nursing*. Putnam, New York.

Pesut, D.J. & Williams, C.A. (1990) The nature of clinical supervision in psychiatric nursing: a survey of clinical specialists. *Archives of Psychiatric Nursing*, 4 (3), 188–94.

Powell, D.J. & Brodsky, A. (1993) *Clinical Supervision in Alcohol and Drug Abuse Counselling: Principles, Models and Methods*. Lexington Books/Macmillan, Inc., New York.

Prime Minister's Strategy Unit (2004) *Alcohol Harm Reduction Strategy*. Strategy Unit, London.

Proctor, B. (1991) On being a trainer. In: *Training and Supervision for Counselling in Action* (Dryden, W. & Thorne, B., eds). Sage, London.

Ramirez III, M. (1991) *Psychotherapy and Counselling with Minorities: a Cognitive Approach to Individual and Cultural Differences*. Pergamon Press, London.

Rassool, G.H. (1993) Substance misuse: responding to the challenge. *Journal of Advanced Nursing*, 18, 9.

Rassool, G.H. (1995) Perception of addiction nurses towards clinical supervision. Centre for Addiction Studies, Department of Addictive Behaviour, St George's Hospital Medical School (unpublished paper).

Rassool, G.H. (1997a) Professional education and training. In: *Addiction Nursing: Perspectives on Professional and Clinical Practice* (Rassool, G.H. & Gafoor, M., eds). Stanley Thornes, Cheltenham.

Rassool, G.H. (1997b) Clinical supervision. In: *Addiction Nursing: Perspectives on Professional and Clinical Practice* (Rassool, G.H. & Gafoor, M., eds). Stanley Thornes, Cheltenham.

Rassool, G.H. (1998) Contemporary issues in addiction nursing. In: *Substance Use and Misuse. Nature, Context and Clinical Interventions* (Rassool, G.H., ed.). Blackwell Science, Oxford.

Rassool, G.H. (1999) Substance use and misuse in nursing: beyond complacency. Editorial in *Association of Nurses in Substance Misuse (ANSA)*, Bulletin 19 (1), 2.

Rassool, G.H. (2000) Addiction: global problem and global response, complacency or commitment? Guest editorial in *Journal of Advanced Nursing*, 32 (3), 505–8.

Rassool, G.H. (2002) Professional education in addiction and mental health issues: a case for less diagnosis and more action? In: *Dual Diagnosis: Substance Misuse and Psychiatric Disorders* (Rassool, G.H., ed.). Blackwell Publishing, Oxford.

Rassool, G.H. & Lind, J. (2000) Perception of addiction nurses towards clinical supervision: an exploratory study. *Journal of Addictions Nursing*, 12 (1), 23–9.

Rich, P. (1993) The form, function and content of clinical supervision: an integrated model. *Clinical Supervisor*, 11 (1), 137–78.

Royal College of Psychiatrists (2001) *Coexisting Problems of Mental Disorder and Substance Misuse ('Dual*

Diagnosis') A Training Needs Analysis. College Research Unit, London.

Royal College of Psychiatrists and Royal College of Physicians (2000) *Drugs: Dilemmas and Choices*. Gashell, London.

Selleck, C.S. & Redding, B.A. (1998) Knowledge and attitudes of registered nurses towards perinatal substance abuse. *Journal of Obstetric, Gynaecologic and Neonatal Nursing*, 27, 70–8.

Staff, A. (1997) Community substance misuse team: management and practice. In: *Addiction Nursing: Perspectives on Professional and Clinical Practice* (Rassool, G.H. & Gafoor, M., eds). Stanley Thornes, Cheltenham.

Tingle, J. (1995) Clinical Supervision is an effective risk management tool. *British Journal of Nursing*, 4 (14), 794–5.

United Kingdom Central Council for Nursing, Midwifery and Health Visiting (1995) *Clinical Supervision for Nursing and Health Visiting*. Registrar's letter, 4/95. 24 January. UKCC, London.

Watkins, C.E. (1995) Psychotherapy supervisor development: on musings, models and metaphor. *Journal of Psychotherapy Practice and Research*, 4 (2), 150–8.

Williams, K. (1999) Attitudes of mental health professionals to co-morbidity between mental health problems and substance misuse. *Journal of Mental Health*, 8 (6), 606–13.

Weaver, T., Charles, V., Madden, P. & Renton, A. (2002) *Co-morbidity of Substance Misuse and Mental Illness Collaborative Study (COSMIC)*. National Treatment Agency, London.

28 The Role and Competencies of Staff in the Treatment of Coexisting Problems of Mental Health and Substance Misuse

R. Edwards

Introduction

There is a high prevalence of dual disorder clients within in-patient mental health services and there is poor detection, liaison between services and treatment for this client group. Overall, it is suggested that 50% of individuals with mental health disorders also have drug and alcohol difficulties at some point in their lives, and between a quarter to a third are currently experiencing difficulties (Menezes *et al.*, 1996; Graham *et al.*, 2004). The screening, detection and treatment of dual disorder are very much 'core business' for mental health services. It is the single most common complication of mental illness (Drake *et al.*, 1993), and yet staff can feel they do not have the skills or confidence to offer effective treatment. It is acknowledged that mental health services need to be far more proactive in placing dual disorder treatment central to the mainstream of mental health service provision (Department of Health, 2002).

There are two reasons why this area of patient care delivery needs urgent attention. The quality of in-patient care generally is poor (Sainsbury Centre for Mental Health, 2004). There are a number of contributing factors to this: busy ward environments, staff shortages, a lack of training and development opportunities, poor quality supervision, uncertainty as to the most effective dual disorder interventions, and ward structures and routines that militate against regular one-to-one interventions (Health Advisory Service, 2003).

The aim of this chapter is to highlight the need for a fundamental shift in the provision of treatment for clients who have a dual disorder in the in-patient setting, and to provide a framework to support change. In addition, an examination of the organisational barriers that may impact on effective in-patient dual disorder treatment is presented. A set of core competencies will be described, which complement the minimum treatment requirements of detection and assessment, engagement, basic care planning and an appropriate liaison on discharge. Second, a set of more advanced competencies are described that include psychosocial interventions. Staff can integrate these into their treatment provision and use them as a framework for continuing professional development. Finally, the training implications for delivering the above skills and competencies for in-patient staff are examined and a number of recommendations are made regarding staff training and development.

Barriers to effective care delivery

There are a number of barriers that may impede effective treatment for clients with dual disorder within acute in-patient settings: the characteristics of the client group, staff skills and attitudes, and the way that care is organised.

Client characteristics

Patients with a dual disorder can present various challenges to an in-patient staff team. As a group, dual disorder clients are often more difficult to treat, as they have higher levels of physical, social and psychological impairment than those with a single diagnosis. They also present challenges when engaging in illicit drug use on the ward, which can be viewed as harmful to both themselves and other patients. Studies have shown higher rates of hospitalisation (Cuffel & Chase, 1994), increased treatment non-compliance (Owen *et al.*, 1996), increased aggression (Scott *et al.*, 1998), increased exacerbation of mental health symptoms (Shumay, 1994), increased psychotic relapse (Linszen *et al.*, 1994) and overall an increase in the use of services (Hipwell *et al.*, 2000). Staff can become frustrated by the perceived 'self-inflicted' nature of the person's drug and alcohol use and the negative consequences on the individual's mental health.

Some studies have shown a high correlation between substance use and personality disorder. The co-morbidity of substance misuse and mental illness collaborative study, a study of co-morbidity amongst adult substance misuse and mental health treatment populations, reported a prevalence of personality disorder of 37% in the drug treatment population and 53% in alcohol treatment (Weaver *et al.*, 2003). There is a risk, however, of diagnosing individuals as suffering from personality disorder as a result of behaviours that can be seen as difficult to manage. Patients often present in crisis, with behaviours that staff can find frustrating. If ward based behaviour from a particular client is problematic, a culture of negativism can develop.

Staff skills and attitudes

The two key barriers that staff report as impacting upon the delivery of effective treatment to this client group are a reported lack of knowledge and a negative attitude towards dual disorder. A training needs analysis carried out by the Royal College of Psychiatrists (Clancy *et al.*, 2001) included staff from four professional groups (psychiatric nurses, psychiatrists, social workers and GPs) and found that '55% of the sample reported feeling inadequately prepared to work with this client group'. Staff may feel that they have inadequate knowledge when discussing drug use with a person who can appear to have a greater understanding of jargon, use, effects and consequences of their drug use. This can be further compounded by an uncertainty as to the most effective treatment response for this client group. In-patient staff often question the legitimacy of their role in the provision of comprehensive substance use interventions. They see the stabilisation of mental health symptoms as the 'key task', and see substance use services as 'specialist'. This perception that substance misuse services have greater expertise, coupled with concerns about their own knowledge deficit presents a real barrier to treatment.

The ability of staff to demonstrate optimism for change and the possibility of positive improvements in an individual's mental and physical health is fundamental to effectively evaluated treatment programmes (Drake *et al.*, 1998). Carers report that it is possible to quickly gauge staff negativity in dealing with this client population. The stereotypical statement from staff is: 'They get well on the ward and then use drugs when discharged, what can you do?' This can decrease self-efficacy and, possibly on an unconscious level, result in withdrawal of the full range of treatment options available.

Finally, there have been found to be variations in attitudes between different professional groups (Williams, 1999) towards the importance of the role of drugs and alcohol in causation of mental illness. This can create tensions within staff teams and may facilitate different treatment. If these attitudes are not recognised and challenged it may impact on the ability of the staff team to build a genuine therapeutic relationship with the individual and carry optimism for positive change in the future. Staff support and supervision must allow staff the opportunity to present and examine complex or difficult case studies; it should be multidisciplinary, working within agreed treatment frameworks and individual client goals.

Organisational barriers

Organisational barriers often compound the barriers experienced by both staff and clients, and include the under resourcing of in-patient care, the structure of in-patient care delivery and poor organisational policy frameworks (Sainsbury Centre for Mental Health, 2004). The reduction in bed capacity within acute in-patient services has increased levels of activity, increasing the in-patient workload. Within some in-patient services there is poor support and supervision, an unclear career structure, and limited opportunities for in-patient focused training.

The nature of an acute care environment militates against the sessional nature of many integrated treatment interventions. The nature and routine of acute care, and the need to respond quickly and effectively to psychiatric emergencies can make regular planned care difficult. Therefore, the challenge facing in-patient staff is how to adapt the ward structure and routines to accommodate sessional treatments. Alternatively, sessional interventions should be adopted to fit the brief, multiple contacts of in-patient client interactions. Multiple, daily interactions could be underpinned by harm reduction, motivational interviewing and relapse prevention interventions, within a framework of specific, planned outcomes. For example, if substance using social networks have been identified as a problem for an individual client, this could be the continued focus of any opportunistic interactions during the course of one or two shifts.

Some in-patient units, recognising the difficulties of having time for care planning, primary nurse sessions and effective liaison have implemented protected engagement time with clients. Wards have ringfenced two or three blocks of time each week, when no visitors are permitted, (including professional workers and carers), no telephone calls are taken and time is set aside solely for client centred activities. Another solution is to manage daily workload planning in a way that protects one-to-one client work. Effective and innovative time management can free staff to provide client centred planned treatment interventions.

The way that mental health services and substance misuse services have been structured has also been problematic. Historically, mental health and substance misuse services have had differing commissioning demands and treatment philosophies. Substance misuse services have focused on opiate treatment in clients who demonstrate a degree of motivation, whilst mental health services see clients with alcohol and cannabis related problems, with a higher degree of ambivalence, requiring a more assertive approach. This can lead to inter-service frustrations, and a reduction in collaborative client work. This has, at best, resulted in duplication of services and poor communication between mental health and substance misuse services, and at worst, access to services being denied altogether because of exclusion criteria.

Mental health and substance misuse service liaison and integrated treatment planning can be improved by developing agreed clear protocols that highlight service roles and responsibilities, shared care planning for clients with complex needs, inter-agency teaching and placements and nominated link workers. The organisation and structure of services should be informed by the presenting needs of the client group.

Basic core competencies

Dual disorder treatment models have predominately focused on community programmes. The core components of approaches that have delivered positive outcomes include assertive community outreach, family interventions, supported employment, skills training, illness self-management and cognitive interventions within an integrated treatment approach (Drake *et al.*, 2001). These approaches now need to be adapted for the in-patient setting.

Engaging with the patient

There is substantial evidence to support the importance of forming an effective therapeutic relationship with clients. The basis of treatment is the formation of a collaborative relationship, in which the clinician, on occasions, has to carry 'hope' of change for the client. As stabilisation with this client group can be slow, with 10–20% gaining stability from their substance use per year, clinicians need to take a longitudinal view of treatment. As both mental health and substance use are relapsing conditions, the clinician/practitioner needs to accept that there may be setbacks and be prepared for them in order to maintain clinical optimism.

The qualities that service users wish to find in staff are respect, understanding, kindness and professionalism in a collaborative framework (McCann, 2004). These qualities are also identified in *Acute In-patient Mental Health Care* (Clarke, 2004), and include working in partnership, practising ethically, promoting safety and positive risk taking, and promoting recovery. These are core interpersonal characteristics and skills and they underpin the remaining competencies.

Brief assessment and risk assessment

The quality of full drug and alcohol history taking for clients with a dual disorder is poor across a range of clinical settings (Farrell & David, 1988). The detection of drug and alcohol problems is a vital step in delivering appropriate treatment. There should be a high index of suspicion for all individuals, but particularly those who are young, male, homeless, have poor family relationships and repeated hospitalisation, or have a history of disruptive behaviour (Mueser *et al.*, 1992). Functional assessment and analysis (Mueser *et al.*, 2003) is recommended as a framework for the identification and treatment planning for clients with a dual disorder, providing an understanding of the interactions between substance use, mental health and physical, psychological and social functioning. The framework for assessment is provided in Chapter 18.

Physical health care

General health screening has been overlooked as part of the assessment process (Health Advisory Service, 2003). Drug users often neglect health care and dental needs, and many are not registered with a GP. An in-patient assessment is an ideal opportunity to address basic health care needs. The following areas could be considered:

- Nutritional needs and possible self-neglect
- Infections due to intravenous drug use
- Blood tests: liver function tests and full blood count
- Hepatitis B and C, and HIV screening (with appropriate counselling)
- Hepatitis B vaccinations
- Dental check-up
- Blood pressure

Mental health symptom stabilisation

Historically this is the primary role of in-patient care, and comprehensive coverage of the interventions associated with this treatment phase is available elsewhere. However, it is important for staff to be aware of the impact of drug and alcohol use on symptom stabilisation and medication compliance, and therefore staff need to be aware of the following:

- Possible interactions of prescribed and non-prescribed drugs, and possible symptom confusion with drug and alcohol withdrawal profiles
- The importance of minimising the prescription of drugs with a high dependency potential
- The impact of potential side effects of prescribed medication on medication compliance
- The possibility of 'self-medication' to reduce symptomatology or unwanted side effects of the medication
- The necessity for the provision of psycho-educational information to clients and families in a collaborative approach in order to maximise medication compliance

Having the conversation

After the detection of a dual disorder, the clinician needs to have the skills and confidence to have a discussion about the person's substance use and its impact on their mental and physical health. At its most basic, this may be no more than a brief intervention, the components of which focus on the feedback of main issues or difficulties, health education, harm reduction advice and a menu of options, with a clear recommendation for change. Studies have shown that brief interventions in the in-patient setting can reduce the level of harmful drinking (Hulse & Tait, 2002).

To engage the client in care planning regarding their drug and alcohol use, the following skills and knowledge are required as outlined in the sections below.

An awareness of the common drugs used by patients

This would include alcohol, cannabis, benzodiazepines, heroin, cocaine and crack cocaine, LSD (lysergic acid diethylamide), hallucinogenic mushrooms, amphetamines, ecstasy, anabolic steroids, khat and nicotine. Staff may feel the patient knows considerably more about drugs and their effects. The provision of basic drug information to people with many years' experience of using substances can feel meaninglessness and highlight their own lack of knowledge; this can result in reluctance by staff to widen discussions further than 'drugs have not been good for your mental health'. It is important to have access to good quality drug and alcohol information that presents a balanced view on the benefits and disadvantages of drug use, if possible written by service users themselves.

An awareness of the common reasons for drug use

There are many reasons why people use drugs, and, particularly, why people with mental illness may use them. A range of factors may need to be considered:

- The alleviation of unpleasant feelings associated with their illness, to counteract sedative or side effects of prescribed antipsychotic medication
- The provision of a social network (to reduce stigma or increase personal acceptance)
- A vulnerability to use substances, either psychological or social predisposition
- A 'supersensivity' to substances, because of a greatly reduced biochemical tolerance
- An understanding of the relationship between substance use and mental health

Mueser *et al.* (2003) suggest that there may be a common factor that has linked both substance use and mental health problems, such as a major trauma. The mental health problem may be followed by substance use problems, or substance use may trigger mental health problems. Finally, a bi-directional model is described in which the substance use and mental health problems maintain each other. Attempting to 'fit' the person into a particular model can detract from understanding individual need; therefore, it is suggested that a flexible hypothesis may be more helpful.

An understanding of how substance use impacts on mental health symptoms

It is important for staff to have basic physiological knowledge of drug actions, and how they impact on mood, thoughts and behaviour of the individual. Common examples are alcohol acting as a depressant and cannabis inducing anxiety.

Raising self-awareness in clients

The conversation is a process to help facilitate the client in the identification of problems associated with their substance use. One technique for assisting that process is the identification of the person's 'relapse signature', that is, the chain of events that have led to their hospitalisation, including the role of their substance use in this. The exploration of 'early warning signs of psychotic relapse' can assist in identifying early changes to thoughts, feelings and behaviours, and also in isolating events that may have triggered illness. The pattern of alcohol and drug use during the relapse process should be explored. As their mental health deteriorated, what impact did their drug and alcohol use have on their relapse? Why did they use substances? The identification of the potential benefits, and negative effects of this, plus the person's beliefs about their substance use as part of the process is also useful. It is important to acknowledge the benefits of some substance use, and to help identify healthier ways of meeting those needs. Finally, it is necessary to explore their use of prescribed medication during this period of relapse, the perceived effectiveness of this, compliance and the impact on their relapse.

The setting of treatment goals on discharge

The clinicians agree realistic goals with the clients, which are underpinned by the principles of harm reduction. Some clients may wish to attempt abstinence; others may identify 'controlled' use as their goal. Agreed goals can be tested with day or overnight leave. Developing an increased knowledge base in the following areas will increase staff confidence in their exploration of the patient's drug and alcohol use; it can often be a shared learning experience. The clinician is unlikely to be an 'expert' in all aspects of the drug lifestyle.

Family and carer involvement

There are several reasons why there should be the provision of services to families and carers of people with mental health problems. Psychoeducation has been found to be effective (Dixon *et al.*, 2001); service users often live with family members who can play an active role in ongoing support. Having a carer's role can be stressful for family members and this may have a negative impact on all family members and increase vulnerability to relapse (Butzlaff & Hooley, 1998).

Staff need to be able to:

- Invite supportive family members to the ward and engage them in the treatment process.
- Provide psycho-educational information about the specific nature of mental health, and drug and alcohol problems, the principles of management and how family members can help.
- Assist the family in their ability to solve problems and develop coping skills, by setting boundaries, encouraging open communication, learning early signs of relapse and getting support for the whole family.

Aftercare, awareness of post-discharge referral and support

A key role for staff is the preparation, facilitation and development of a discharge plan that will provide structure and support to enable the individual to maintain the stability achieved in the in-patient setting, and build on the foundations of self-management. Ideally, meeting new community workers, making first appointments and beginning new activities should be commenced prior to discharge. Providing a comprehensive aftercare package requires effective liaison with a range of community based services. The early identification and referral to community service treatment may minimise the difficulties of providing a seamless service. It is important to ensure that both substance use and mental health needs have been assessed and provided for. If the allocated care coordinator is within the mental health domain, it is important to ensure that the individual's substance use needs will be met. Likewise, if substance use is viewed as the main problem, it is important to ensure that mental health needs are being met. A named worker should be identified, and contact should be established prior to discharge. This may require accompanying the individual to the relevant service, or the community worker attending the in-patient unit to engage with the client, prior to discharge. Self-help organisations and groups could be considered, such as Alcoholics Anonymous/ Narcotics Anonymous. Again, attendance is encouraged prior to discharge, so that support mechanisms are already in place. A crisis plan, with emergency contacts, should also be part of the discharge plan.

Advanced competencies

An awareness of the transtheoretical model of change

It is important to assess whether the client views their drug and alcohol use as problematic, and whether they wish to change their behaviour. Developing the necessary level of motivation required to achieve behaviour change that we may feel ambiguous about can be difficult. The 'assessment of the readiness to change measure' (Heather *et al.*, 1999) may be helpful in identifying the person perspective at that moment, but the process of change is fluid and it should be viewed as a possible guide only. It may be helpful to view a dual cycle of change, one relating to substance use and the other to mental health. Each can operate independently, but will often be linked; staff should assess and facilitate awareness as to where in each part of the cycle of change the patient may be, and its potential impact on behaviour change (Law *et al.*, 2002). In-patient staff should create space for clients to feel comfortable talking about and exploring their drug use. It is important that clients feel that previous lapses and relapses are not going to be judged negatively, but will be seen as opportunities to learn and revise future attempts. Developing motivational change is enhanced by the clients themselves highlighting drug and alcohol related difficulties and staff supporting realistic harm related goals, building on previous small successes and making links between poorer mental health and their substance use. Below is an example of a more detailed approach in enhancing motivation.

Enhancing motivation: MI and MET skills

Motivational enhancement therapy (MET) is a more practical application of the client centred motivational interviewing (MI) approach (Miller & Rollnick, 1991) that can be used as part of an integrated treatment approach. Its strength is that it can be used as a three-session, brief intervention that can be utilised within the in-patient setting. A word of caution is needed. Although studies broadly support MI in the population with a dual disorder (Martino *et al.*, 2000; Baker *et al.*, 2002), the clinician needs to be aware of the possible implications that individuals presenting with mental health disorder may have, when applying both MI and MET interventions. The underlying principle of increasing internal dissonance to facilitate change may be contraindicated in such individuals. For those who are vulnerable to stress it may exacerbate psychotic or neurotic symptomatology.

Therefore, elements of an adapted approach have been shown to be helpful. Martino *et al.* (2002) recommend the following modifications to primary MI skills: simplifying open-ended questions, refining reflective listening skills, heightening emphasis on affirmations, integrating psychiatric issues into personalised feedback and decisional balance matrices (the pros and cons of substance use). Outlined below is an example of a three-session MET approach that could be used in an in-patient setting (Squires & Moyers, 2002). It comprises feedback, a decision balance exercise, which links identified drug and alcohol related problems to an exploration of client values, and an agreed change plan.

Session 1: feedback about drink or drug use behaviour

Levels of use, consequences of use, and risk factors, such as level of tolerance, age of onset or HIV risk behaviour might be included. Standardised tools can provide more objective evidence, for example liver function tests, the AUDIT or the addiction severity index (ASI). The feedback can be difficult for the client, and there is a risk of the individual denying or minimising the consequences of their substance use. The MI principle of 'rolling with resistance' can minimise confrontation. The object of the first session is to increase the client's awareness of the degree to which substance use is affecting their lives. If possible, a supportive carer should be present, as studies have shown an increase in treatment efficacy with such involvement. A summary should cover the main points raised, reflect the seriousness of the problem, highlight the person's strengths and demonstrate optimism for the possibility of positive change.

Session 2: exploration of personal values and decisional balance

This exercise is to help the client 'define' their true self-values, which can feel lost or unobtainable. The client is asked to list, in as concrete terms as possible, things that they value for themselves in everyday life. Values should be placed in order of importance and then discussed individually. Areas that might be discussed could include why they are important, the impact of substance use on values, raising awareness as to the impact of short-term behaviour on longer-term value driven goals, and a refocusing away from 'problematic' behaviour towards a more rewarding lifestyle.

The second part of the session is the completion of the 'good' and 'not so good' aspects of an individual's substance use. The individual lists all the positive aspects of their substance use first; this may include physical, psychological and social aspects of their lifestyle. This can then facilitate the identification of disadvantages from the client, so that they are providing the negative consequences themselves. The clinician can facilitate an expansion and more in-depth exploration of the 'not so good' things. For example, 'You said your partner doesn't like you when you are drunk; can you tell me about a time when that might have happened?' The clinician can help develop discrepancies between the 'good' and the 'not so good', and the values and goals that have been identified. For example, 'On one hand, you say that you enjoy drinking because it gives you confidence and helps you socialise; however, on the other you have said you have had arguments with friends after drinking, which has upset you and stopped you going out.' This introduces a discrepancy for the client to consider.

Session 3: developing a change plan

This is the development of an agreed change plan that is based on an intervention outlined by Miller *et al.* (1995). It highlights areas of change and breaks them down into specific goals.

The following areas are covered:

- The changes I want to make are . . .
- The most important reasons I want to make these changes are . . .
- The steps I plan to take in changing are . . .
- The ways that people can help me are . . .
- I will know if my plan is working if . . .
- Some things that could interfere with my plan are . . .

To try to minimise a premature focus on the action stage in the model of change, this form could record a number of different agreed actions. It might simply be to think more about a particular aspect of use, or in the community, maintaining diaries that record levels of use and their consequences. Commitment to the change plan is asked for and the client should then sign and date their copy.

An awareness of the relapse prevention model

The in-patient environment, away from the usual daily routine, pressures and substance availability, is an ideal opportunity to raise awareness of the cognitive model of substance use, identifying the person's own pattern of use and formulating an initial relapse plan (Marlatt & Gordon, 1985). The clinician can explain the events that a person may go through that contribute to potential lapse or relapse. Linking the thoughts, feelings and behaviour can be summarised in the following five stages and then a plan developed to support abstinence (Beck *et al.*, 1993; Liese & Franz, 1996): triggers and high-risk situations, drug and alcohol related beliefs, automatic thoughts, urges and cravings, actively seeking drugs and alcohol. See Chapter 26 on relapse prevention.

Developing social networks

It is common for clients to feel that their entire social network is comprised of friends and acquaintances who use alcohol and drugs. Without some form of supportive or non-using network clients are going to find it difficult to reduce their use. It is helpful to identify everyone in the client's social network and map this out. Then discuss the significance of the individuals, their role in the client's life, and drug and alcohol use. Individuals who are identified as being supportive of change can be highlighted, and, if appropriate, they can be included in discharge planning. A similar mapping exercise could be completed for how the person is going to manage their time. A list of interests and activities, personal goals, training and occupational goals can be identified. The ward should have a comprehensive list of ideas and contact details to support an agreed plan. A proactive supportive approach to assist initial contact is important; staff should assist in telephoning or form filling to facilitate engagement. Attending first appointments before discharge in order to have support in place can increase social stability.

Skills training for this client group

The cognitive behavioural integrated treatment (C-BIT) model (Graham *et al.*, 2004) highlights six areas where specific skill building strategies could be introduced. These could include:

- Communication
- Refusing alcohol and drugs
- Strengthening alternative activities/networks
- Money management
- Mood management
- Goal planning and problem solving

Staff need to develop the necessary skills and knowledge to be aware of the treatment models, identify particular deficits and teach strategies to improve them.

Addressing in-patient training needs

The development of knowledge and skills in the treatment of dual diagnosis needs to have greater prominence in pre-registration training. It should also be part of continuing professional development (CPD). Drug and alcohol knowledge and, by association, dual diagnosis knowledge has been viewed as a specialism for clinicians to develop an interest in if they wish, rather than the major contributory presentation associated with mental disorder. There is an urgent need for educationalists to provide practical, skills based interventions that newly qualified clinicians can feel confident in applying within the clinical setting. Two of the main barriers to training are a lack of availability, and a lack of time. In-patient staff, and in particular non-qualified staff, have lower attendance at CPD training than community based or substance misuse staff. Short training packages have been found to be effective at raising awareness and knowledge, but poorer at facilitating changes to clinical practice. Training needs that were identified in the *Training Needs Analysis* by the Mears *et al.* (2001) included psychological interventions, issues of diagnosis/classification/recognition, and treatment/management issues in general.

Training approaches need to be innovative and employ a variety of approaches and styles to accommodate differing levels of staff knowledge and needs. Medical staff that are completing the admission process will have different training needs from occupational therapists or health care assistants working with this client group. Ideally, the whole staff team should undergo a training module, which would then be supported by ward based instruction, practice and supervision that will facilitate actual change to clinical practice. The development of lead clinicians and link workers, inter-agency and interdisciplinary teaching, the use of structured work books to assist practice and e-learning could all be considered in the development of the workforce.

Conclusion

This chapter is an attempt to highlight core and advanced competencies and skills for in-patient staff to consider in the development of providing more meaningful, focused interactions for individuals with a dual diagnosis. The list of competencies does not profess to be exhaustive, and some readers may have different views or preferences. It is, however, an attempt to highlight an area that requires a more comprehensive package of teaching and support, in developing in-patient specific adaptations of evidence based dual disorder treatments, within ward regimes that enable staff protected time to deliver these interventions.

References

Baker, A., Lewin, T., Reichler, H. *et al.* (2002) Motivational interviewing among psychiatric in-patients with substance use disorders. *Acta Psychiatrica Scandinavica*, 106, 233–40.

Beck, A.T., Wright, F.D., Newman, C.F. & Liese, B.S. (1993) *Cognitive Therapy of Substance Abuse*. Guilford, New York.

Butzlaff, R.L. & Hooley, J.M. (1998) Expressed emotion and psychiatric relapse: a meta-analysis. *Archives of General Psychiatry*, 55, 547–52.

Clancy, C., Mears, A., Banerjee, S., Crome, I. & Agbo-Quaye, S. (2001) *Coexisting Problems of Mental Disorder and Substance Misuse (Dual Diagnosis): a Training Needs Analysis*. College Research Unit, London.

Clarke, S. (2004) *Acute In-patient Mental Health Care: Education, Training and Continuing Professional Development for All*. Sainsbury Centre for Mental Health and National Institute for Mental Health in England, London.

Cuffel, B.J. & Chase, P.C. (1994) Remission and relapse of substance use disorders in schizophrenia. *Journal of Nervous and Mental Disease*, 182, 342–8.

Department of Health (2002) *Mental Health Policy Implementation Guide: Adult In-patient Care Provision*. Department of Health, London.

Dixon, L., McFarlane, W., Lefley, H. *et al.* (2001) Evidence based practices for services to family members of people with psychiatric disabilities. *Psychiatric Services*, 52: 903–10.

Drake, R.E., Bartels, S.J., Teague, G.B., Noordsy, D.L. & Clarke, R.E. (1993) Treatment of substance abuse in severe mental illness patients. *Journal of Nervous and Mental Disease*, 181, 606–11.

Drake, R.E., Mercer-McFadden, C., Mueser, K., McHugo, G.J. & Bond, G.R. (1998) Review of integrated mental health and substance abuse treatment for patients with dual disorders. *Schizophrenia Bulletin*, 26, 441–9.

Drake, R.E., Essock, S.M., Shaner, A. *et al.* (2001) Implementing dual diagnosis services for clients with severe mental health problems. *Journal of Nervous and Mental Disease*, 181, 298–305.

Evans, K. & Sullivan, J.M. (2001) *Dual Diagnosis. Counselling the Mentally Ill Substance Abuser*, 2nd edn. Guilford Press, New York.

Farrell, M.J. & David, A.S. (1988) Do psychiatric registrars take a proper drinking history? *British Medical Journal*, 6, 296 (6619), 395–6.

Graham, H., Copello, A., Birchwood, M. *et al.* (2004) *Cognitive Behaviour Integrated Treatment (C-BIT): a Treatment Manual for Substance Misuse in People with Severe Mental Health Problems*. Wiley and Sons, Chichester.

Health Advisory Service (2003) *Improving the Quality of Psychiatric In-patient Care in London (IQPIL)*. Health Advisory Service, London.

Heather, N., Luce, A., Peck, D., Dunbar, B. & James, I. (1999) Development of a treatment version of the readiness to change questionnaire. *Addiction Research*, 7, 63–83.

Hipwell, A.E., Singh, K. & Clark, A. (2000) Substance misuse among clients with a severe and enduring mental illness: service utilisation and implications for clinical management. *Journal of Mental Health*, 9, 37–50.

Hulse, G. & Tait, R. (2002) Six-month outcomes associated with a brief alcohol intervention for adult in-patients with psychiatric disorders. *Drug and Alcohol Review*, 21, 105–12.

Law, F., McEvoy, J., Cottee, H. & Petersen, T. (2002) *The Bi-cycle Model of Dual Diagnosis*. Poster presentation at the Annual Meeting of the Society for Study of Addiction (SSA), Leeds.

Liese, B.S. & Franz, R.A. (1996) Treating substance use disorders with cognitive therapy: lessons learned and implications for the future. In: *Frontiers of Cognitive Therapy* (Salkovskis, P., ed.), pp. 470–508. Guilford, New York.

Linszen, D.H., Dingemans, P.M. & Lenior, M.E. (1994) Cannabis abuse and the course of recent onset schizophrenic disorders. *Archives of General Psychiatry*, 51, 273–9.

McCann, J. (2004) What users want. Chapter 15. In: *From Toxic Institutions to Therapeutic Environments: Residential Settings in Mental Health Services* (Campling, P., Davies, S. & Farquharson, G., eds), p. 164. Gaskell, London.

Marlatt, G.A. & Gordon, G.R. (1985) *Relapse Prevention: Maintenance Strategies in the Treatment of Addictive Behaviours*. Guilford, New York.

Martino, S., Carroll, K.M., O'Malley, S.S. & Rounsaville, B.J. (2000) Motivational interviewing with psychiatrically ill substance abusing patients. *American Journal of Addictions*, 9, 88–91.

Martino, S., Carroll, K.M., Kostas, D., Perkins, J. & Rounsaville, B. (2002) Dual diagnosis motivational interviewing: a modification of motivational interviewing for substance abusing patients with psychotic disorders. *Journal of Substance Abuse Treatment*, 23, 297–308.

Mears, A., Clancy, C., Banerjee, S., Crome, I. & Agbo-Quaye, S. (2001) *Co-existing Problems of Mental Disorder and Substance Misuse (Dual Diagnosis): A Training Needs Analysis. Final Report to the Department of Health*. Royal College of Psychiatrists' Research Unit, London.

Menezes, P.O., Johnson, S., Thornicroft, G. *et al.* (1996) Drug and alcohol problems among individuals with severe mental illness in South London. *British Journal of Psychiatry*, 168, 612–19.

Miller, W.R. & Rollnick, S. (1991) *Motivational Interviewing*. Guilford Press, New York.

Miller, W.R., Zweben, A., DiClemente, C.C. & Rychtarik, R.G. (1995) *Motivational Enhancement Therapy Manual: a Clinical Research Guide for Therapists Treating Individuals with Alcohol Abuse and Dependence*. Project MATCH Monograph Series, Vol 2. NIH Pub. No. 94-3723. National Institute on Alcohol Abuse and Alcoholism, Rockville, Md.

MIND (2000) *Environmentally Friendly? Patients' Views on Conditions in Psychiatric Wards* (MIND Report). MIND, London.

Mueser, K.T., Yarnold, P.R. & Bellack, A.S. (1992) Diagnostic and demographic correlates of substance abuse in schizophrenia and major affective disorder. *Acta Psychiatrica Scandinavica*, 85, 48–55.

Mueser, K.T., Noordsy, D.L., Drake, R.E. & Fox, L. (2003) *Integrated Treatment for Dual Disorders: Effective Intervention for Severe Mental Illness and Substance Abuse*. Guilford, New York.

Owen, R.R., Fischer, E.P., Booth, B.M. & Cuffel, B.J. (1996) Medication non-compliance and substance abuse among patients with schizophrenia. *Psychiatric Services*, 47, 853–8.

Sainsbury Centre for Mental Health (2004) *Acute Care 2004: a National Survey of Adult Psychiatric Wards in England*. SCMH Publications, London.

Saunders, J.B., Aasland, O.G., Babor, T.F., de la Fuente, J.R. & Grant, M. (1993) Development of the alcohol use disorders identification test (AUDIT): WHO collaborative project on early detection of persons with harmful alcohol consumption. *Addiction*, 88, 791–804.

Scott, H., Johnson, S., Menezes, P. *et al.* (1998) Substance misuse and the risk of aggression and offending among the severely mentally ill. *British Journal of Psychiatry*, 172, 345–50.

Shumay, M., Chouljian, T.L. & Hargreaves, W.A. (1994) Patterns of substance misuse in schizophrenia: a Markov modelling approach. *Journal of Psychiatric Research*, 28, 277–87.

Skinner, H.A. (1982) The drug abuse screening test. *Addictive Behaviours*, 7, 363–71.

Squires, D.D. & Moyers, T. (2002) *Motivational Enhancement for Dually Diagnosed Consumers. The Behavioural Health Recovery Management Project*. University of New Mexico on Alcoholism, New Mexico.

Weaver, T., Madden, P., Charles, V. *et al.* (2003) Comorbidity of substance misuse and mental illness in community mental health and substance misuse services. *British Journal of Psychiatry*, 183, 304–13.

Williams, K. (1999) Attitudes of mental health professionals to co-morbidity between mental health problems and substance misuse. *Journal of Mental Health*, 8 (6), 605–13.

Index

abstinence, 29, 32, 101, 122, 155
  oriented, 172
  syndrome, 190
  total, 214, 227
abstinence-violation effect, 234
abstinent, 261
abuse, 97
  childhood, 108
  physical, 48
  sexual, 48
acceptance, 249
action plans, 156
active treatment, 9, 11, 12
actualising tendency, 243
acupuncture, 217
acute alcohol withdrawal, 196
acute in-patient settings, 150
addiction, 150, 165
  addictive behaviour, 7
  nursing, 121, 196, 197
  services, 13
addiction nurses, 121, 123
  perception, 280
  roles, 123
adolescence, 97, 171
adult and child services, 108
adult drug misusers, 10
aetiological, 4
  models, 47
affective disorders, 5, 6
after-care and follow-up, 103
aggression, 51, 54
alcohol, 5, 7, 25, 34, 150, 162
  aggression, 54, 55
  anxiety, 54
  assessment, 57, 58
  bipolar disorders, 50, 55
  dependence, 6, 25, 57
  depression, 50, 54, 58
  detoxification, 60, 172
  diaries, 57
  dual diagnosis, 54
  education, 58
  hallucinations, 60
  hopelessness, 58
  intoxication, 54, 58
  medication, 58
  mental health, 55, 58
  misuse, 6
  models of care, 56
  mood disorders, 50
  non-problematic, 57
  panic attacks, 58
  personality disorders, 55
  reduction, 57
  relapse assessment, 57
  risk, 58
  schizophrenia, 55
  screening tools, 57
  self-harm, 55, 58

services, 55
substance misuse services, 55
suicidal behaviour, 54
suicide, 58
use, 143
withdrawal symptoms, 58
withdrawal syndrome, 190–91
violence, 55
Alcohol Harm Reduction Strategy, 26, 55
Alcoholics Anonymous, 66, 155, 166, 218
alienation, 152
alleviation of dysphoria model, 7
ambivalence, 215, 254
amphetamines, 7, 43, 51, 98
amplification, 236
anabolic steroids, 36
anaemia, 36
anger management, 183
angina, 35
anorexia nervosa, 62
biological, 62
psychological, 62
socio-cultural factors, 62
suicide, 62
antidepressants, 9
antidote, 189
anti-psychotic, 9
anti-social personality, 165
anxiety, 5, 6, 45, 46
disorders, 5, 151
panic attacks, 47
assertive outreach, 8, 20, 119
assessment, 52, 57, 99, 120, 123, 143, 161, 215, 225, 235
accurate, 153
comprehensive, 59
functional, 288
in-depth, 267
multidimensional, 177
risk, 179
routine, 274
and screening, 179
staged, 104
successful, 163
asylums, 16
Ativan, 39
attachment, 112
attitudes, 6, 119, 165, 178, 276
authenticity, 251

barbiturates, 39
bed capacity, 287
behaviour, 243
behavioural
approach, 224
therapy, 101
benzodiazepines, 39, 193
binge, 30
bingeing, 63
bio-psychosocial approach, 218
bipolar disorder, 49, 108
affective disorder, 45
black and ethnic
alcohol misuse, 86
cannabis psychosis, 86
discrimination, 83
drug misuse, 85
groups, 82, 173
mental health, 82, 84
minority, 13
suicide, 85
tobacco, 87
blood pressure, 60
blood tests, 182
boundaries, 246
boundary setting, 229
breathalysers, 123
brief
focused approaches, 156
interventions, 102, 143, 288
British system, 17
bulimia, 63
bingeing, 63
diagnosis, 64
features, 63
prevalence, 63
self-medication hypothesis, 67
buprenorphine, 193

caffeine, 25
cannabis 7, 25, 36, 51, 98, 150, 162, 169
psychosis, 86
carbon dioxide, 35
cardiovascular
diseases, 45
problems, 36
care
coordinator, 131
plan, 121, 131, 224

plan approach, 141–2
planning, 287
care programme approach (CPA), 20, 131
carers, 6, 13
definition, 222
involvement, 290
Cartesian dualism, 210
case
example, 246
management, 127, 131
chaotic use, 31
child
centred philosophy, 108
protection, 110, 111
childhood, 98
Children Act 1989, 108
class A, B and C drugs, 27
classical conditioning, 233
client centred, 172
clinical management plan, 199
clinical supervision, 68, 132, 155, 206, 276
approaches, 278
concept, 277
co-supervision, 278
one-to-one, 278
purpose, 277
self-supervision, 278
clonidine, 143, 193
close monitoring, 9
clozapine, 232
cocaine, 4, 7, 17, 42, 50, 51
induced psychosis, 48
intoxication, 59
withdrawal, 51
codeine, 41
co-existing psychiatric disorder, 3
cognitive behavioural integrated treatment (C-BIT), 292
cognitive impairments, 262
behaviour therapy, 12, 67, 101, 224
behavioural, 232
behavioural treatment, 235
in schizophrenia, 51
cognitive model of problem substance misuse, 262–3
collateral information, 189
Commission for Racial Equality, 83
communication, 113
systems, 200
community
care, 18
engagement, 83
interventions, 120
models, 152
psychiatric nurses, 135
Community Drug and Alcohol Teams (CDATs), 197
Community Mental Health Teams (CMHTs), 124, 132
community programme approach (CPA), 120, 232
comorbidity, 3, 97
complex
health needs, 206
needs, 6, 131
compliance with medications, 151, 224
compulsion, 29
confidentiality, 136, 223
conflict resolution, 133
confrontation, 12
congruence, 245
context, 34
continuing professional development, 205
convulsions, 39
coping strategies, 267
core competencies, 275, 285
counselling, 9, 102, 147
crack/cocaine, 25, 98
cravings, 234, 267
criminal
behaviour, 163
problems, 170
criminal justice
agencies, 11
agendas, 120
system, 6, 170
crisis management, 68
cue exposure, 233
therapy, 267
cultural
appropriateness, 89
awareness, 89
competence, 81, 89, 282
expectations, 186
influences, 34
model, 91
needs, 209
sensitivity, 89
specificity, 89

culture, 81, 113
cycle of change, 156
  model, 122

dance culture, 98
dangerousness, 266
DANOS, 22
decision-balance matrix, 254
degeneration theory, 17
de-institutionalisation, 8
delirium, 16, 43
  tremens, 35
delusional beliefs, 7
delusions, 50, 144
denial, 6
dental services, 144
dependence syndrome, 29
dependent users, 30
depression, 5, 7, 45, 48, 98, 108, 110
depressive disorders, 103
deprivation, 170
detoxification, 127, 166, 189
  home, 190
developing discrepancy, 255
diabetes, 45
diamorphine, 199
diazepam, 39
Diconal, 41
dihydrocodeine, 41
discrepancy, 236
disorientation, 44
dissociative states, 243
diversity, 81, 89, 97
drug
  addiction, 74
  dependence, 27
  detoxification, 172
  experience, 99
  overdose, 188
  related deaths 187
  screening, 182
  tolerance, 34
  using careers, 101
drug and alcohol liaison teams, 197
drug experience, 34
drug taking
  oral, 31
  inhalation 31
  injecting, 31
  smoking, 31
  subcultures, 118
dual diagnosis, 6, 10, 108, 150, 240
  concept, 3
  good practice guide, 13, 21
dual diagnosis nursing, 126
dysthymia, 49

early intervention, 154
eating disorders, 62, 241
  aetiology, 65
  anorexia nervosa, 62
  boundaries, 69
  bulimia, 63
  carbohydrate consumption, 67
  clinical obesity, 66
  craving, 66
  dual diagnosis, 66
  family characteristics, 65
  nursing care, 67
  re-feeding, 68
  self-harm, 66
  self-help groups, 67
  sexual abuse, 65
  sexual promiscuity, 66
  substance misuse, 66
  treatment, 67
Eating Disorders Association, 67
ecstasy, 37, 98
education, 104, 165, 167, 237
  and training, 205, 273
educational development, 197, 273
electrocardiogram, 189
emergency clinic, 6
empathic contact, 247
empathy, 236, 243, 255, 262
engagement, 9, 11, 127, 152, 156, 288
environmental
  factors, 97
  stress, 7
epileptic fits, 29, 40
escalation theory, 37
ethnic
  Bangladeshi, 86
  black Caribbeans, 86
  minorities, 91, 144
  Pakistani, 86
  South Asians, 86
ethnicity, 81

ethnocentric, 6, 88
evaluation, 268
evidence based
  practice, 121, 206, 238
  research, 141, 206
examination
  physical, 144
  mental state, 144
exclusion, 119
expectations, 235
experimental users, 30

family, 6, 222
  assessment tools, 226
  dynamics, 225
  history, 144
  interventions, 223
  involvement, 290
  problems, 6
  therapy, 67, 101, 103
fetal alcohol syndrome, 111
flashback, 41
forensic, 161
  history, 144

genetic, 7
  disposition, 112
GHB, 38
Glasgow coma scale, 187
glaucoma, 36
ground rules, 226
group
  therapy, 103
  work, 69, 183

hallucinations, 16, 39, 43, 50, 144
hallucinogens, 7, 25, 51
harm minimisation, 20, 77, 143
harm reduction, 20, 32, 101, 155, 165, 166, 214, 287, 289
  measures, 187
  skills, 203
  strategies, 177
head injuries, 187
healing, 214
  interventions, 216
  process, 249
health
  education, 177
  information, 198
helping alliance, 246
hepatitis B and C, 25, 143, 182
heroin, 17, 25, 42, 98, 163
HIV (human immunodeficiency virus), 18, 143, 151, 182
  prevalence, 25
HIV infections, 6
holistic, 28
  approach, 12, 209
  care, 209
homeless, 98, 143
  populations, 127
homelessness, 6, 12, 108, 120
Home Office regulations, 196
hopelessness, 257
hospital admission, 157
hostels, 9
housing, 8, 9
Human Rights Act 1999, 69
hypno-sedatives, 39
hypomania, 7

iatrogenic, 206
illegal behaviour, 137
illicit drug use, 108
imagery techniques, 77
individual psychological therapies, 102
information strategies, 100
injecting, 143
in-patient training needs, 292
institutions, 17
integrated
  care pathway, 11
  treatment, 76, 141
integrated treatment interventions, 287
integration, 9
inter-agency
  intervention, 99
  training, 275
inter-disciplinary tension, 135
inter-personal violence, 161
inter-professional practice, 131
interventions, 127
  strategies, 11
intoxication, 4, 12, 101, 153
  acute, 186
  alcohol, 161
Islam, 214

Judeo-Christian, 212
junkie syndrome, 75

ketamine, 40
Korsakoff's syndrome, 163

learning
  by association, 233
  biological, 97
  difficulty, 162
  disability, 3
  psychological, 97
  sociological, 97
legal needs, 6
life stressors, 156
locus of control, 74
lofexidine, 193
low threshold prescribing, 171
LSD (lysergic acid diethylamide), 40, 98

manic depression, 151
maternal deaths, 49, 109
medical
  model, 248
  needs, 6
medication, 6, 51, 60, 246, 253
  antidepressants, 51, 52
  antipsychotics, 51, 52, 164
  anxiolytics, 51, 52
  errors, 201
  management, 154, 196, 198, 202
  mood stabilisers, 51, 52
medico-nursing practice, 123
meditation, 217
mental
  health assessment, 180
  health nurses, 202
  health nursing, 196
  health policy, 16
  health problems, 108, 170
  health services, 13, 52
  health status, 177
  health symptom stabilisation, 288
  state examination, 180
Mental Health Act, 59, 67, 128, 161, 169
mental illness, 4
methadone, 9, 41, 42, 145, 192, 199
  maintenance, 102
  overdose, 189
midwives, 144, 199
Mind, 22
minimal interventions, 121
miscarriages, 17
misdiagnosis, 166
Misuse of Drug Act 1971, 17
mobile methadone clinics, 197
Model of Change, Transtheoretical, 155
models, 7, 10
  alleviation of dysphoria model, 7
  behavioural, 29
  biological, 29
  of change, 155
  integrated, 10
  multiple risk factor, 7
  parallel, 10
  serial, 10
  shared care, 10
  supersensitivity model, 7
modelling, 234
models of care, 19, 20, 26, 142, 170
moral
  reasoning, 234
  therapy, 17
morphine, 17, 41, 199
motivation, 123,
  for change, 11
  lack, 10
motivation for change, 58
motivational enhancement therapy (MET), 291
motivational interviewing, 11, 67, 156, 253, 255, 264–5, 287
multi-cultural, 91, 214
multi-dimensional approach, 13
multi-ethnic, 214
multiple morbidity, 141
multiple needs, 170
multiple risk factor model, 7
multi-professional training, 197
mushrooms, 40

naloxone, 102, 189,
  hydrochloride, 199
  take home, 199
National Health Service, 17
National Prescribing Centre, 196
National Service Framework for Mental Health, 18
National Treatment Agency, 10, 82, 169, 196
National Treatment Outcome Research Study (NTORS), 5, 21
needle exchanges, 20, 33, 171, 197

needs, 19
  medical, 187
  physical, 187
  psychosocial, 187
neuroleptic, 225
nicotine, 25
  addiction, 51
  withdrawal, 29, 51
nitrite
  amyl, 35
  butyl, 35
  isobutyl, 35
non-compliance, 45
non-pharmacological therapies, 204
non-prescribed medications, 206
nurse roles, 126
nurse prescribing
  independent nurse prescribers, 197
  nurse prescribers' formulary, 197
  patient group directions, 197
  supplementary prescribers, 197
nursing
  assessment, 177
  care, 177
  interventions, 177
  practice, 202
Nursing and Midwifery Council, 205

observation, 164
obsessive-compulsive disorder, 45, 47
occupational therapy, 12
Office of Population Censuses and Surveys, 5
older people, 173
operant conditioning, 233
operational management, 136
opiates, 41
  abuse, 50
  detoxification, 192
  use, 50
opioids, 41
organic, 16
  model, 226
  services, 18
  work, 197
organisations, 130
overdose, 20, 187
  awareness, 143
  drug, 188
  methadone, 189
  nursing interventions, 188
Overeaters Anonymous, 66

pain management, 205
panic, 43
  disorder, 5, 45
parallel
  model, 10
  treatment, 141
paranoia, 5, 250
paranoid delusions, 4
paranoid psychosis, 43
paraphernalia, 267
parenthood, 99
patient-centred approach, 123, 240, 245, 253
PCP, 40
personality, 34
  development, 242
personality disorders, 5, 73, 10, 162, 249, 286
  anti-social personality, 73, 74
  assessment, 74, 76
  criminal activities, 73
  harm minimisation, 77
  illicit drug use, 73
  integrated treatment models, 76
  management, 77
  vulnerability hypothesis, 74
persuasion, 9
pharmacist, 199
pharmacological, 12, 34
  treatment, 173
pharmacotherapy, 102
phobias, 47
  social, 48
phobic disorder, 5
physical
  abuse, 48
  complications, 155
  dependence, 7, 27, 28
  health care, 288
  health problems, 170
  illnesses, 151
polydrug
  substance misuse, 151
  use, 145
  user, 178
post-natal depression, 49
post-traumatic stress, 173
  disorder, 47
poverty, 7, 107

pregnancy, 99, 109
prejudice, 6, 127
prescribing, 102
  authority, 196
  legislation, 196
  multiple, 200
  role of nurse, 196
  supplementary, 196
pre-therapy, 247
prevalence, 5
prevention, 45, 112, 165
  activities, 100
primary care services, 140
prisons, 6, 161
  service, 110
problem drug user definition, 27–8
problem solving, 227, 236–7
process of change model, 258
professional development, 282, 285
prostitution, 17
psychiatric
  disorder, 4
  diagnosis, 248
  institutions, 7
  morbidity, 45
psychoactive substances, 5, 7, 34, 186, 200
  irrational use, 200
  rational use, 200
psychodynamic psychotherapy, 67
psycho-education, 226
psycho-educational strategies, 123
psychological
  approaches, 232
  dependence, 27, 28
  needs, 6
  treatments, 173
psychopharmacology, 120, 205
psychosis, 6, 7, 37, 151, 154, 222, 250
psychosocial
  approach, 156
  interventions, 198, 241
psychosomatic reactions, 29
psycho-stimulant, 7
psychotic illness, 5
psychoticism, 5
psychotropic medication, 109, 201

QuADS, 21
qualitative research, 152
quality assurance, 206

race, 81
racial harassment, 244
racism, 6
rapport, 165
recreational
  drug use, 124
  user definition, 30
referral, 171
reflective listening, 236
  skills, 265
reflective teams, 133
reframing, 12,
rehabilitation, 127, 190
reinforcement, 233
  external, 233
  intermittent, 233
  secondary, 233
  self, 233
  vicarious, 233
relapse, 7, 124, 166, 219, 224, 261
relapse prevention, 9, 11, 12, 123, 124, 152, 237, 261, 287
  model, 292
  planning, 264
  in practice, 263–4
relaxation, 204
religion, 212
religious
  beliefs, 16
  faiths, 213
research, 4
residential
  settings, 103
  rehabilitation, 172, 197
resilience, 112
resistance, 11
revolving door
  pathology, 151
  syndrome, 128
risk, 127
  assessment, 107, 145, 179, 182, 288
  factors, 29, 98
  management, 111, 122, 127
  of overdose, 40
  of violence, 6
  of victimisation, 6
Road Traffic Act 1988, 26
roll with resistance, 236, 255
route of administration, 31
rule violation experience, 263

safe drinking levels, 35
safer sex, 33
satellite clinics, 197
schizo-affective disorder, 52
schizophrenia, 5, 6, 12, 45, 50, 108, 150, 162, 165, 224, 235, 248
screening, 99, 143, 171, 177
  instruments, 163
  tests, 120
  tools, 153, 181
seasonal affective disorder (SAD), 49
seizures, 38, 187
self, 243
self-awareness model, 68
self-efficacy, 234, 236, 256, 262, 286
self-esteem, 58
self-fulfilling prophecy, 34
self-harm, 6, 124, 145
self-help groups, 66, 100
self-medication, 25, 145, 164, 288
self-medication hypothesis, 7
self-neglect, 145
self-regulation, 234
self-reinforcement, 234
self-starvation, 68
sensation seeking, 99
sense of identity, 97
serial treatment, 141
service providers/provision, 100, 119, 172
service users, 12, 23, 223
setting, 34
sexual
  abuse, 48, 65
  activity, 99
  behaviour, 144
  experiences, 65
  problems, 52
sexuality, 97
sexually transmitted diseases, 152
shared care, 141, 142
skills based training, 275
smoking cessation clinics, 197
snow ball effect, 33
social
  competence, 98
  control, 21
  custom, 25
  drift hypothesis, 8
  exclusion, 6, 152, 156, 170, 262
  inclusion, 19, 22
  isolation, 7, 45, 107, 120
  learning theory, 233
  needs, 6
  outcomes, 6
  problems, 170
  skills, 12
  status, 107
  stigma, 262
  support, 12
  withdrawal, 51
sodium pentathol therapy, 251
solution focused therapy, 257
spirituality, 211
  concept, 211
spiritual needs, 6, 209
stable living situation, 9
staff training, 13
stage of change, 152
stages of treatment, 9
state benefits, 8
stepped care model, 68
stereotyped perception, 178
stigma, 6
stigmatisation 119, 152
stimulants, 25, 42, 193
street agencies, 197
stress, 97
stress-vulnerability model, 224
subculture, 7
substance
  misuse, 4, 5, 98, 150
  misuse disorder, 5
substance misuse , 4, 5, 98, 150
  assessment, 180
  services, 52, 130
substitute medications, 140
suicidal thoughts, 5
suicide, 5, 12, 45, 49, 52, 98, 108, 131, 183, 187, 266
suicide attempts, 113
supervision, 8, 246, 286
symptom management, 241
symptomatology, 241

team leadership, 133
teamwork, 130
temazepam, 39
therapeutic
  optimism, 10
  relationship, 147
  techniques, 10

tobacco, 87
tolerance, 44, 186
toxicity, 35
toxicology, 164
training, 13
  needs, 146, 152
  needs analysis, 274, 286, 293
  staff, 166
  strategy, 173
tranquillisers, 25
transcultural
  approach, 91
  counselling, 91
trauma, 187
treatment, 99
  approaches, 123
  compliance, 101, 122, 145
  plan, 164
Twelve-step approach, 103

unemployment, 108
upstream approach, 206
urine
  analysis, 182

violence, 12, 162
  domestic, 107
  risk of, 184
  sexual, 107
virtual team, 9
volatile substances, 25, 44
vulnerability, 120
vulnerable, 97
  populations, 141

withdrawal, 12, 153
  symptoms, 154
women, 13, 143

young people, 13, 97, 143, 171
  conduct disorders, 98
  depression, 98
  disengagement, 99
  risk factors, 98
  school drop out, 98
  self-harm, 99
  set, 99
  sexual activity, 99
  suicide, 98, 99